# Medical Informatics Handbook

# Medical Informatics Handbook

Editor: Patrick Garter

AMERICAN
MEDICAL PUBLISHERS
www.americanmedicalpublishers.com

AMERICAN
MEDICAL PUBLISHERS
www.americanmedicalpublishers.com

**Cataloging-in-Publication Data**

Medical informatics handbook / edited by Patrick Garter.
p. cm.
Includes bibliographical references and index.
ISBN 978-1-63927-717-9
1. Medical informatics. 2. Medical care--Technological innovations. 3. Medicine--Data processing.
4. Information storage and retrieval systems--Medicine. 5. Medical innovations. 6. Medical technology.
I. Garter, Patrick.
R858 .M43 2023
610.285--dc23



American Medical Publishers,
41 Flatbush Avenue,
1st Floor, New York,
NY 11217, USA

ISBN 978-1-63927-717-9 (Hardback)

# Contents

# Preface

Medical informatics is concentrated on information technology, which provides effective collection of data by utilizing technological tools for enhancing medical knowledge and smooth delivery of patient medical care. Health data is linked with the health of a person or collective population. This information is collected through a series of health information systems (HIS), as well as from other technological tools used by professionals and healthcare providers involved in healthcare systems. Medical informatics makes use of data analytics, which is a process of investigating raw datasets for discovering trends, drawing conclusions and recognizing the potential needed for enhancement of healthcare. Analytics in healthcare utilizes historical and current data for understanding and supporting decision-making on both business and patient level. The usage of data analytics results in improvements in patient care, finding preventive measures, decision-making, as well as more accurate diagnosis and more personalized treatment. The various advancements in medical informatics are glanced at and their applications as well as ramifications are looked at in detail within this book. The readers would gain knowledge that would broaden their perspective in this area.

The information contained in this book is the result of intensive hard work done by researchers in this field. All due efforts have been made to make this book serve as a complete guiding source for students and researchers. The topics in this book have been comprehensively explained to help readers understand the growing trends in the field.

I would like to thank the entire group of writers who made sincere efforts in this book and my family who supported me in my efforts of working on this book. I take this opportunity to thank all those who have been a guiding force throughout my life.

**Editor**

# Development of a Mobile Personal Health Record Application Designed for Emergency Care in Korea: Integrated Information from Multicenter Electronic Medical Records

**Yuri Choi [1,†], June-sung Kim [2,†], In Ho Kwon [1,*], Taerim Kim [3], Su Min Kim [4], Wonchul Cha [3,4,5], Jinwoo Jeong [1] and Jae-Ho Lee [2,6]**

1 Department of Emergency Medicine, Dong-A University Hospital, Dong-A University College of Medicine, Busan 49201, Korea; yurichoi@damc.or.kr (Y.C.); jinwoo@dau.ac.kr (J.J.)
2 Department of Emergency Medicine, Asan Medical Center, University of Ulsan College of Medicine, Seoul 05505, Korea; jstyle06@amc.seoul.kr (J.-s.K.); jaeholee@amc.seoul.kr (J.-H.L.)
3 Department of Emergency Medicine, Samsung Medical Center, Sungkyunkwan University School of Medicine, Seoul 06351, Korea; taerimi.kim@samsung.com (T.K.); wc.cha@samsung.com (W.C.)
4 Department of Digital Health, Samsung Advanced Institute for Health Sciences & Technology, Sungkyunkwan University, Seoul 06355, Korea; ksm1003@g.skku.edu
5 Health Information and Strategy Center, Samsung Medical Center, Seoul 06351, Korea
6 Department of Information Medicine, Asan Medical Center, University of Ulsan College of Medicine, Seoul 05505, Korea
* Correspondence: kwoninho@dau.ac.kr
† Yuri Choi and June-sung Kim equally contributed to this study.

**Abstract:** Collecting patient's medical data is essential for emergency care. Although hospital-tethered personal health records (PHRs) can provide accurate data, they are not available as electronic information when the hospital does not develop and supply PHRs. The objective of this research was to evaluate whether a mobile app can assemble health data from different hospitals and enable interoperability. Moreover, we identified numerous barriers to overcome for putting health data into one place. The new mobile PHR (mPHR) application was developed and evaluated according to the four phases of the system development life cycle: defining input data and functions, developing a prototype, developing a mobile application, and implementation testing. We successfully introduced the FirstER (First for Emergency Room) platform on 23 September 2019. Additionally, validation in three tertiary hospitals has been carried out since the launch date. From 14 October to 29 November 2019, 1051 cases registered with the FirstER, and the total download count was 15,951 records. We developed and successfully implemented the mPHR service, which can be used as a health information exchange tool in emergency care, by integrating medical records from three different tertiary hospitals. By recognizing the significance and limitations of this service, it is necessary to study the development and implementation of mPHR services that are more suitable for emergency care.

**Keywords:** emergency medicine; interoperability; mobile applications; personal health records; electronic medical records

## 1. Introduction

Collecting data about underlying diseases, food or drug allergies, and prescribed medications is essential whenever physicians see patients [1]. These data make it possible to efficiently diagnose and treat patients by reducing unnecessary laboratory or imaging tests [2]. When patients go to an emergency department (ED) that they regularly visit, physicians can obtain medical information without any additional effort [3]. In South Korea, medical records are transferred by paper or telephone when patients decide to move from one hospital to the other. Meanwhile, in the case of an unexpected visit to a nearby hospital, especially in an emergency, it is hard to know a patient's detailed history because patients do not remember exactly their prior illnesses, doses, or types of drugs taken [4]. Although hospital-tethered personal health records (PHRs) can provide accurate data, they are not available as electronic information when the hospital does not develop and supply PHRs [5].

Although the need for convenient access to medical information has been increasing, several factors have limited the development of a PHR platform: related laws, ownership of data, privacy, and security [6]. The patient Privacy Act states that electronic medical records (EMRs) must not be leaked or stored outside of hospitals [7]. However, on account of the high penetration rate of EMRs and the elevated usage rate of smartphones in the country, there has been sufficient social consensus for developing PHRs [8]. Meanwhile, established policies and systems for collecting and utilizing individual medical records have been implemented that have enabled the storage of EMR data in cloud systems outside the boundaries of hospitals. Additionally, operable PHR apps have become available that tether EMRs and link several hospitals [9].

In this context, the Korean government announced a voluntary program called "MyData" in 2019, which gives consumers increased access to their data in portable electronic devices, such as smartphones. This program is a paradigm shift of personal data storage and management that propels the current institution-centric system to a person-centric system, which has already been adopted in medical fields in numerous countries [10]. The MyData program has been applied to various fields, including the health industry, and enables individuals to manage their own health data more actively and efficiently. The development of a new PHR application for emergencies was carried out as the medical part of this program. This PHR application was designed to enable medical information to be owned by patients, not hospitals, and for patients to provide that information to healthcare providers by appropriately utilizing it when necessary. Two tertiary hospitals (Asan Medical Center (AMC) and Samsung Medical Center (SMC)) already have applications for PHR-tethered EMRs (My chart in my hand, SMC mobile) since 2015 and 2013 [11]. However, there are no applications that could link different hospitals across the country. Therefore, we formed a consortium that consisted of one application developer, called value through Technology and Wisdom (vTW) and three tertiary hospitals (AMC, SMC, and Dong-A Medical Center (DAMC)) and developed a new PHR platform that especially targets emergency situations.

The objective of this research was to evaluate whether a mobile app can assemble health data from different hospitals and enable interoperability. Moreover, we identified numerous barriers to overcome when putting health data into one place.

## 2. Methods

To develop a mobile PHR (mPHR) application for use in emergency situations, a consortium was formed consisting of data-providing hospitals, data-utilizing hospitals, and an application developer. Three academic tertiary hospitals (AMC, SMC, and Dong-A Medical Center (DAMC)) with integrated full-scale hospital information systems, which were essential for providing data to build a system, participated as data-providing and data-utilizing centers. These hospitals are located in two large metropolitan cities, Seoul and Busan, and have different EMR systems that were established in 2003, 2005, and 2013. The annual numbers of visits to the EDs of these centers are 100,000, 130,000, and 35,000, respectively. These centers have about 2000, 2000, and 990 inpatient beds. The application developer (vTW) designed a service model, built a platform and cloud service, and operated the mPHR service. The three hospitals built the foundation for the extraction of personal data from the EMRs, standardized medical records, and data to be used in the application. In addition, two local secondary-care hospitals (Hyemin Hospital, Chung Hospital) that are closely related to the three hospitals were offered the data provided.

### *2.1. Design of the mPHR Service for Emergency Situations*

#### 2.1.1. Functions and Input Data That Were Considered Necessary

Prior to the development of the mPHR application, there was consensus among the participating researchers that the input data, screen, and functions should emphasize two main aspects: (1) patient ownership to generate and review their own health data and (2) utilization of the PHR data by healthcare providers in cases of emergency. The general design and development process are presented in Figure 1.

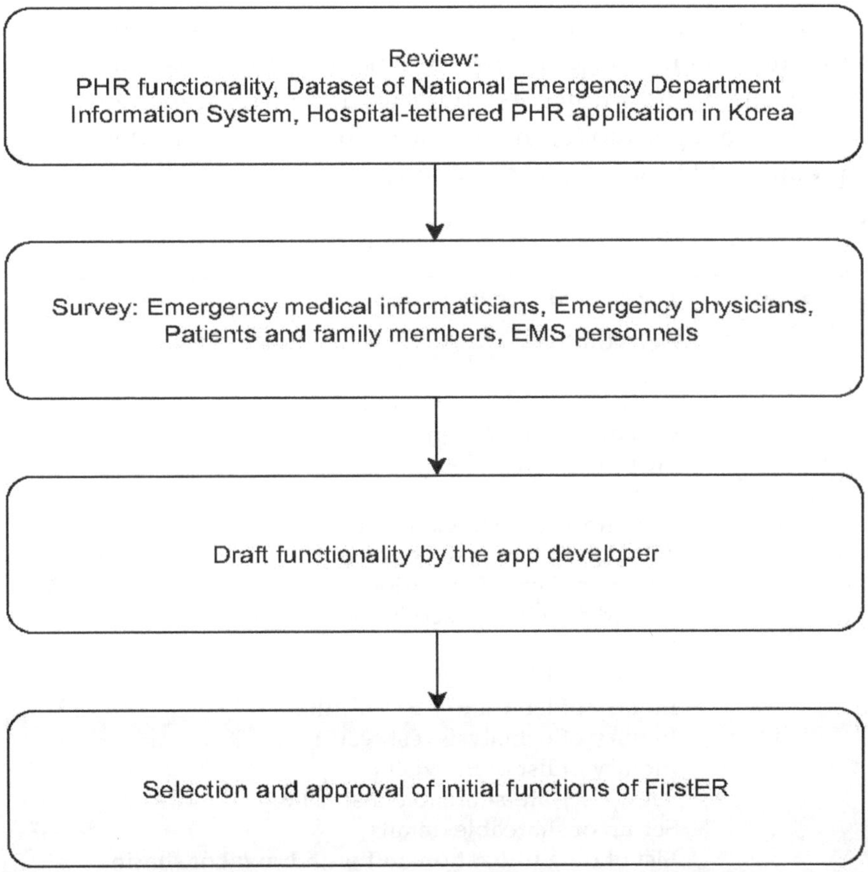


**Figure 1.** Process overview for mPHR for emergency departments (PHR: personal health record, EMS: emergency medical service, mPHR: mobile PHR).

The data structure and functionality design of the mPHR were based on the PHR and Emergency Department Information System (EDIS) functionality standards of Health Level Seven (HL7). Essential functions and data for inclusion in the mPHR were adopted from existing PHR applications developed by the participating researchers at AMC and SMC [11]. The data structure and formats were standardized to the National ED Information System (NEDIS) registry, which is a national database of prospectively collected ED patient data from all emergency medical institutions in Korea [12,13]. Essential items for inclusion in the mPHR were chosen based on a survey collected from potential users, including ED staff, EMS personnel, and ED patients and their family members, using a structured questionnaire.

The final decision on the inclusion of functionality and data items was made through discussion between participating researchers in the three hospitals based on previous research and the survey results mentioned above. The functionalities were categorized into patient information, previous ED visit information, and patient-generated health data (PGHD). There were disagreements about the items for inclusion in the application; therefore, the decision was made to limit the number of items at the initial development and expand later as necessary.

After the basic function of the PHR application was established, to make the mPHR useful in an emergency situation, a novel application service should provide not only a PHR function with which a user can review his or her previous medical records in ED, but also a "disclosure" function that enables ED staff to access a user's previous ED records in an emergency situation. A server for integrating and transferring multicenter data was built, and a private cloud with protected privacy that was verified for compliance with the relevant laws was used outside the three hospitals.

Prior to the new development, the expected user groups for the user-centered interface configuration were specified as being three groups: patients and caregivers, medical staff, and managers. Because the required functions are different depending on who the user is, the interface and main functions are configured differently by applying them when a user logs in. When patients and caregivers log in, the function to check and manage health records is implemented, while medical staff authenticate themselves and implement the function to receive and view patient records by URL. In addition, in the manager mode, the notification function and dashboard function for user management is implemented as the interface (Table 1).

**Table 1.** Functionalities required for targeted user groups.

| Targeted User Groups | Functionalities Required |
|---|---|
| Patient | Registration |
| | Log-in |
| | Personal information management |
| | Customer service center |
| | Health records (Home) |
| | Medication alarm |
| | Download of medical record |
| | "Disclosure" of medical record |
| | Record of health condition |
| | Record of self-checked blood pressure |
| | Emergency ID |
| | Inquiry of ED records |
| | Inquiry of laboratory test results |
| | Inquiry of urinalysis test result |
| | Inquiry of list of ED visits |
| | Set-up of data-shareable institution |
| | Set-up of shareable details |
| | List of data utilization and withdrawal of sharing |
| | SOS to care-taker |
| ED staff | Receiving temporary URL of "ED record summary" via e-mail or SNS |
| | Authentication |
| | Inquiry of "ED record summary" |
| | Inquiry of details of ED records |
| Manager | Management of service usage |
| | Management of notice |
| | Dashboard |
| Others | Easy-to-read terms |
| | Selective sharing method |
| | Safe data collection and utilization process |
| | Explicit consent before downloading |
| | Receipt of utilized data |

ID: identification, ED: emergency department, URL: uniform resource locator, SNS: social network service.

The patient's information includes name, age, gender, blood type, allergy history, and each hospital's identification numbers. Previous ED history consists of hospital visited, visiting date, visiting time, vital signs at the time of visit, the International Classification of Disease-10 (ICD-10) code diagnosed in the ED, medication prescribed, and results of laboratory tests. The three hospitals have different EMR systems and data recorded, which are coded in different ways for each hospital. For interoperability and standardization of data, an NEDIS conversion method was used. The coding method used to send data to the NEDIS is universal in all EDs across the country. This method enabled various information that existed in different forms at each hospital to be converted into one form.

Similarly, data on medications prescribed in the ED are sent to the National Health Insurance, which also uses the electronic data interchange (EDI) code of the country's single insurer. Further, information for each medication was mapped using data from the Korea Pharmaceutical Information Center.

There are technical limitations when trying to include all the laboratory tests; thus, the most frequent test items were extracted from the three hospitals' data. Two ED doctors from each hospital (Y.C., I.H.K., J.K., J.-H.L., T.K., and W.C.) reviewed the whole list of extracted laboratory tests and discussed the clinical importance of the laboratory tests for making treatment decisions in the ED.

The items of the PGHD were determined by considering those items that are valuable for suspecting and diagnosing a disease in the ED.

#### 2.1.2. Development of the System and Server

A server for each data-providing hospital linked to a main server and a private cloud was planned for the system. When selecting the private cloud, legal considerations and the system's suitability were taken into account. There were several discussions with the computer experts of the three hospitals and the app developer, leading to the building of the MyData server, which connects to the main server.

### *2.2. Development of the Prototype*

Based on the previous arrangement of the core data and function, the application developer (vTW) developed a prototype of the PHR application by laying out the screen, modeling the data, constructing the technical architecture, and designing the interface using a design toolkit (Sketch© 2020, online. Sketch B.V.). Through several meetings, the participating researchers from the three hospitals corrected and supplemented the prototype by providing feedback on the user interface, correcting typos, and showing how to indicate the reference values of the laboratory test results.

### *2.3. Development of the mPHR Application*

The new mPHR application was developed and evaluated according to the four phases of the system development life cycle. According to this method, it proceeded as a process consisting of planning, analysis, design, and implementation. Each phase was reviewed and advised on by the participating researchers and revised by the application developers. Based on the modified prototype, standards for details were defined, and each unit module was developed. To design a user-centered screen, we targeted three groups of users: patients, ED staff, and program managers. Mobile Application Content Accessibility Guideline 2.0, a modification of the Web Content Accessibility Guideline 2.0 for implementation in Korea, was complied with by vTW. The mPHR application was developed with the Android Software Development Kit 28 using Android Studio 3.5 (Google LLC) and Swift 4.0 using Xcode 11© (1999–2020 Apple Inc.). The Spring tool suite 4© (2020 VMware, Inc.) was used to program the web service.

In order to comply with the Privacy Act of Korea, legal advice was sought at the time of app development.

### *2.4. Testing the New mPHR Application*

The developed application was subjected to unit tests and integration tests. Unit tests were conducted twice by the computer experts of the three hospitals and the app developer on 20–27 September. The integration test was conducted twice on 4–11 October in the same way.

## 3. Results

We successfully introduced the FirstER (First for Emergency Room) platform on 23 September 2019. Moreover, it has been implemented in three tertiary hospitals since the launch date.

### *3.1. Services Provided by the Novel PHR Application for Emergency Situations: FirstER*

#### 3.1.1. Main Function

The user-centered screen was designed considering the main functions (Figure 2). The essential functions for the patient as the owner of the entire set of information include registration, management of his or her health record, download and viewing, disclosure of the PHR-tethered EMR of the hospital, contact with care providers, and setting of the degree of information disclosure. ED staff receive a temporary URL so that a patient's information could be viewed within the limits allowed by him or her.

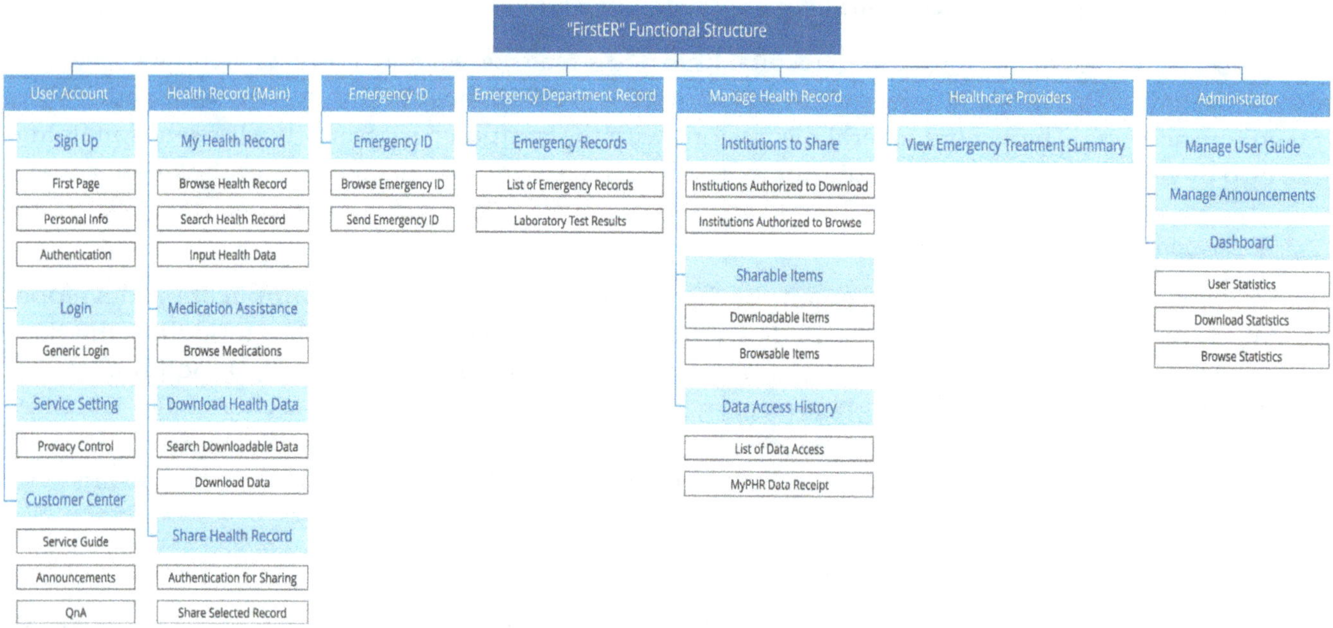


**Figure 2.** The functional structure of FirstER. The main functions for patients were categorized into registration, management of health records and emergency ID, download and view, disclosure of the PHR-tethered EMR of the hospital, and setting of the degree of information disclosure. (ID: identification, PHR: personal health record)

#### 3.1.2. Data Provided by FirstER

Patients' ED records (name, gender, age, diagnosis, vital signs, hospital visited, visiting date and time, etc.) coded by the NEDIS method were integrated among the three data-providing tertiary hospitals. Medication information coded by the EDI mapped with different drug codes from each hospital was successfully extracted. Twenty-nine items most frequently referred to by emergency physicians were selected for the most frequent test categories (Table 2). These data extracted from the hospital information system constituted a "core dataset" to be sent to the private cloud.

**Table 2.** Extraction and standardization of the most frequent laboratory examinations.

| Sample | Name of Laboratory Test |
|---|---|
| Blood | White blood cell count |
| Blood | Hemoglobin |
| Blood | Platelet count |
| Blood | Absolute neutrophil count |
| Blood | Prothrombin time |
| Blood | Activated prothrombin time |
| Blood | Blood urea nitrogen |
| Blood | Creatinine |
| Blood | Total bilirubin |
| Blood | Gamma glutamyl transpeptidase |
| Blood | Alkaline phosphatase |
| Blood | Alanine transaminase |
| Blood | Aspartate transaminase |
| Blood | Amylase |
| Blood | Lipase |
| Blood | Sodium |
| Blood | Potassium |
| Blood | Uric acid |
| Blood | Hemoglobin A1c |
| Blood | Creatine kinase |
| Blood | Creatine kinase-myocardial band fraction |
| Blood | Troponin I |
| Blood | C-reactive protein |
| Blood | N-terminal pro-B-type natriuretic peptide |
| Blood | Brain natriuretic peptide |
| Urine | pH |
| Urine | Occult hematuria |
| Blood | ABO blood typing |
| Others | Influenza antigen immunoassay |

#### 3.1.3. Developed System and Server of FirstER

Based on privacy legislation, the medical cloud zone, an IaaS (Infrastructure as a Service) provided by Samsung Data System (Seoul, Korea), met the facilities and equipment standards necessary for the management and preservation of EMRs, which is a requirement for the remote storage of EMRs. Data transmission and reception between the hospitals and the MyData cloud servers were linked by RESTful API (Representational State Transfer Application Programming Interface), SSL (Secure Socket Layer, https), and JSON (JavaScript Object Notation, data format). (Figure 3).

A patient sends subscriber information (patient hospital ID) to the hospital information system (HIS) through the private cloud platform when the patient agrees to subscribe to the mobile app and to the collection/use of their personal information. After validation of the subscriber information, the ED core data of the patient are extracted from the HIS server to the MyData-linked server in the hospital. Afterwards, when a patient requests "download", the core data of the patient are transferred from the connected server in the hospital to the MyData cloud platform.

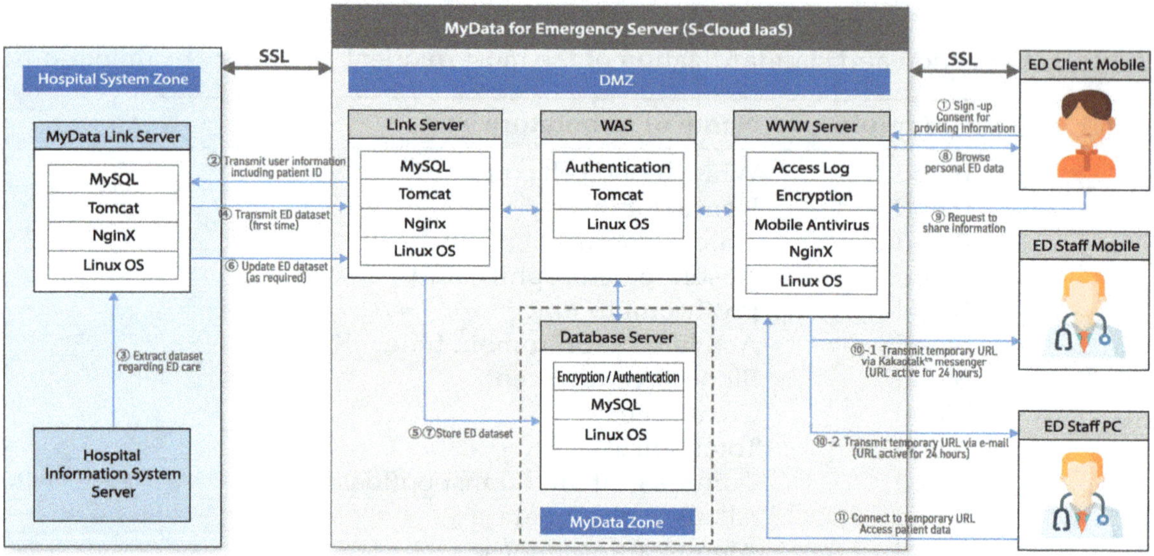


**Figure 3.** System and server architecture for FirstER. Data transmission and reception between the hospitals and the MyData cloud servers were linked by RESTful API, SSL, and JSON. A patient sends his or her hospital ID to the HIS through the private cloud platform when the patient agrees to subscribe to the mobile app and the collection/use of their personal information. After validation of the subscriber information, the ED core data of the patient are extracted from the HIS server to the MyData-linked server in the hospital. Afterwards, when a patient requests "download", the core data of the patient are transferred from the connected server in the hospital to the MyData cloud platform (OS: operating system, ED: emergency department, SSL: Secure Socket Layer, ID: identification, IaaS: Infrastructure as a Service, DMZ: demilitarized zone, WAS: web application server, WWW: World Wide Web, URL: uniform resource locator, PC: personal computer, HIS: hospital information system).

### *3.2. Pre-Operation Testing*

Unit testing and integrated testing were conducted two times each. Twenty-two items out of a total of 79 in the first unit test were evaluated as inadequate, and all these items were supplemented and corrected in the second unit test. In the first integrated test, 81 items from seven categories (registration, PHR function, ED record, management, etc.) were accessed, and 18 items were evaluated as inappropriate. All items passed in the second integrated test.

### *3.3. Flow of Services*

An app user who is a patient or caretaker launches this app and registers using his or her e-mail and password after consent of privacy (Figure 4A).

After login, the main page shows the user's picture, name, blood type, drug allergies, and recent visits to the ED at a glance. Additionally, there are four items linked on the main page: details of medical records from recent ED visits, medication that has to be taken today, "My recent health condition", and recent self-checked blood pressure. Additionally, there is an SOS button to directly call the patient's care provider on the top left and a plus-shaped button that included items associated with the ED records at the bottom right (Figure 4B).

When the user inputs "My recent health condition", the most recent record is displayed on the main page. The user can choose a part of the body that is uncomfortable and add a note. In the same way, a record of self-checked blood pressure is shown. The systolic and diastolic blood pressures can be entered separately (Figure 4C).

Upon touching a button labeled "I have to take medicines today", the screen displays the hospital and department, day, medication and dosage, and frequency prescribed. Each medication button is linked to a page with a description of it (Figure 4D).

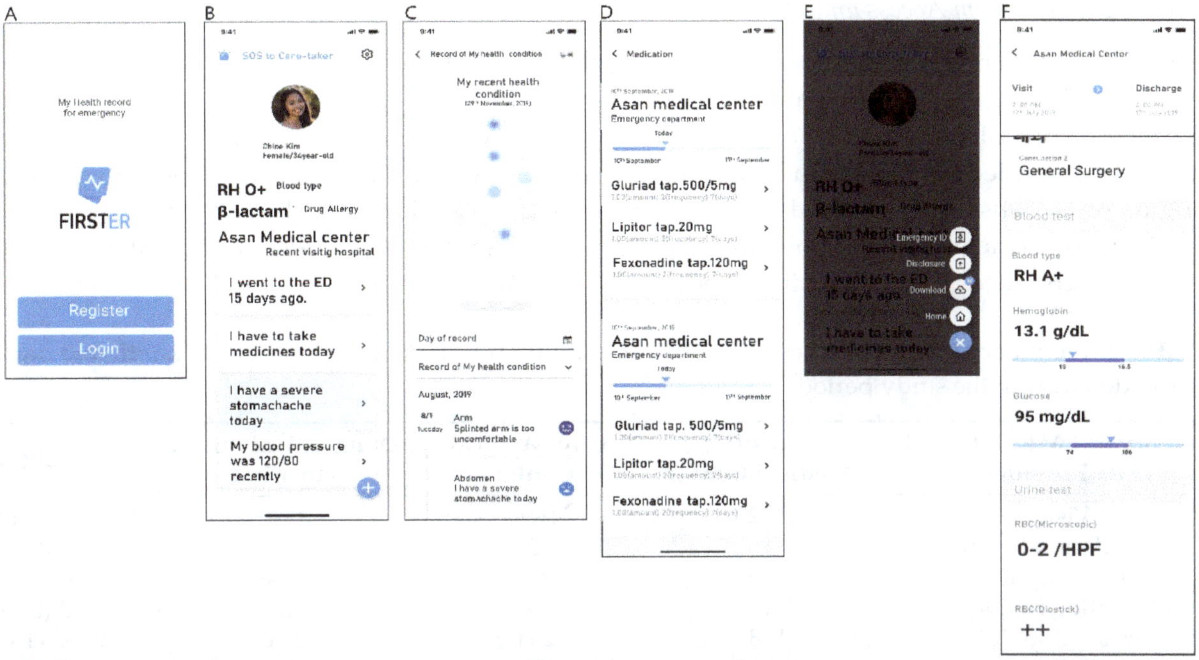


**Figure 4.** Screenshots of the FirstER user interface (translated to English). (**A**) Introduction page for registration and log-in; (**B**) main page for user's information, ED visiting history, medication alarms and PGHD at a glance; (**C**) details of PGHD contents: "My recent health condition"; (**D**) prescribed medication (duration, amount, and frequency) and buttons linked to detailed drug information; (**E**) emergency ID, useful information when a user visits an emergency department, and buttons linked to download and "disclosure" PHR data; (**F**) details of My ED records: visiting time, department consulted, and results of blood tests and urine tests. (ED: emergency department, PGHD: patient-generated health data, ID: identification, PHR: personal health record).

To use the functions of the EMR-tethered PHR, the user touches the plus-shaped button on the main page and then touches the "Download" button. When the user selects the hospital and inputs the hospital ID number, the existence of newly generated data is checked and any such data are downloaded. Downloaded data are displayed as a button labeled "I went to the ED several days ago" on the main page. When the user touches the button, details of the ED records from the EMR system of the selected hospital are seen. The user can see the time of the visit and discharge from the ED, diagnosis, department, results of blood and urine tests, and medications prescribed at discharge. If the user has several ED visit records, the user can press the "List" button at the bottom and check each entry (Figure 4B,E).

When the button labeled "Emergency ID" in the plus-shaped button on the main page is touched, it shows at a glance the information—namely, the patient's name, gender, age, blood type, drug allergies, hospitals recently visited, caretaker information, and a document on the decision to withdraw from life-sustaining treatment—that is needed immediately in an emergency situation (Figure 4D).

Upon touching a button labeled "disclosure" in the plus-shaped logo on the main page, the user enters his or her password for authentication and then selects the institution and items to share. After that, the user sends a temporary URL (limited to 24 h) of their previous ED records via SNS or e-mail (Figure 4D).

By adding a function of selecting the institution and items to share in his or her medical record to the fundamental setting function, the user can choose whether to share sensitive medical information.

Based on advice from a legal executive, the patient is required to provide consent for several steps of installing, using, and withdrawing FirstER. Accordingly, there are no major legal problems in installing and utilizing FirstER.

### 3.4. *Frequency of System Access and Utilization*

From 14 October to 29 November 2019, the registration desks were operated in three EDs. While the desks were running, about 5100 patients were discharged at the EDs, and about 20% of the patients (1051 patients) installed the mobile app with informed consent. The number of EMR-tethered records that were downloaded per user request was 15,951 records in total. These records were categorized into visiting records, consultation records, laboratory records, operation records, and prescription records (Table 3). In two local secondary hospitals that only received data, there were a total of 22 downloads. Additionally, 265 cases had PGHD inputted.

**Table 3.** Frequency of system access and utilization. Numbers indicate counts of EMR-tethered data provided during the study period.

| Category of EMR-Tethered Data Provided | Samsung Medical Center | Asan Medical Center | Dong-A University Hospital | Total (%) |
|---|---|---|---|---|
| Visit | 4523 | 1694 | 2398 | 8615 (54.0) |
| Consultation history | 16 | 0 | 0 | 16 (0.0) |
| Laboratory test | 2699 | 886 | 1636 | 5221 (32.7) |
| Operation history | 10 | 0 | 2 | 12 (0.0) |
| Prescription data | 1285 | 241 | 561 | 2087 (13.1) |
| Total | 8533 | 2821 | 4597 | 15,951 |

EMR: electronic medical record.

## 4. Discussion

In this study, we introduced a newly developed mobile app, called FirstER, which enables the aggregation of data from three hospitals and yields PHRs to others if needed. Even though FirstER needs further validation, it demonstrates that mobile apps can enable interoperability between different sources of PHRs from different hospitals.

Medical record interoperability has been recognized to improve convenience and clinical outcomes for patients. With the rapid uptake of smartphones and the digitalization of medical records, healthcare services have planned the development of mobile health apps. Jung et al. previously introduced a mobile application to provide diabetes self-management, including cardio-cerebrovascular risk evaluation, stress evaluation, and an exercise tutor [14]. Wagner et al. evaluated the usefulness of PHRs for patients with hypertension and concluded that they might have a limited impact. However, these studies focused on non-emergency situations [15]. One pilot study announced the development of a mobile emergency app to improve interoperability between pre-hospital services and hospitals in a mass-casualty situation [16]. Although this application might be useful for emergency physicians, it was not intended for patients. To the best of our knowledge, FirstER is the first mobile app prototype for patients who visit the ED and use their PHRs at other hospitals in an emergency. Whenever patients unintentionally first visited nearby hospitals, FirstER enabled medical personnel to know about the patients' previous underlying diseases, the reasons why they visited other hospitals, and what they were prescribed [17]. Furthermore, we also enabled patients to input their health records (i.e., patient-generated health data), such as conditions and blood pressure results, into FirstER, which then provided physicians with these data to help understand patients' conditions [18]. Using wearable devices with FirstER could provide more expansive and diverse datasets to help clinicians with decision-making about care plans [19,20].

In this investigation, we focused on variables that are commonly useful for emergencies by analyzing the frequencies of prescriptions. Furthermore, emergency medicine physicians discussed with each other the clinical importance of the variables and reached a consensus on which ones to include. The parameters needed to be reliable, accurate, and easy to access. Regarding the selection of such parameters, we considered numerous issues. At first, we attempted to insert radiologic examinations, which could be helpful for efficient diagnosis and treatment. Nevertheless, the final version of the app did not contain such data because of storage and bandwidth issues. Radiologic reports without images were not provided because these frequently mislead both patients and physicians. Secondly, we also did not include the results of bacterial or viral cultures, including those for multi-resistance bacteria, sexually transmitted diseases, or new emerging infections. We thought that hiding such data could be problematic in specific situations. However, after reviewing Korean Privacy Act issues, we decided to exclude sensitive health records, including those relating to sexually transmitted diseases. This was largely because there tends to be a stigma in our country around revealing delicate past medical histories. Even though there were several limitations, as we mentioned above, FirstER is well-designed and developed for our initial purpose. The usability of this prototype may be expanded by having more participating hospitals, containing admission records, and having other medical data, such as radiological examinations. Moreover, further updates would focus on covering detailed data on chronic medical illnesses and recent emerging infectious diseases.

Research about the validity and reliability of FirstER has been progressing in another study with survey analyses from both healthcare providers and patients. It is promising that FirstER has already been downloaded more than 1000 times, and most responses to questions about usability in the pilot surveys have shown user satisfaction. Meanwhile, dissatisfaction, because the app was hard to use the first time, was one of the most common answers on the surveys, especially for those patients who were not familiar with using a smartphone. After developing FirstER and installing the app on a user's device, there were some cases in which the app did not work due to conflicts between the app and certain versions of mobile phones. Most such problems were solved by stabilizing the cloud server and updating the app. However, the app did not work in very remote versions in a few mobile phones despite continuously updating the app. Furthermore, the patients need to follow multiple steps with many instances of giving informed consent to provide their records to physicians. These complicated processes are largely to protect the patients' privacy; however, involving patients' caregivers to introduce manuals for the app and further updates would improve usability.

With the developing platform for the mPHR, ED physicians could diagnose and treat their patients more quickly and efficiently, because problems similar to previous ones could be solved without duplicated tests. Fewer clinical tests due to decreased duplicated tests might have a positive effect on improving overcrowding in EDs, though this needs further evaluation. Previous studies reported that the turnaround time for laboratory and radiologic tests negatively impacts ED overcrowding and length of stay [21,22]. Improving the quality of care and enhancing the safety of patients is multifactorial, and one of the most effective ways to diminish overcrowding can be by avoiding unnecessary laboratory and imaging examinations [23]. Future studies need to focus on which information on the PHRs can improve patient outcome. Also, research on PHR-based emergency medical services can further progress by expanding the mobile app.

Categorizing the data provided, it was found that the app users requested their laboratory results in addition to the visit data that are provided by default.

We noticed several limitations while developing and applying FirstER. First, the patients' usability and satisfaction might be lower than expected because a relatively small number of hospitals participated. If the clinical data could be connected between tertiary hospitals and primary clinics, the app's usability would be improved. For example, patients with mild infectious illnesses or simple minor trauma cases could provide their laboratory results and prescriptions to their primary healthcare provider through this app after adequate treatment in the emergency department. However, FirstER is the first platform in an emergency to support interoperability between hospitals, and further study could make it possible to share PHRs at many hospitals. Second, data for radiologic examinations, such as simple radiographs, computed tomography, and magnetic resonance imaging, could not be provided because of limited storage and bandwidth. Third, there were some reports of errors during the uploading and downloading of data in the mobile app. These errors were mostly because of the different existing platforms between hospitals and different data types with test codes. However, these technical challenges were recognized in the early phase and fixed by standardizing the data from each hospital. Fourth, this app only covered the clinical data from the emergency department. Information during admission could be more informative, especially for patients admitted for a long duration. Regretfully, this app was a prototype and only included the medical records from the emergency department, including laboratory results, presumed diagnosis, and prescriptions at time of discharge from the emergency department. A future study is planned to update the app to include clinical data during admission. Lastly, we could not evaluate the clinical impacts of the mobile application, such as mortality or length of ED stay, due to the short study period.

## 5. Conclusions

In this study, we developed and successfully implemented an mPHR service that can be used as a health information exchange tool in emergencies by integrating medication information from three different tertiary hospitals. By recognizing the significance and limitations of this service, it is necessary to study the development and implementation of mPHR services that are more suitable for emergency medical services.

**Author Contributions:** Y.C., I.H.K., W.C. and J.-H.L. contributed to conceptualization of new application and platform: S.M.K. helped conduct the data curation and formal analysis. I.H.K., W.C. and J.-H.L. contributed to funding acquisition. Y.C., J.-s.K., I.H.K., T.K. and S.M.K. initiated this study as principle investigators of this project. Y.C., J.K., I.H.K., T.K., W.C. and J.-H.L. contributed to application of the research methodology. Y.C., I.H.K. and T.K. administrated the project. Y.C., I.H.K. and J.-H.L. supervised the entire process; J.J. helped visualize the figures and tables; Y.C., J.-s.K. and I.H.K. drafted the manuscript as first and corresponding authors. T.K. and J.J. reviewed and edited for completion of the manuscript. All authors have read and agreed to the published version of the manuscript.

**Acknowledgments:** This study included some results of 1st year product of research project supported by a grant from the PHR based personalized health management system development project through the Korea Evaluation Institute of Industrial Technology, funded by the Ministry of Trade, Industry and Energy, Korea (grant number:20004503 Project principal investigator: Seok Jae Heo of vTW).

## References

1. Hudson, P.; Ekholm, J.; Johnson, M.; Langdon, R. Early identification and management of the unstable adult patient in the emergency department. *J. Clin. Nurs.* **2015**, *24*, 3138–3146. [CrossRef]
2. Abel, G.A.; Mendonca, S.C.; McPhail, S.; Zhou, Y.; Elliss-Brookes, L.; Lyratzopoulos, G. Emergency diagnosis of cancer and previous general practice consultations: Insights from linked patient survey data. *Br. J. Gen. Pract.* **2017**, *67*, e377–e387. [CrossRef] [PubMed]
3. Alimenti, D.; Buydos, S.; Cunliffe, L.; Hunt, A. Improving perceptions of patient safety through standardizing handoffs from the emergency department to the inpatient setting. *J. Am. Assoc. Nurse Pract.* **2019**, *31*, 354–363. [CrossRef] [PubMed]
4. Shapiro, J.S.; Kannry, J.; Lipton, M.; Goldberg, E.; Conocenti, P.; Stuard, S.; Wyatt, B.M.; Kuperman, G. Approaches to patient health information exchange and their impact on emergency medicine. *Ann. Emerg. Med.* **2006**, *48*, 426–432. [CrossRef] [PubMed]
5. Bouayad, L.; Ialynytchev, A.; Padmanabhan, B. Patient health record systems scope and functionalities: Literature review and future directions. *J. Med. Internet Res.* **2017**, *19*, e388. [CrossRef]
6. Bouri, N.; Ravi, S. Going mobile: How mobile personal health records can improve health care during emergencies. *JMIR Mhealth Uhealth* **2014**, *2*, e8. [CrossRef] [PubMed]
7. Zhao, J.Y.; Song, B.; Anand, E.; Schwartz, D.; Panesar, M.; Jackson, G.P.; Elkin, P.L. Barriers, facilitators, and solutions to optimal patient portal and personal health record use: A systematic review of the literature. *AMIA Annu. Symp. Proc.* **2018**, *2017*, 1913–1922.

8. Ro, H.J.; Jung, S.Y.; Lee, K.; Hwang, H.; Yoo, S.; Baek, H.; Lee, K.; Bae, W.K.; Han, J.-S.; Kim, S.; et al. Establishing a personal health record system in an academic hospital: One year's experience. *Korean J. Fam. Med.* **2015**, *36*, 121–127. [CrossRef]
9. Andrikopoulou, E.; Scott, P.J.; Herrera, H. Important design features of personal health records to improve medication adherence for patients with long-term conditions: Protocol for a systematic literature review. *JMIR Res. Protoc.* **2018**, *7*, e159. [CrossRef]
10. Koivumäki, T.; Pekkarinen, S.; Lappi, M.; Väisänen, J.; Juntunen, J.; Pikkarainen, M. Consumer adoption of future MyData-based Preventive eHealth Services: An acceptance model and survey study. *J. Med. Internet Res.* **2017**, *19*, e429. [CrossRef]
11. Park, J.-Y.; Lee, G.; Shin, S.-Y.; Kim, J.H.; Han, H.-W.; Kwon, T.-W.; Kim, W.S.; Lee, J.H. Lessons learned from the development of health applications in a tertiary hospital. *Telemed. J. E Health* **2014**, *20*, 215–222. [CrossRef] [PubMed]
12. Ryu, J.-H.; Min, M.-K.; Lee, D.-S.; Yeom, S.-R.; Lee, S.-H.; Wang, I.-J.; Cho, S.-J.; Hwang, S.-Y.; Lee, J.-H.; Kim, Y.H. Changes in relative importance of the 5-level triage system, Korean Triage and Acuity Scale, for the disposition of emergency patients induced by forced reduction in its level number: A multi-center registry-based retrospective cohort study. *J. Korean Med. Sci.* **2019**, *34*, 1–12. [CrossRef]
13. Ham, S.; Min, Y.-G.; Chae, M.K.; Kim, H.-H. Epidemiology and regional differences of acute poisonings of eight cities in Gyeonggi-do province in Korea using data from the National Emergency Department Information System of Korea. *Clin. Exp. Emerg. Med.* **2020**, *7*, 43–51. [CrossRef] [PubMed]
14. Jung, E.-Y.; Kim, J.; Chung, K.-Y.; Park, D.K. Mobile healthcare application with EMR interoperability for diabetes patients. *Cluster Comput.* **2013**, *17*, 871–880. [CrossRef]
15. Wagner, P.J.; Dias, J.; Howard, S.; Kintziger, K.W.; Hudson, M.F.; Seol, Y.H.; Sodomka, P. Personal health records and hypertension control: A randomized trial. *J. Am. Med. Inform. Assoc.* **2012**, *19*, 626–634. [CrossRef]
16. Bellini, P.; Boncinelli, S.; Grossi, F.; Mangini, M.; Nesi, P.; Sequi, L. Mobile emergency, an emergency support system for hospitals in mobile devices: Pilot study. *JMIR Res. Protoc.* **2013**, *2*, e19. [CrossRef] [PubMed]
17. Zhou, L.; DeAlmeida, D.; Parmanto, B. Applying a user-centered approach to building a mobile personal health record app: Development and usability study. *JMIR Mhealth Uhealth* **2019**, *7*, e13194. [CrossRef] [PubMed]
18. Nittas, V.; Mütsch, M.; Ehrler, F.; Puhan, M.A. Electronic patient-generated health data to facilitate prevention and health promotion: A scoping review protocol. *BMJ Open* **2018**, *8*, e021245. [CrossRef] [PubMed]
19. Abdolkhani, R.; Gray, K.; Borda, A.; DeSouza, R. Patient-generated health data management and quality challenges in remote patient monitoring. *JAMIA Open* **2019**, *2*, 471–478. [CrossRef] [PubMed]
20. Jung, S.Y.; Kim, J.-W.; Hwang, H.; Lee, K.; Baek, R.-M.; Lee, H.-Y.; Yoo, S.; Song, W.; Han, J.-S. Development of comprehensive personal health records integrating patient-generated health data directly from Samsung S-health and Apple health apps: Retrospective cross-sectional observational study. *JMIR Mhealth Uhealth* **2019**, *7*, e12691. [CrossRef]
21. Perotte, R.; Lewin, G.O.; Tambe, U.; Galorenzo, J.B.; Vawdrey, D.K.; Akala, O.O.; Makkar, J.S.; Lin, D.J.; Mainieri, L.; Chang, B.C. Improving emergency department flow- reducing turnaround time for emergent CT scans. *AMIA Annu. Symp. Proc.* **2018**, *2018*, 897–906. [PubMed]
22. Kaushik, N.; Khangulov, V.S.; O'Hara, M.; Arnaout, R. Reduction in laboratory turnaround time decreases emergency room length of stay. *Open Access Emerg. Med.* **2018**, *10*, 37–45. [CrossRef] [PubMed]
23. Stang, A.S.; Crotts, J.; Johnson, D.W.; Hartling, L.; Guttmann, A. Crowding measures associated with the quality of emergency department care: A systematic review. *Acad. Emerg. Med.* **2015**, *22*, 643–656. [CrossRef] [PubMed]

# 2

# A Machine Learning Approach to Predicting Readmission or Mortality in Patients Hospitalized for Stroke or Transient Ischemic Attack

**Ling-Chien Hung [1,†], Sheng-Feng Sung [1,2,3,†] and Ya-Han Hu [4,5,*]**

1 Division of Neurology, Department of Internal Medicine, Ditmanson Medical Foundation Chia-Yi Christian Hospital, Chiayi 600, Taiwan; 07177@cych.org.tw (L.-C.H.); sfsung@cych.org.tw (S.-F.S.)
2 Department of Information Management and Institute of Healthcare Information Management, National Chung Cheng University, Chiayi 621, Taiwan
3 Department of Nursing, Min-Hwei Junior College of Health Care Management, Tainan 736, Taiwan
4 Department of Information Management, National Central University, Taoyuan 320, Taiwan
5 MOST AI Biomedical Research Center at National Cheng Kung University, Tainan 701, Taiwan
* Correspondence: yhhu@mgt.ncu.edu.tw
† Ling-Chien Hung and Sheng-Feng Sung contributed equally to this work.

**Abstract:** Readmissions after stroke are not only associated with greater levels of disability and a higher risk of mortality but also increase overall medical costs. Predicting readmission risk and understanding its causes are thus essential for healthcare resource allocation and quality improvement planning. By using machine learning techniques on initial admission data, this study aimed to develop prediction models for readmission or mortality after stroke. During model development, resampling methods were implemented to balance the class distribution. Two-layer nested cross-validation was used to build and evaluate the prediction models. A total of 3422 patients were included for analysis. The 90-day rate of readmission or mortality was 17.6%. This study identified several important predictive factors, including age, prior emergency department visits, pre-stroke functional status, stroke severity, body mass index, consciousness level, and use of a nasogastric tube. The Naïve Bayes model with class weighting to compensate for class imbalance achieved the highest discriminatory capacity in terms of the area under the receiver operating characteristic curve (0.661). Despite having room for improvement, the prediction models could be used for early risk assessment of patients with stroke. Identification of patients at high risk for readmission or mortality immediately after admission has the potential of enabling early discharge planning and transitional care interventions.

**Keywords:** machine learning; prediction models; readmission; risk assessment; stroke

---

## 1. Introduction

Stroke is a leading cause of mortality and adult disability worldwide [1,2]. It causes a huge financial burden on the healthcare system [3]. Stroke survivors are prone to recurrence of stroke. Approximately 7% to 12% of patients with a first ischemic stroke have stroke recurrence within one year [4,5]. In addition, patients with stroke are likely to develop complications such as pneumonia, urinary tract infection, falls, etc., which may have a deleterious effect on the outcome of stroke [6]. As a result, a substantial proportion of stroke survivors are readmitted for various reasons after the initial hospitalization. In Taiwan, the 30-day readmission rate in patients with stroke was around 10% [7,8], and the 1-year readmission rate was between 30% and 43% [7–10]. Moreover, nearly 30% of the first-year medical cost for patients with stroke was spent on readmission [9]. Therefore, readmission after stroke is costly and needs more attention.

Patients with stroke who are readmitted have greater levels of disability, a higher risk of mortality, and more medical resource utilization than those not readmitted [11,12]. At the same time, risk-standardized mortality and readmission rates are used as indicators for hospital performance [13]. Even though it is arguable to link these indicators to reimbursement [14], the US Centers for Medicare & Medicaid Services (CMS) has implemented a program to reduce payments to hospitals with excess readmissions [15]. Specifically, for stroke care, CMS uses a hospital-level 30-day risk-standardized all-cause readmission measure to determine payments to hospitals [16]. Hospitals would thereby be penalized if their risk-standardized readmission rates were higher than expected [17]. Similarly, in Taiwan, the rate of unplanned 14-day readmission for the same or a related diagnosis and crude mortality rate are among the continuous monitoring indicators of care quality of Taiwan's hospital accreditation system [18]. While the hospital level is determined based on the results of hospital accreditation, it in turn determines the reimbursement a hospital will receive from the National Health Insurance program in Taiwan.

Thorough knowledge of the risk and causes of readmission or mortality is thus essential for both quality improvement planning and healthcare resource allocation. Because the occurrence of medical complications increases the risk of readmission or mortality, aggressive management, and treatment of complications that are potentially modifiable might be able to reduce readmissions or mortality following stroke [6,8,19]. Furthermore, early risk assessment using information available upon admission might help identify high-risk patients for targeted interventions, which could possibly prevent avoidable readmissions, reduce mortality and improve functional outcomes, and even enhance the financial health of hospitals.

Because machine learning (ML) techniques have been widely used in clinical decision support, this study aimed to use ML-based techniques to explore the predictive factors and to develop prediction models for readmission or mortality in patients hospitalized for stroke or transient ischemic attack (TIA). Specifically, this study compared prediction models that were developed using various ML techniques based on initial admission data from a large teaching hospital in Taiwan.

## 2. Materials and Methods

### 2.1. Study Population

The study hospital is a 1000-bed teaching hospital serving a city and its adjoining rural areas of approximately 500,000 inhabitants. The study population was identified from the hospital stroke registry, which enrolled consecutive patients hospitalized for ischemic stroke, hemorrhagic stroke, or TIA within 10 days of symptom onset. Ischemic stroke, hemorrhagic stroke, and TIA were defined in accordance with the criteria of the Taiwan Stroke Registry [20]. Adult patients admitted with the principal diagnosis of stroke or TIA between October 2007 and January 2016 who were discharged alive were identified. Only those who gave informed consent to participate in the stroke registry were included. Patients who were lost to follow-up at 90 days were excluded. The earliest admission during the study period was designated as the index hospitalization. The study protocol was approved by the Ditmanson Medical Foundation Chia-Yi Christian Hospital Institutional Review Board (CYCH-IRB No.104098).

### 2.2. Variables

The dependent variable of the dataset was a combined outcome of readmission or mortality within 90 days after discharge from the index hospitalization. While previous studies mainly focused on 30-day readmission models [21,22], around half of the first readmissions within one year after stroke occurred within 90 days [8]. The prediction of 90-day readmission after stroke has gained attention in recent years [23,24].

As a standard operating protocol for the stroke registry, each patient was interviewed in person or by telephone at 90 days. Information was obtained from a proxy for patients who could not be interviewed because of neurological deficits or death. The reason to use a combined outcome was to avoid underestimation of readmission rates. Patients who did not survive until hospitalization because of critical illness or sudden death might be recorded as dead rather than readmission during the telephone interview.

The independent variables included variables that were available upon admission, such as demographic data, initial vital signs and laboratory results, past medical history and comorbidities, treatment-seeking behavior, pre-stroke functional status as assessed using the modified Rankin Scale (mRS), and initial stroke severity as assessed using the National Institutes of Health Stroke Scale (NIHSS). Age, pre-stroke mRS, and initial NIHSS were treated as continuous variables. The frequency of prior emergency department (ED) visits within one year was categorized into 0, 1, or ≥2 visits. Prior hospitalizations within one year before the index hospitalization were categorized as yes or no. Physiological measurements and laboratory values were categorized into meaningful groups to align with clinical practice (Table S1). For example, the body mass index (BMI) status was categorized according to the local standard as follows: underweight (<18.5 kg/m$^2$), normal (18.5–23.9 kg/m$^2$), overweight (24–26.9 kg/m$^2$), and obese (≥27 kg/m$^2$) [25].

### *2.3. Machine Learning Techniques*

Various ML algorithms, including C4.5, classification, and regression tree (CART), *k*-nearest neighbor (*k*NN), logistic regression (LR), multilayer perceptron (MLP), Naïve Bayes (NB), random forest (RF), and support vector machines (SVM) were used to build classifiers for prediction of readmission or mortality. Specifically, the J48, SimpleCart, IBK, Logistic, MultilayerPerceptron, NaiveBayes, RandomForest, and SMO modules of Weka 3.8.3 open-source data mining software (Hamilton, New Zealand, www.cs.waikato.ac.nz/ml/weka) were used.

Class imbalance is common in health-related datasets and may distort the performance evaluation of ML methods because of their preference towards the majority class. Therefore, cost-sensitive learning and data resampling have been widely used to address this problem [26,27]. This study implemented several resampling methods, including undersampling, oversampling, synthetic minority oversampling technique (SMOTE), and class weighting, to investigate their effect on the performance of classifiers. Specifically, the SpreadSubsample, Resample, SMOTE, and ClassBalancer filters in Weka were used.

### *2.4. Experiments*

Experiments were conducted using Python 3.7 with the python-weka-wrapper3 package version 0.1.7 running on the MacOS 10.15 operating system. The scripts can be downloaded from Supplementary Material. Figure 1 illustrates the process of the classifier building. Two-layer nested cross-validation was used to build and evaluate the classifiers. In the outer loop, the dataset was split into 10 folds containing a training set and a holdout test set in a 9:1 ratio using stratified random sampling. The process of data splitting was repeated three times by varying the random seed, thus generating 30 training and test set pairs. In the inner loop, the training set was used to build classifiers, for which another 10-fold cross-validation was used to find the optimal hyperparameters (Table 1). The classifiers with the optimal hyperparameters were tested on the holdout test set. Then the evaluation metrics from the 30 training and test set pairs were averaged to estimate the generalization performance of classifiers. This approach ensures that the training, validation, and evaluation data are completely separated.

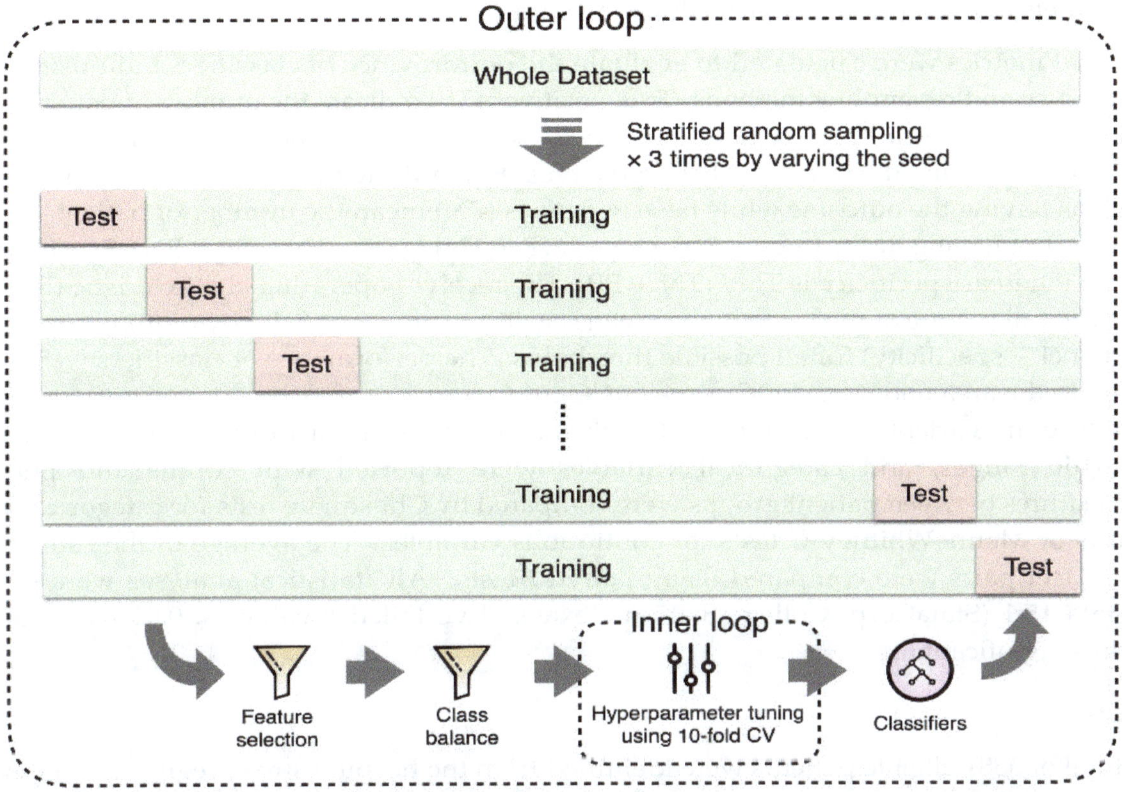


**Figure 1.** The process of classifier building. In the outer loop, 10-fold cross-validation (CV) was used to estimate the performance of the classifiers. In the inner loop, another 10-fold CV was used to find the optimal hyperparameters.

**Table 1.** Machine learning (ML) techniques and hyperparameter tuning. NA = not applicable.

| Techniques | Hyperparameters | Range | Increment |
|---|---|---|---|
| NB | NA | NA | NA |
| LR | Ridge value | Default | NA |
| RF | Number of trees | 10–200 | 10 |
| *k*NN | Number of neighbors | 1–20 | 1 |
| SVM | Complexity | 0.5–1.0 | 0.5 |
| | Kernel | PolyKernel, RBFKernel | NA |
| C4.5 | Confidence factor | 0.20–0.45 | 0.05 |
| | Minimum of number of instances per leaf | 2–20 | 1 |
| CART | Minimum number of instances per leaf | 2–20 | 1 |
| MLP | Learning rate | 0.1–0.5 | 0.2 |
| | Momentum | 0.1–0.3 | 0.1 |

Feature selection is a common ML technique. It has the potential of improving training efficiency, result comprehensibility, and prediction performance. Therefore, during the experiments, feature selection was applied to the training sets mainly to filter out redundant and/or irrelevant features from the original data to build a more explainable model. In this study, the correlation-based feature subset selection (CfsSubsetEval module in Weka) with the BestFirst search method was used to perform the feature selection procedure. A correlation-based feature selection method was used to evaluate the correlations between feature subsets and the dependent variable. The optimal feature subset contains features that are highly correlated with the dependent variable, but uncorrelated with each other [28]. The best first search strategy was used to find an optimal feature subset from the feature space. This approach does not specify a threshold to determine the most important features. Instead, the search terminates when the limit of the number of fully expanded subsets that result in no improvement is reached [28].

### 2.5. *Evaluation Metrics and Statistical Analysis*

Several metrics were calculated to evaluate the performance of classifiers built using different ML techniques and resampling methods. True positives (TP) indicate the number of patients correctly classified as having the outcome whereas true negatives (TN) mean the number of patients correctly classified as not having the outcome. False positives (FP) indicate the number of patients incorrectly classified as having the outcome while false negatives (FN) mean the number of patients incorrectly classified as not having the outcome. Accuracy is (TP + TN) / (TP + TN + FP + FN). Sensitivity is TP / (TP + FN) whereas specificity is TN / (TN + FP). The receiver operating characteristic (ROC) curve displays the full picture of the trade-off between sensitivity and specificity by plotting sensitivity as a function of (1 − specificity) for all possible thresholds. The performance of classifiers was compared according to the area under the ROC curve (AUC).

Continuous variables were reported with means and standard deviations or medians with interquartile ranges, and categorical variables were reported with counts and percentages. Clinical features between patient groups were compared by Chi-square tests for categorical variables and *t*-tests or Mann–Whitney U tests for continuous variables. The average of the estimates from the 30 dataset pairs were compared using paired *t*-tests. All statistical analyses were performed using Stata 15.1 (StataCorp, College Station, Texas). Two-tailed $p$ values $< 0.05$ were considered statistically significant.

## 3. Results

A total of 5581 eligible patients were identified from the hospital stroke registry. After excluding patients who did not give informed consent ($n$ = 1384) and those who were lost to follow-up at 90 days ($n$ = 775), the remaining 3422 patients comprised the study population. The study population did not differ statistically from those who were excluded in age (68.3 ± 12.6 versus 68.3 ± 12.9, $p$ = 0.928), sex (female 39.9% versus 41.3%, $p$ = 0.317), and stroke severity (NIHSS median 4, interquartile range [IQR] 2–9 versus 5, IQR 2–11, $p$ = 0.056). Table 2 gives the demographics and characteristics of the stroke of the study population. Patients with the combined outcome were older, more likely to be female, and had greater stroke severity. The 90-day rate of readmission or mortality was 17.6% (602/3422). Table S1 lists the independent variables considered to build the models. Most of the variables were significantly different between groups.

**Table 2.** Demographics and characteristics of stroke of the study population. TIA = transient ischemic attack. ICH = intracerebral hemorrhage. NIHSS = National Institute of Health Stroke Scale. SD = standard deviation. IQR = Interquartile range.

| Clinical Feature | Total ($n$ = 3422) | Readmission or Mortality within 90 Days ($n$ = 602) | No Readmission or Mortality within 90 Days ($n$ = 2820) | $p$ |
|---|---|---|---|---|
| Age, years, mean (SD) | 68.3 (12.6) | 71.3 (12.3) | 67.7 (12.6) | <0.001 |
| Female, n (%) | 1366 (39.9) | 264 (43.9) | 1102 (39.1) | 0.030 |
| Stroke type, n (%) | | | | 0.924 |
| Ischemic stroke | 2622 (76.6) | 465 (77.2) | 2157 (76.5) | |
| TIA | 467 (13.7) | 80 (13.3) | 387 (13.7) | |
| ICH | 333 (9.7) | 57 (9.5) | 276 (9.8) | |
| NIHSS, median (IQR) | 4 (2–9) | 6 (3–14) | 4 (2–8) | <0.001 |

### 3.1. *Important Features*

Correlation-based feature selection was applied to the 30 training sets to find the optimal feature subset. Table 3 lists the features and the times that each feature was selected from the training sets. Among them, age, prior ED visits within one year, pre-stroke functional status as assessed by the mRS, initial stroke severity as assessed by the NIHSS, BMI, consciousness level as assessed by the Glasgow Coma Scale, and use of nasogastric tube were the most important features that predict readmission or mortality at 90 days after stroke. These features were constantly selected by the feature selection algorithm from the 30 different training sets. In addition, failed dysphagia screening test, coronary artery disease, cancer, heart failure, atrial fibrillation, recent infection, prior hospitalization within one year, the stage of renal dysfunction as assessed by the estimated creatinine clearance rate, and use of Foley catheter, which were selected in more than 20 out of the 30 feature selection processes, were also key features.

**Table 3.** Features selected among 30 training sets. BMI = body mass index. CAD = coronary artery disease. eCCr = estimated creatinine clearance rate. ED = emergency department. ESRD = end-stage renal disease. GCS = Glasgow Coma Scale. mRS = modified Rankin Scale. NIHSS = National Institutes of Health Stroke Scale.

| Features | Selection Times (out of 30) |
|---|---|
| Age | 30 |
| Prior ED visits within one year | 30 |
| Pre-stroke mRS | 30 |
| NIHSS | 30 |
| BMI group | 30 |
| GCS group | 30 |
| Use of nasogastric tube | 30 |
| Failed dysphagia screening test | 29 |
| CAD | 29 |
| Cancer | 29 |
| Heart failure | 28 |
| Atrial fibrillation | 27 |
| Recent infection | 25 |
| Prior hospitalization within one year | 23 |
| eCCr stage | 22 |
| Use of Foley catheter | 22 |
| Hematocrit | 18 |
| ESRD | 18 |
| Hemoglobin | 18 |
| Diabetes mellitus | 7 |
| ED arrival mode | 4 |
| Occupation | 2 |
| Cared by attendant | 2 |
| Education | 1 |
| Use of birth control pill | 1 |

### 3.2. Evaluation Results

Table 4 gives the average AUC, sensitivity, specificity, and accuracy of various prediction models. The average AUC values across the ML techniques and resampling methods are displayed as a heatmap in Figure 2. In general, the AUC values of NB (0.602–0.661) and LR models (0.539–0.659) were higher than those of the other ML techniques, whereas MLP models (0.545–0.563) had the lowest AUC values. Among the data resampling methods, the undersampling method improved the performance of prediction for most of the ML techniques. On the contrary, the SMOTE method resulted in lower performance for all the ML techniques. Figure 3 shows the average AUC values ordered from the highest to the lowest. NB models with class weighting, undersampling, imbalanced, and oversampling, and LR with class weighting ranked the top five. The AUC values between the top five models were not significantly different according to paired $t$-tests.

**Table 4.** The average performance of various models. AUC = area under the receiver operating characteristic curve.

| | AUC | Sensitivity | Specificity | Accuracy |
|---|---|---|---|---|
| Imbalanced | | | | |
| C4.5 | 0.583 | 0.097 | 0.960 | 0.808 |
| CART | 0.568 | 0.071 | 0.965 | 0.808 |
| *k*NN | 0.585 | 0.044 | 0.980 | 0.815 |
| LR | 0.649 | 0.075 | 0.983 | 0.823 |
| MLP | 0.547 | 0.188 | 0.884 | 0.762 |
| NB | 0.660 | 0.328 | 0.868 | 0.773 |
| RF | 0.607 | 0.070 | 0.956 | 0.800 |
| SVM | 0.500 | 0.000 | 1.000 | 0.824 |
| Undersampling | | | | |
| C4.5 | 0.600 | 0.531 | 0.642 | 0.623 |
| CART | 0.599 | 0.526 | 0.657 | 0.634 |
| *k*NN | 0.611 | 0.434 | 0.740 | 0.686 |
| LR | 0.653 | 0.553 | 0.680 | 0.657 |
| MLP | 0.563 | 0.494 | 0.621 | 0.599 |
| NB | 0.660 | 0.503 | 0.742 | 0.700 |
| RF | 0.599 | 0.578 | 0.575 | 0.575 |
| SVM | 0.614 | 0.465 | 0.763 | 0.711 |
| Oversampling | | | | |
| C4.5 | 0.581 | 0.472 | 0.656 | 0.624 |
| CART | 0.588 | 0.516 | 0.643 | 0.620 |
| *k*NN | 0.587 | 0.482 | 0.646 | 0.617 |
| LR | 0.652 | 0.550 | 0.688 | 0.663 |
| MLP | 0.552 | 0.395 | 0.708 | 0.653 |
| NB | 0.659 | 0.511 | 0.739 | 0.699 |
| RF | 0.598 | 0.346 | 0.772 | 0.697 |
| SVM | 0.616 | 0.484 | 0.748 | 0.701 |
| SMOTE | | | | |
| C4.5 | 0.542 | 0.238 | 0.796 | 0.698 |
| CART | 0.544 | 0.263 | 0.780 | 0.689 |
| *k*NN | 0.532 | 0.313 | 0.724 | 0.652 |
| LR | 0.539 | 0.369 | 0.696 | 0.638 |
| MLP | 0.545 | 0.291 | 0.774 | 0.689 |
| NB | 0.602 | 0.431 | 0.740 | 0.686 |
| RF | 0.588 | 0.162 | 0.870 | 0.745 |
| SVM | 0.540 | 0.397 | 0.682 | 0.632 |
| Class weighting | | | | |
| C4.5 | 0.584 | 0.486 | 0.657 | 0.627 |
| CART | 0.586 | 0.502 | 0.636 | 0.613 |
| *k*NN | 0.598 | 0.488 | 0.660 | 0.630 |
| LR | 0.659 | 0.558 | 0.693 | 0.669 |
| MLP | 0.550 | 0.364 | 0.738 | 0.673 |
| NB | 0.661 | 0.499 | 0.744 | 0.701 |
| RF | 0.603 | 0.239 | 0.844 | 0.737 |
| SVM | 0.618 | 0.486 | 0.751 | 0.704 |

| | C4.5 | CART | *k*NN | LR | MLP | NB | RF | SVM |
|---|---|---|---|---|---|---|---|---|
| **Imbalanced** | 0.583 | 0.568 | 0.585 | 0.649 | 0.547 | 0.660 | 0.607 | 0.500 |
| **Undersampling** | 0.600 | 0.599 | 0.611 | 0.653 | 0.563 | 0.660 | 0.599 | 0.614 |
| **Oversampling** | 0.581 | 0.588 | 0.587 | 0.652 | 0.552 | 0.659 | 0.598 | 0.616 |
| **SMOTE** | 0.542 | 0.544 | 0.532 | 0.539 | 0.545 | 0.602 | 0.588 | 0.540 |
| **Class weighting** | 0.584 | 0.586 | 0.598 | 0.659 | 0.550 | 0.661 | 0.603 | 0.618 |

**Figure 2.** Heat map showing the area under the receiver operating characteristic curve (AUC) across the ML techniques and resampling methods. In the heat map, the red color indicates high, yellow intermediate, and green low values of AUC.

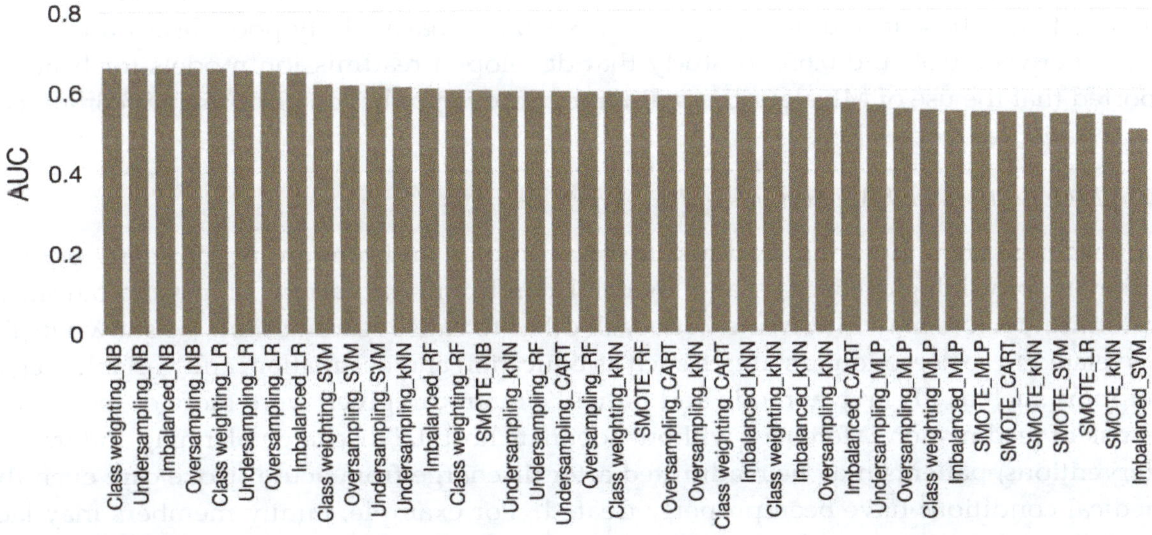


**Figure 3.** Performance of various ML models in predicting 90-day readmission or mortality in patients hospitalized for stroke or transient ischemic attack. Prediction models are ordered according to the area under the receiver operating characteristic curve (AUC).

## 4. Discussion

### *4.1. Principal Findings*

By analyzing a hospital stroke registry, this study found a rate of readmission or mortality of 17.6% at 90 days after stroke or TIA. The most important features that predict readmission or mortality included age, prior ED visits within one year, pre-stroke functional status, initial stroke severity, BMI, consciousness level, and use of nasogastric tube. Several ML techniques were applied to build prediction models. NB and LR models performed better than the other models in terms of AUC. The best model, i.e., the NB model with class weighting, achieved an AUC of 0.661. Although data resampling was expected to improve the performance of prediction, not all resampling methods performed equally well. Among them, the undersampling method improved prediction performance for most of the ML techniques.

### *4.2. Comparisons with Past Studies*

Previous studies that examined 90-day readmissions after stroke have found readmission rates ranging from around 18% to 26% [12,24,29,30] even though the inclusion criteria and outcome measures varied slightly across studies. The rate of readmission or mortality in this study was similar to those in previous reports. However, this study differed from previous readmission models in that only the variables available upon stroke admission were used to build the prediction models.

Several prior studies have investigated readmissions in patients with stroke admitted to post-acute-care or inpatient rehabilitation facilities [21,22,31]. Even though their predictor variables were more informative and generally included past medical history, comorbidities, complications during acute care, and factors related to post-acute care [21,22,31], their values of AUC were not much different from those in this study. For example, a large retrospective study of 803,124 patients with stroke using inpatient rehabilitation facility functional outcome data achieved AUC values ranging from 0.553 to 0.694 in predicting 30-day readmissions [21]. In other words, the prediction of readmission after stroke is not a trivial task. This is probably because various patient clinical and social characteristics are associated with readmission and these characteristics are not always routinely collected in clinical databases [32].

In addition to readmission models for stroke, a systematic review found that readmission models for various disease populations based on administrative data, clinical data, or both generally performed inadequately [33]. Those tested in large populations had a particularly poor discriminative ability with AUCs between 0.55 and 0.65. A study that developed readmission models for heart failure also reported that the use of ML algorithms did not improve prediction performance compared with traditional statistical models [34].

### *4.3. Clinical Implications and Applications in Real-World Settings*

The mechanisms underlying readmission are complex and remain incompletely understood. In addition to physiological factors and medical conditions, a variety of psychological, social, and economical factors may intertwine with each other to cause readmission. As shown in Table 3, variables related to socioeconomic statuses such as education and occupation, and variables regarding social support such as ED arrival mode and patient's main caregiver, were more or less associated with the risk of readmission. Moreover, without adequate hospital discharge planning and transitional care interventions, patients may be readmitted after discharge from acute stroke care even though their medical conditions have been properly treated. For example, family members may lack the training, skills, and support services to provide caregiving for disabled stroke survivors, and therefore, bring patients back to the hospital. Adequate preparation and support for transition from acute stroke care to home may be required to reduce readmissions [24].

Previous studies have shown that a substantial proportion (up to 12.9%) of readmissions were potentially preventable [16,35]. Even though hospital discharge planning has the potential of preventing readmissions [36], one of the key steps is to identify patients at risk of readmission, preferably in the early stage of admission. The prediction models in this study were developed using only variables available upon admission and, therefore, can be used to estimate the probability of readmission soon after patients are admitted to the hospital. A clinical decision support system employing the ML prediction models developed in this study can facilitate clinicians to identify patients likely to experience readmission upon hospital admission. In this way, early targeted interventions for patients at high risk of readmission can be enabled. Certainly, these predischarge interventions should be tailored to the individual patient according to the estimated risk of readmission and may include patient needs assessment, patient education, medication reconciliation, the arrangement of early outpatient follow-up, and referrals to home health rehabilitation [37–39]. Furthermore, after hospital discharge, at-risk patients identified by the prediction models can be closely monitored to detect in time whether they are having problems and about to bounce back [40].

### 4.4. Future Directions

Several approaches may be attempted to improve the performance of prediction models for readmission. First, high-dimensional information in administrative claims data may be used to supplement clinical information in the development of prediction models. Readmission models for patients with chronic pancreatitis using standardized billing codes and basic patient characteristics were found to perform reasonably with AUCs ranging from 0.65 to 0.73 [41]. Second, in addition to structured clinical information, significant determinants of readmission, such as social factors, can be extracted from clinical notes through natural language processing [42], and in turn, used to build prediction models. Third, other ML algorithms can be explored. For example, extreme gradient boosting models were shown to have higher AUCs than traditional statistical models in predicting 90-day readmissions due to recurrent ischemic events in patients with ischemic stroke [23].

### 4.5. Limitations

First, this is a single-hospital study and the generalizability of the study findings should therefore be made with caution. Second, about 39% (2159/5581) of patients were excluded from the analysis because of declining informed consent or missing 3-month data. However, the possibility of selection bias might not be a concern because the study population did not differ from excluded patients in age, sex, and stroke severity. Third, the dependent variable of interest, i.e., readmission or mortality, was obtained through interviews with patients or their proxies. Therefore, recall bias might cause underestimation of the dependent variable. Fourth, this study did not use variables related to the process of acute care or post-acute care hospitalizations to develop prediction models, thus possibly undermining the prediction performance. On the other hand, prediction models using only information available upon admission might be advantageous in delivering the early targeted intervention to patients at high risk of readmission or mortality.

## 5. Conclusions

This study developed ML-based models to predict readmission or mortality in patients hospitalized for stroke or TIA. Several important predictive factors that increase the risk of readmission or mortality were identified, including age, prior ED visits within one year, pre-stroke functional status, initial stroke severity, BMI, consciousness level, and use of nasogastric tube. Various resampling methods were implemented to balance the class distribution. Nevertheless, they did not always improve predictive performance. The NB model with class weighting to compensate for class imbalance achieved the highest prediction performance in terms of the AUC. Even though the prediction models did not have a high discriminatory capacity, these models could be useful for identifying patients at high risk for readmission or mortality immediately after admission and enable early discharge planning and transitional care interventions. Future studies may explore previously unrecognized predictive factors in clinical text or high-dimensional electronic medical records.

**Author Contributions:** Conceptualization, L.-C.H. and S.-F.S.; methodology, S.-F.S., and Y.-H.H.; software, S.-F.S.; validation, L.-C.H. and S.-F.S.; formal analysis, L.-C.H. and S.-F.S.; investigation, L.-C.H., S.-F.S., and Y.-H.H.; resources, S.-F.S.; data curation, L.-C.H.; writing—original draft preparation, L.-C.H. and S.-F.S.; writing—review and editing, S.-F.S. and Y.-H.H.; visualization, S.-F.S.; supervision, Y.-H.H.; project administration, Y.-H.H.; funding acquisition, S.-F.S. All authors have read and agreed to the published version of the manuscript.

**Acknowledgments:** We would like to thank Li-Ying Sung for English language editing.

## References


1. Roth, G.A.; Abate, D.; Abate, K.H.; Abay, S.M.; Abbafati, C.; Abbasi, N.; Abbastabar, H.; Abd-Allah, F.; Abdela, J.; Abdelalim, A.; et al. Global, regional, and national age-sex-specific mortality for 282 causes of death in 195 countries and territories, 1980–2017: A systematic analysis for the Global Burden of Disease Study 2017. *Lancet* **2018**, *392*, 1736–1788. [CrossRef]
2. Kyu, H.H.; Abate, D.; Abate, K.H.; Abay, S.M.; Abbafati, C.; Abbasi, N.; Abbastabar, H.; Abd-Allah, F.; Abdela, J.; Abdelalim, A.; et al. Global, regional, and national disability-adjusted life-years (DALYs) for 359 diseases and injuries and healthy life expectancy (HALE) for 195 countries and territories, 1990–2017: A systematic analysis for the Global Burden of Disease Study 2017. *Lancet* **2018**, *392*, 1859–1922. [CrossRef]
3. Johnson, C.O.; Nguyen, M.; Roth, G.A.; Nichols, E.; Alam, T.; Abate, D.; Abd-Allah, F.; Abdelalim, A.; Abraha, H.N.; Abu-Rmeileh, N.M.; et al. Global, regional, and national burden of stroke, 1990–2016: A systematic analysis for the Global Burden of Disease Study 2016. *Lancet Neurol.* **2019**, *18*, 439–458. [CrossRef]
4. Bergström, L.; Irewall, A.-L.; Söderström, L.; Ögren, J.; Laurell, K.; Mooe, T. One-Year Incidence, Time Trends, and Predictors of Recurrent Ischemic Stroke in Sweden From 1998 to 2010. *Stroke* **2017**, *48*, 2046–2051. [CrossRef]
5. Hsieh, C.-Y.; Wu, D.P.; Sung, S.-F. Trends in vascular risk factors, stroke performance measures, and outcomes in patients with first-ever ischemic stroke in Taiwan between 2000 and 2012. *J. Neurol. Sci.* **2017**, *378*, 80–84. [CrossRef]
6. Kumar, S.; Selim, M.H.; Caplan, L.R. Medical complications after stroke. *Lancet Neurol.* **2010**, *9*, 105–118. [CrossRef]
7. Li, H.-W.; Yang, M.-C.; Chung, K.-P. Predictors for readmission of acute ischemic stroke in Taiwan. *J. Formos. Med. Assoc.* **2011**, *110*, 627–633. [CrossRef]
8. Lin, H.-J.; Chang, W.-L.; Tseng, M.-C. Readmission after stroke in a hospital-based registry: Risk, etiologies, and risk factors. *Neurology* **2011**, *76*, 438–443. [CrossRef]
9. Lee, H.-C.; Chang, K.-C.; Huang, Y.-C.; Hung, J.-W.; Chiu, H.-H.E.; Chen, J.-J.; Lee, T.-H. Readmission, mortality, and first-year medical costs after stroke. *J. Chin. Med. Assoc.* **2013**, *76*, 703–714. [CrossRef]
10. Hsieh, C.-Y.; Lin, H.-J.; Hu, Y.-H.; Sung, S.-F. Stroke severity may predict causes of readmission within one year in patients with first ischemic stroke event. *J. Neurol. Sci.* **2017**, *372*, 21–27. [CrossRef]
11. Kind, A.; Smith, M.; Liou, J.-I.; Pandhi, N.; Frytak, J.R.; Finch, M.D. The price of bouncing back: One-year mortality and payments for acute stroke patients with 30-day bounce-backs. *J. Am. Geriatr. Soc.* **2008**, *56*, 999–1005. [CrossRef] [PubMed]
12. Bjerkreim, A.T.; Thomassen, L.; Brøgger, J.C.; Waje-Andreassen, U.; Næss, H. Causes and Predictors for Hospital Readmission after Ischemic Stroke. *J. Stroke Cerebrovasc. Dis.* **2015**, *24*, 2095–2101. [CrossRef] [PubMed]
13. Fonarow, G.C.; Smith, E.E.; Reeves, M.J.; Pan, W.; Olson, D.; Hernandez, A.F.; Peterson, E.D.; Schwamm, L.; for the Get With the Guidelines Steering Committee and Hospitals. Hospital-Level Variation in Mortality and Rehospitalization for Medicare Beneficiaries With Acute Ischemic Stroke. *Stroke* **2011**, *42*, 159–166. [CrossRef] [PubMed]
14. Axon, R.N.; Williams, M.V. Hospital Readmission as an Accountability Measure. *JAMA* **2011**, *305*, 504–505. [CrossRef] [PubMed]
15. Daras, L.C.; Ingber, M.J.; Carichner, J.; Barch, D.; Deutsch, A.; Smith, L.M.; Levitt, A.; Andress, J. Evaluating Hospital Readmission Rates After Discharge From Inpatient Rehabilitation. *Arch. Phys. Med. Rehabil.* **2018**, *99*, 1049–1059. [CrossRef]
16. Lichtman, J.H.; Leifheit-Limson, E.C.; Jones, S.B.; Wang, Y.; Goldstein, L.B. Preventable Readmissions Within 30 Days of Ischemic Stroke Among Medicare Beneficiaries. *Stroke* **2013**, *44*, 3429–3435. [CrossRef]
17. Fisher, S.R.; Graham, J.E.; Krishnan, S.; Ottenbacher, K.J. Predictors of 30-Day Readmission Following Inpatient Rehabilitation for Patients at High Risk for Hospital Readmission. *Phys. Ther.* **2016**, *96*, 62–70. [CrossRef]
18. Chiu, W.-T.; Yang, C.-M.; Lin, H.-W.; Chu, T.-B. Development and implementation of a nationwide health care quality indicator system in Taiwan. *Int. J. Qual. Health Care* **2006**, *19*, 21–28. [CrossRef]
19. Shah, S.V.; Corado, C.; Bergman, D.; Curran, Y.; Bernstein, R.A.; Naidech, A.M.; Prabhakaran, S. Impact of Poststroke Medical Complications on 30-Day Readmission Rate. *J. Stroke Cerebrovasc. Dis.* **2015**, *24*, 1969–1977. [CrossRef]

20. Hsieh, F.-I.; Lien, L.-M.; Chen, S.-T.; Bai, C.-H.; Sun, M.-C.; Tseng, H.-P.; Chen, Y.-W.; Chen, C.-H.; Jeng, J.-S.; Tsai, C.-F.; et al. Get With The Guidelines-Stroke Performance Indicators: Surveillance of Stroke Care in the Taiwan Stroke Registry: Get With The Guidelines-Stroke in Taiwan. *Circulation* **2010**, *122*, 1116–1123. [CrossRef]
21. Slocum, C.; Gerrard, P.; Black-Schaffer, R.; Goldstein, R.; Singhal, A.; Divita, M.A.; Ryan, C.M.; Mix, J.; Purohit, M.; Niewczyk, P.; et al. Functional Status Predicts Acute Care Readmissions from Inpatient Rehabilitation in the Stroke Population. *PLoS ONE* **2015**, *10*, e0142180. [CrossRef] [PubMed]
22. Fehnel, C.R.; Lee, Y.; Wendell, L.C.; Thompson, B.B.; Potter, N.S.; Mor, V. Post–Acute Care Data for Predicting Readmission After Ischemic Stroke: A Nationwide Cohort Analysis Using the Minimum Data Set. *J. Am. Hear. Assoc.* **2015**, *4*, e002145. [CrossRef] [PubMed]
23. Xu, Y.; Yang, X.; Huang, H.; Peng, C.; Ge, Y.; Wu, H.; Wang, J.; Xiong, G.; Yi, Y. Extreme Gradient Boosting Model Has a Better Performance in Predicting the Risk of 90-Day Readmissions in Patients with Ischaemic Stroke. *J. Stroke Cerebrovasc. Dis.* **2019**, *28*, 104441. [CrossRef]
24. Kilkenny, M.F.; Dalli, L.L.; Kim, J.; Sundararajan, V.; Andrew, N.E.; Dewey, H.M.; Johnston, T.; Alif, S.M.; Lindley, R.I.; Jude, M.; et al. Factors Associated With 90-Day Readmission After Stroke or Transient Ischemic Attack. *Stroke* **2020**, *51*, 571–578. [CrossRef]
25. Chu, N.-F. Prevalence of obesity in Taiwan. *Obes. Rev.* **2005**, *6*, 271–274. [CrossRef]
26. Rao, R.R.; Makkithaya, K. Learning from a Class Imbalanced Public Health Dataset: A Cost-based Comparison of Classifier Performance. *Int. J. Electr. Comput. Eng. (IJECE)* **2017**, *7*, 2215. [CrossRef]
27. Chen, J.; Lalor, J.; Liu, W.; Druhl, E.; Granillo, E.; Vimalananda, V.G.; Yu, H.; Cronin, R.; Sulieman, L. Detecting Hypoglycemia Incidents Reported in Patients' Secure Messages: Using Cost-Sensitive Learning and Oversampling to Reduce Data Imbalance. *J. Med. Internet Res.* **2019**, *21*, e11990. [CrossRef]
28. Hall, M.A. Correlation-based feature selection for machine learning. Ph.D. Thesis, The University of Waikato, Hamilton, New Zealand, April 1999.
29. Ottenbacher, K.J.; Graham, J.E.; Lee, J.; Al Snih, S.; Karmarkar, A.; Reistetter, T.; Ostir, G.V.; Ottenbacher, A.J. Hospital Readmission in Persons With Stroke Following Postacute Inpatient Rehabilitation. *J. Gerontol. Ser. A Biomed. Sci. Med. Sci.* **2012**, *67*, 875–881. [CrossRef]
30. Andrews, A.W.; Li, D.; Freburger, J.K. Association of Rehabilitation Intensity for Stroke and Risk of Hospital Readmission. *Phys. Ther.* **2015**, *95*, 1660–1667. [CrossRef]
31. Ottenbacher, K.J.; Smith, P.M.; Illig, S.B.; Linn, R.T.; Fiedler, R.C.; Granger, C.V. Comparison of logistic regression and neural networks to predict rehospitalization in patients with stroke. *J. Clin. Epidemiol.* **2001**, *54*, 1159–1165. [CrossRef]
32. Hu, J.; Gonsahn, M.D.; Nerenz, D.R. Socioeconomic Status and Readmissions: Evidence From An Urban Teaching Hospital. *Health Aff.* **2014**, *33*, 778–785. [CrossRef] [PubMed]
33. Kansagara, D.; Englander, H.; Salanitro, A.; Kagen, D.; Theobald, C.; Freeman, M.; Kripalani, S. Risk Prediction Models for Hospital Readmission. *JAMA* **2011**, *306*, 1688. [CrossRef] [PubMed]
34. Frizzell, J.D.; Liang, L.; Schulte, P.J.; Yancy, C.W.; Heidenreich, P.A.; Hernandez, A.F.; Bhatt, D.L.; Fonarow, G.C.; Laskey, W.K. Prediction of 30-Day All-Cause Readmissions in Patients Hospitalized for Heart Failure: Comparison of Machine Learning and Other Statistical Approaches. *JAMA Cardiol.* **2017**, *2*, 204–209. [CrossRef]
35. Vahidy, F.; Donnelly, J.; McCullough, L.D.; Tyson, J.E.; Miller, C.C.; Boehme, A.K.; Savitz, S.I.; Albright, K.C. Nationwide Estimates of 30-Day Readmission in Patients With Ischemic Stroke. *Stroke* **2017**, *48*, 1386–1388. [CrossRef]
36. Henke, R.M.; Karaca, Z.; Jackson, P.; Marder, W.D.; Wong, H.S. Discharge Planning and Hospital Readmissions. *Med. Care Res. Rev.* **2016**, *74*, 345–368. [CrossRef] [PubMed]
37. Kripalani, S.; Theobald, C.; Anctil, B.; Vasilevskis, E.E. Reducing hospital readmission rates: Current strategies and future directions. *Annu. Rev. Med.* **2013**, *65*, 471–485. [CrossRef]
38. Leppert, M.; Sillau, S.; Lindrooth, R.C.; Poisson, S.N.; Campbell, J.D.; Simpson, J.R. Relationship between early follow-up and readmission within 30 and 90 days after ischemic stroke. *Neurology* **2020**, *94*, e1249–e1258. [CrossRef]
39. Hong, I.; Knox, S.; Pryor, L.; Mroz, T.M.; Graham, J.; Shields, M.F.; Reistetter, T.A. Is Referral to Home Health Rehabilitation Following Inpatient Rehabilitation Facility Associated With 90-Day Hospital Readmission for Adult Patients With Stroke? *Am. J. Phys. Med. Rehabil.* **2020**. [CrossRef]

40. Bates, D.W.; Saria, S.; Ohno-Machado, L.; Shah, A.; Escobar, G. Big Data In Health Care: Using Analytics To Identify And Manage High-Risk And High-Cost Patients. *Health Aff.* **2014**, *33*, 1123–1131. [CrossRef]
41. He, D.; Mathews, S.C.; Kalloo, A.N.; Hutfless, S.M. Mining high-dimensional administrative claims data to predict early hospital readmissions. *J. Am. Med. Informatics Assoc.* **2014**, *21*, 272–279. [CrossRef]
42. Navathe, A.S.; Zhong, F.; Lei, V.J.; Chang, F.Y.; Sordo, M.; Topaz, M.; Navathe, S.B.; Rocha, R.A.; Zhou, L. Hospital Readmission and Social Risk Factors Identified from Physician Notes. *Health Serv. Res.* **2017**, *53*, 1110–1136. [CrossRef] [PubMed]

# 3

# Machine Learning in High-Alert Medication Treatment: A Study on the Cardiovascular Drug

**Chun-Tien Tai [1,2,3], Kuen-Liang Sue [4] and Ya-Han Hu [4,5,*]**

1. Department of Information Management and Institute of Healthcare Information Management, National Chung Cheng University, Chiayi 621, Taiwan; flamquit@cgmh.org.tw
2. Chiayi Chang Gung Memorial Hospital, Chiayi 613, Taiwan
3. Department of Information Management, Shu Zen College of Medicine and Management, Kaohsiung 821, Taiwan
4. Department of Information Management, National Central University, Taoyuan 320, Taiwan; klsue@mgt.ncu.edu.tw
5. MOST AI Biomedical Research Center, National Cheng Kung University, Tainan 701, Taiwan

* Correspondence: yhhu@mgt.ncu.edu.tw

**Abstract:** The safety of high-alert medication treatment is still a challenge all over the world. Approximately one-half of adverse drug events (ADEs) are related to high-alert medications, which motivates us to improve the predicament faced in clinical practice. The purpose of this study is to use machine-learning techniques to predict the risk of high-alert medication treatment. Taking the cardiovascular drug digoxin as an example, we collected the records of 513 patients who received the pertinent therapy during hospitalization at a tertiary medical center in Taiwan. Considering serum digoxin concentration (SDC) is the primary indicator for assessing the risk of digoxin therapy, patients with SDC being controlled at the recommended range before their discharge were defined as a low-risk population; otherwise, patients were defined as the high-risk population. Weka 3.9.4—an open source machine learning software—was adopted to develop binary classification models to predict the risk of digoxin therapy by a number of machine-learning techniques, including k-nearest neighbors (kNN), decision tree (C4.5), support vector machine (SVM), random forest (RF), artificial neural network (ANN) and logistic regression (LGR). The results showed that the performance of RF was the best, followed by C4.5 and ANN; the remaining classifiers performed poorly. This study confirmed that machine-learning techniques can yield favorable prediction effectiveness for high-alert medication treatment, thereby decreasing the risk of ADEs and improving medication safety.

**Keywords:** machine learning; high-alert medication; cardiovascular drug; adverse drug events; decision tree

---

## 1. Introduction

Since To Err is Human published by the Institute of Medicine (IOM) in 1999, patient safety has become a global concern [1]. Although governments, nonprofit organizations and medical institutions have proposed various measures and invested much resources to improve patient safety in the past 20 years, incidents of patients being injured due to improper medical care continue to occur every day around the world [2]. Therefore, the avoidance of medical injuries to maintain patient safety is still a difficult problem to solve [3].

The World Health Organization (WHO) and the World Alliance for Patient Safety have jointly proposed two Global Patient Safety Challenges, which provide improvement measures and methods for patient safety issues to reduce the possible harm to patients during medical care. In 2017, the WHO released the third global patient safety challenge which indicates that if medication errors occur in the medical system, it may cause serious harm to patients [4].

In the United States, medication errors cause at least one death each day and injure nearly 1.3 million people each year [4]. It is estimated that the additional medical costs worldwide caused by medication errors amount to US $42 billion per year, accounting for 0.7% of global healthcare expenditure [5].

Compared with ordinary drugs, high-alert medications carry greater risks of adverse drug events (ADEs) and have received widespread attention [6]. The definition of high-alert medications is drugs that bear a heightened risk of causing significant patient harm when they are used in error [7]. Therefore, although high-alert medications account for only a small portion of all therapeutic drugs, they are the main cause of adverse drug events (ADEs). Recent studies have shown that up to 50% of ADEs are related to high-alert medications [8].

Medication errors will not only lead to an increase in medical costs, but also cause varying degrees of harm to patients, especially high-alert medications. To date, clinical decision support systems (CDSS) have been widely and maturely applied to most drugs. However, the current application of CDSS in high-alert medications is mainly based on the recommendations of the Clinical Practice Guideline (CPG) to establish prompts in the system, rather than generating predictions of treatment results. Therefore, some scholars have begun to use machine-learning techniques to conduct research on specific high-alert medications [9,10]. The purpose is to provide better clinical decision support to enhance the safety of high-alert medication treatment.

Cardiovascular disease (CVD) is currently the main cause of death in the world [11]. According to WHO statistics, approximately 17.65 million people worldwide died of CVD in 2016, accounting for 31% of all deaths, indicating that approximately one in three people died of CVD. The number of people who have died of CVD is not only twice as high as that of cancer, but more than the sum of all deaths from infectious diseases [12]. Similarly, CVD is also the most common cause of death in Europe. Although the mortality rate of CVD has gradually decreased, more than four million Europeans die each year.

Because of the high mortality rate of CVD, the treatment of this disease has received considerable attention. In terms of medication therapy, cardiovascular drugs can effectively control the symptoms of CVD, but such drugs are also prone to severe ADEs. Levy et al. pointed out that nearly half of ADEs are related to the use of cardiovascular drugs [13].

Among all cardiovascular drugs, digoxin is classified as a high-alert medication. Because of the complex pharmacological properties, the use of digoxin is more likely to cause serious injury to patients. In the treatment process of CVD with digoxin, inappropriate decisions may affect treatment outcome, cause drug toxic reactions and severely lead to death. When physicians decide to prescribe high-alert medications, more careful decision-making is needed. However, physicians need to interpret a large amount of information within a limited time, including the patient's physiology, disease status and laboratory data to determine the treatment regimen. The risk of medication therapy needs to be assessed during decision-making process to reduce the incidence of ADEs. For a busy medical environment, these goals are not easy to achieve.

In the past, the applications of machine-learning techniques in medical domain covered a wide range of ordinary drugs and only a few studies focused on the high-alert medications [14–28]. On the other hand, those related studies used relatively few variables or adopted techniques lacking interpretability. We intend to apply machine-learning techniques, including *k*-nearest neighbors (kNN), decision tree (C4.5), support vector machine (SVM), random forest (RF), artificial neural network (ANN) and logistic regression (LGR), to build binary classification models and enhance the safety of high-alert medication treatment.

In order to improve the predicament faced in practice, this study attempts to focus on high-alert medication treatment and investigate cardiovascular drugs that have attracted much attention worldwide. We will take digoxin as an example, retrieve the data needed for research from the medical record database of a tertiary medical center in Taiwan and then adopt the method of machine learning to construct a risk prediction model. It is hoped that the results will help physicians to make better clinical decisions and thus improve patient medication safety.

## 2. Materials and Methods

### 2.1. Data Source

The source of research data were received from a patient records database of a tertiary medical center in Taiwan. Patients who had accepted digoxin therapy during hospitalization between January 2004 and December 2013 were included in this study. Exclusion criteria were that the patient had taken digoxin within 3 months before hospitalization. Because the half-life of the drug is 36 to 48 h with normal renal function, a 3 month clearance period was applied to ensure the accuracy of the prediction models [29].

The experimental data for this study were collected from 513 clinical cases. According to the variables mentioned in the previous literature, each clinical record included initial dose of digoxin, demographic data and laboratory data related to liver function, renal function and serum K+. In addition, a specific disease congestive heart failure (CHF) was also included.

Finally, we considered another important variable known as drug-to-drug interaction (DDI). The variable cannot only affect treatment outcome, but also increase the incidence of ADEs. For this reason, we included DDI in our experiment before constructing the prediction models. According to Thomson Micromedex Database [30], the clinical significance of DDI can be divided into three degrees (major, moderate and minor), the major degree being the most severe DDI. In addition to drug interaction facts, we compared DDI information published by the Ministry of Health and Welfare in Taiwan with the drugs used at the case hospital. Table S1 shows the drugs that induce the major degree DDI when combined with digoxin. During the treatment of digoxin, patients who used any of the drugs listed in Table S1 will be considered to be at risk of DDI.

### 2.2. Variable

The dependent variable (DV) of this study was the risk of digoxin treatment, which can be determined by serum digoxin concentration (SDC). In clinical practice, physicians judge the therapeutic effect of digoxin mainly based on SDC. To eliminate the ADEs rates of digoxin, SDC value is recommended at the range of 0.5–0.9 ng/mL [28,31]. Therefore, patients with SDC being controlled at recommended range before their discharge were defined as a low-risk population; otherwise, patients were defined as the high-risk population. Moreover, a total of 12 independent variables (IVs) were considered in our study (Table 1).

**Table 1.** Definition of variables.

| Category | | Name | Definition | Type |
|---|---|---|---|---|
| IV | Demographic | Gender | Male/female | Categorical |
| | | Age | Actual age on the day of hospitalization | Numeric |
| | | Weight | Body weight measured on the day of hospitalization | Numeric |
| | Laboratory | ALT * | The record measured before digoxin therapy | Numeric |
| | | AST * | The record measured before digoxin therapy | Numeric |
| | | SCr * | The record measured before digoxin therapy | Numeric |
| | | BUN * | The record measured before digoxin therapy | Numeric |
| | | ALB * | The record measured before digoxin therapy | Numeric |
| | | $K^+$ * | The record measured before digoxin therapy | Numeric |
| | History | CHF | The diagnostic records of CHF noted in the past year | Categorical |
| | Medication | Dose | Initial dose of digoxin during hospitalization | Numeric |
| | | DDI | Patients who used any of the drugs listed in Table S1 during hospitalization. | Categorical |
| DV | Treatment outcome | Risk | $0.5 \leqq SDC \leqq 0.9$ ng/mL: low risk<br>SDC < 0.5 or SDC > 0.9 ng/mL: high risk | Categorical |

* ALB—albumin; ALT/AST—alanine aminotransferase/aspartate aminotransferase; BUN—blood urea nitrogen; $K^+$—serum potassium; SCr—serum creatinine.

## 2.3. *Investigated Classification Techniques*

Six well-known classification techniques were considered, including *k*NN, C4.5, SVM, RF, ANN and LGR. Table 2 lists the primary applications of these techniques in previous studies in medical domain [14–28].

**Table 2.** Applications of classification techniques in medical domain.

| Techniques | Applications |
|---|---|
| *k*NN | Modeling liver-related adverse effects of drugs [14].<br>Predicting drug side effects [15].<br>Personalized drug concentration predictions [16]. |
| C4.5 | Detecting adverse drug events [17].<br>The analysis of adverse drug reactions [18].<br>Expert system for adverse drug reaction detection [19]. |
| SVM | Antidiabetic drug failure prediction [20].<br>Prediction models for drug-induced hepatotoxicity [21].<br>Prediction of drug-induced eosinophilia adverse effect [22]. |
| RF | Prediction of cardiovascular outcomes [23].<br>Adverse drug reaction detection [19].<br>Prediction of drug-induced nephrotoxicity [24]. |
| ANN | Predicting the serum digoxin concentrations of infants [25].<br>Prediction of the serious adverse drug reactions [26]. |
| LGR | Clinical decision support system to toxicity in patients treated with digoxin [27].<br>Analysis of patients with digoxin serum concentration [28]. |

*k*-nearest neighbors (*k*NN) is a well-known case learning method that classifies new cases based on distance functions. For a test case, *k*NN first finds its top *k*-nearest neighbors in the vector space; the class label of the test case is assigned to the majority class among its neighbors [32]. The Euclidean distance and the Hamming distance are usually used for numeric and categorical variables, respectively.

Decision tree (C4.5) is a commonly used classification technique. The growth of the decision tree is a recursive process. First, an attribute with the best gain ratio is selected as the split node of the tree, and the corresponding branches are generated according to its attribute values. Then, the dataset can be partitioned into subsets, and each subsets can be used for next round of tree partition. The decision tree grows until the termination condition is met. The rules generated by the decision tree are easy to understand and can be applied in practice [33]. Because gain ratio is proposed to measure the improvement of data purity in C4.5, it is also used to measure the importance of IVs [34].

Support vector machine (SVM) is a supervised learning method that maps IVs and a DV to a high-dimensional vector space by using structural risk minimization. Then, it attempts to find a hyperplane to separate the data into two categories. Therefore, a new test case can be mapped into one subspace based on the determined hyperplane [35].

Random forest (RF) is a tree-based ensemble learning algorithm, which adopts bagging and random feature selection techniques [36]. Each decision tree is constructed from bootstrap samples of training data, and the final predicted result is determined by a majority vote. When building multiple trees, a random sample with replacement and the random selection of feature of the training set are used, which reduce the possibility of overfitting in tree growing process.

Artificial neural network (ANN) consists of an input- and an output- layer with a number of hidden layers. Artificial neurons between two adjacent layers are connected; the neurons receive the inputs from the outputs of the front adjacent neurons and convert them into an output value through the transfer functions. The key component in the learning procedure is the connection weights between two neurons. In training phase, it iteratively tunes the connection weights between neurons for minimizing the difference between the estimated output value and the actual output. The learning process repeatedly executes the feedforward and backward phases until any stop criteria is reached [37].

Logistic regression (LGR) is a statistical learning method that uses the dataset to develop a mathematical model for predicting the DV. LGR is a nonlinear regression model that can be applied when the DV is binomial category data; it can find the relationships between the binomial DV and a group of IVs [38]. Specifically, it puts the values of IVs into the logistic function to get a probability value.

## 2.4. Experimental Setup and Performance Measure

To construct the risk prediction models for digoxin treatment, this study adopted Weka 3.9.4 (www.cs.waikato.ac.nz/mL/weka), an open source machine learning software to investigate the performance of the selected techniques, including IBk (kNN in Weka), J48 (C4.5 in Weka), SMO (SVM in Weka), random forest (RF in Weka), multilayer perceptron (ANN in Weka), simple logistic (LGR in Weka). To optimize the prediction performance of the models, we used the CV parameter selection meta-learner module implemented in Weka to search the best parameter settings. Table 3 lists the tests of parameter tuning for each classification technique and the final best parameter settings found in this study.

**Table 3.** Parameter settings in Weka.

| Technique | WEKA Module | Parameters | Test Range | Best Parameter Setting |
|---|---|---|---|---|
| *k*NN | IBk | Number of neighbors | 1–10 | 1 |
| C4.5 | J48 | Confidence factor | 0.1–0.3 | 0.3 |
| | | Minimum number of instances per leaf | 2–10 | 2 |
| SVM | SMO | Kernel | Polykernel, RBF Kernel | Polykernel |
| RF | Random forest | Number of trees | 10–100 | 60 |
| | | Number of attributes to be used in random selection | 2–10 | 10 |
| ANN | Multilayer perceptron | Number of hidden nodes | 3–10 | 9 |
| | | Learning rate | 0.1–0.5 | 0.3 |
| | | Momentum factor | 0–0.5 | 0 |
| | | Maximum number of epochs | 300–1000 | 1000 |
| LGR | Simple logistic | None | | N/A |

The classification performance of the prediction models was compared to find out the optimal classifier. We split the data into training and testing datasets in a proportion of 70:30 and applied 10-fold cross-validation method in the training dataset to search the best parameter settings. In addition, previous research indicated that the class imbalance problem can significantly affect learning performance [39]. To improve the classification performance, the resample module (spread subsample module in Weka) is used in this study to modify the distribution of instances of two classes in the training set. Finally, we used the best parameter setting to construct the binary classification models and reported the classification results of testing set.

By using a confusion matrix (Table 4), the precision, recall and F-measure were adopted to analysis the performance of each prediction models. These three metrics were defined by the following Formulas:

$$Precision = TP/(TP + FP), \quad (1)$$

$$Recall = TP/(TP + FN), \quad (2)$$

$$F\text{-}measure = 2.\ Precision.\ Recall/(precision + recall) \quad (3)$$

**Table 4.** Confusion matrix.

| Classes | | Predicted Class | |
|---|---|---|---|
| | | High Risk | Low Risk |
| Actual Class | High risk | TP | FN |
| | Low risk | FP | TN |

Precision is the ratio of correctly predicted high risk patients to the total predicted high risk patients. Recall is the ratio of correctly predicted high risk patients to all of the high risk patients in the dataset. F-measure is the harmonic mean of precision and recall. In addition, our study also included the area under the curve (AUC) as a performance indicator. To evaluate the performance of the models, we referred to the guidelines proposed by Hosmer and Lemeshow [38]. The performance is defined as "outstanding" if AUC $\geq$ 0.9, "excellent" if 0.9 > AUC $\geq$ 0.8, "acceptable" if 0.8 > AUC $\geq$ 0.7, "fair to poor" if 0.7 > AUC $\geq$ 0.5.

## 3. Results

### 3.1. Descriptive Statistics

According to the aforementioned definitions of variables, our research collected and preprocessed the medical records of all patients. Finally, 513 cases were enrolled in this study and the statistical information is shown in Table 5.

**Table 5.** Statistical information for the collected cases.

| | Category | Name | Range | Unit | Summary Statistics |
|---|---|---|---|---|---|
| IV | Demographic | Gender | Male/female | - | Male: 278 (54.19%)<br>Female: 235 (45.81%) |
| | | Age | 19 to 101 | years | $\mu = 74.03, \sigma = 12.08$ |
| | | Weight | 32 to 105 | kg | $\mu = 56.26, \sigma = 12.01$ |
| | Laboratory | ALT | 5 to 1754 | U/L | $\mu = 78.33, \sigma = 161.58$ |
| | | AST | 11 to 2615 | U/L | $\mu = 88.25, \sigma = 215.26$ |
| | | SCr | 0.27 to 12.1 | mg/dL | $\mu = 1.466, \sigma = 1.387$ |
| | | BUN | 2 to 237 | mg/dL | $\mu = 34.33, \sigma = 28.53$ |
| | | ALB | 1 to 4.3 | g/dL | $\mu = 2.625, \sigma = 0.639$ |
| | | K+ | 1.9 to 6.7 | meq/L | $\mu = 3.987, \sigma = 0.726$ |
| | History | CHF | Yes/no | - | Yes: 278 (54.19%)<br>No: 235 (45.81%) |
| | Medication | Dose | 0.125 to 2 | mg | $\mu = 0.504, \sigma = 0.232$ |
| | | DDI | Yes/no | - | Yes: 364 (70.96%)<br>No: 149 (29.04%) |
| DV | Treatment outcome | Risk | Low/high | - | Low: 169 (32.94%)<br>High: 344 (67.06%) |

### 3.2. Experimental Results

In experimental evaluations, six binary classification models were developed to identify high risk patients. The experimental results are reported in Table 6. AUC, F-measure, precision, and recall were used to assess the performance of the prediction models.

**Table 6.** Results of classification performance.

| Classifier | AUC | Precision | Recall | F-Measure |
|---|---|---|---|---|
| *k*NN | 0.569 | 0.722 | 0.691 | 0.706 |
| C4.5 | 0.719 | 0.803 | 0.734 | 0.767 |
| SVM | 0.554 | 0.698 | 0.536 | 0.607 |
| RF | 0.836 | 0.852 | 0.742 | 0.794 |
| ANN | 0.688 | 0.795 | 0.682 | 0.734 |
| LGR | 0.551 | 0.689 | 0.532 | 0.600 |

Regarding the AUC values ranged from 0.551–0.836. The results showed that the performance of RF classifier was the best (0.836; excellent discrimination), followed by C4.5 (0.719) and ANN (0.688); the remaining classifiers performed poorly. Figure 1 illustrates the receiver operating characteristic (ROC) curve of RF classifier. In addition, F-measure is the harmonic mean of precision and recall, so it is commonly adopted to compare the whole performance. Regarding the F-measure of the prediction models, the RF result was still the best (0.794), followed by C4.5 (0.767) and ANN (0.734); the other classifiers performed poorly. Overall, the decision tree-based methods including RF and C4.5 exhibited markedly superior prediction performance in our study.

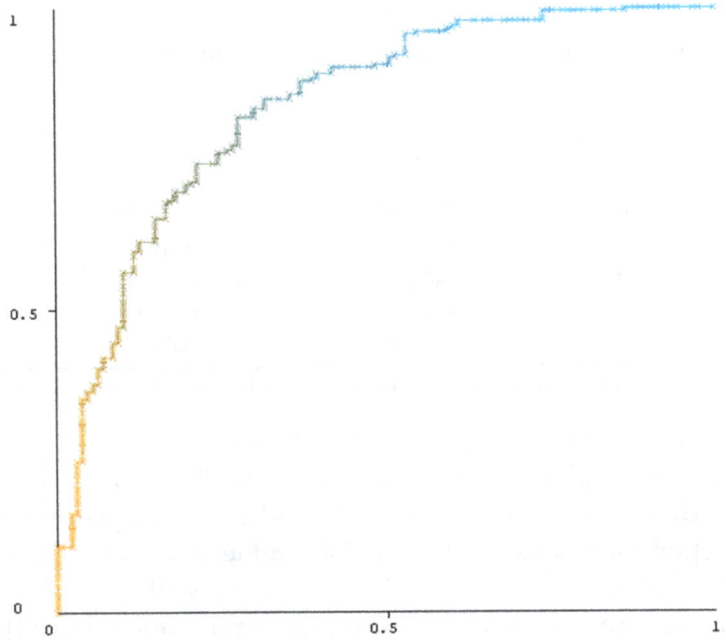


**Figure 1. The receiver operating characteristic** (ROC) curve of RF classifier.

To understand the performance of the model in more specific realistic scenarios, we further adopted the best classifier RF to investigate the changes when controlling for specific variables, including gender, CHF and DDI. The experimental results are shown in Table 7. The highest AUC value was 0.848 in the female and patients with DDI datasets; the model for patients without DDI was the only one that yielded the result below 0.8.

**Table 7.** Results of classification performance in specific scenarios.

| Dataset | AUC | Precision | Recall | F-measure |
|---|---|---|---|---|
| Male | 0.834 | 0.875 | 0.824 | 0.848 |
| Female | 0.848 | 0.901 | 0.753 | 0.820 |
| With CHF * | 0.804 | 0.845 | 0.803 | 0.824 |
| Without CHF * | 0.809 | 0.866 | 0.640 | 0.736 |
| With DDI * | 0.848 | 0.840 | 0.794 | 0.816 |
| Without DDI * | 0.750 | 0.793 | 0.676 | 0.730 |

* CHF—congestive heart failure; DDI—drug-to-drug interaction.

## 4. Discussion

In recent years, the patient safety of high-alert medication treatment is an urgent issue, especially cardiovascular drugs [1,3]. Previous studies have employed various methods, such as statistical models and pharmacokinetics, to enhance the safety of using high-alert medications. In addition, machine-learning techniques (e.g., ANN) have lately been used to enhance the predictive power of models. However, because the decision-making process of ANN cannot be known and lack of explanatory power, its use in clinical applications is still limited.

Our study investigated various well-known machine-learning techniques. The results indicated that, compared with other techniques (kNN, LGR and SVM), the average performance of decision tree-based methods was superior to that of other techniques. In addition, decision tree-based methods yielded the information of decision rules that can support physicians in making treatment decision of high-alert medications.

In addition to comparing the prediction capabilities of different classification techniques, we further analyzed the influence of each variable on the occurrence of ADEs to provide a reference for clinicians. By computing gain ratios, we disclosed that the most important variables affecting the outcome of the treatment are shown in Table 8. After discussion with the medical specialists, including 2 cardiologists, 1 clinical nurse specialists and 3 clinical pharmacists, the validity of the results is discussed as follows:

**Table 8.** Ranking of the selected variables.

| Rank | Variables | Gain Ratios |
|---|---|---|
| 1 | BUN * | 0.0182 |
| 2 | SCr * | 0.0151 |
| 3 | DDI * | 0.0103 |
| 4 | Dose | 0.0085 |

* BUN—blood urea nitrogen; SCr—serum creatinine; DDI—drug-to-drug interaction.

First, BUN and SCr are commonly used indicators of kidney function. A raised BUN/SCr ratio will increase the hospitalization risk and mortality of CHF patients [40]. Doherty et al. found that the higher the BUN value, the more digoxin is accumulated in the body. Because digoxin is primarily excreted by kidneys, low kidney function may cause the rise of SDC and lead to ADEs such as digoxin toxicity [41]. Our study confirmed that kidney function is highly correlated with the risk of ADEs. This finding is similar with the outcomes of previous studies about digoxin treatment [42,43]. Therefore, physicians need to adjust the dose when decided to prescribe digoxin to patients with renal insufficiency.

Furthermore, we also found that DDI is a significant factor of treatment outcome in high-alert medications. DDI has long received considerable attention in the field of medicine, especially involving high-alert medications, which has a complex pharmacological mechanism [16,17,44–49]. The digoxin related DDIs can easily cause toxicity reaction and ADEs [50]. Although our study only considered drugs that will produce major degree DDI with digoxin, these results are still adequate to confirm the significance of DDI.

Finally, the adequacy of the initial dose is important in high-alert medication therapy. Inappropriate doses resulting in high plasma drug concentrations can lead to severe ADEs that influence the treatment outcome, particularly digoxin [51]. Therefore, previous studies have focused on novel approaches to predict the adequate dose of digoxin [44–49,51]. In practice, the initial dose is considerably different from the maintenance dose, which may increase the risk of ADEs before reaching a stable maintenance dose. In this study, we investigated the initial dose instead of the maintenance dose and demonstrated the influence of initial dose on the treatment outcome.

To further clarify the dependencies between the top four important IVs and the predicted binary outcome, four feature sets were formulated in this study: BUN only, BUN + SCr, BUN + SCr + DDI, BUN + SCr + DDI + Dose. The classification performance results for each feature set are shown in Table 9. Among the four feature sets, the highest AUC value was 0.796 in BUN + SCr + DDI + Dose. The experiment results reveal that the combination of two or more IVs would make better predictions than just one IV alone.

**Table 9.** Classification performance results for each feature set.

| Selected IVs | AUC | Precision | Recall | F-measure |
|---|---|---|---|---|
| BUN | 0.702 | 0.789 | 0.579 | 0.668 |
| BUN, SCr | 0.766 | 0.825 | 0.708 | 0.762 |
| BUN, SCr, DDI | 0.788 | 0.833 | 0.747 | 0.787 |
| BUN, SCr, DDI, Dose | 0.796 | 0.851 | 0.708 | 0.773 |

## 5. Conclusions

The issue of medication safety has received considerable attention and discussion over the past few decades [1]. It is especially critical for high-alert medications that have complex pharmacological properties and easily cause ADEs. Digoxin is not only a high-alert medication, but also a widely used cardiovascular drug in clinical practice. When making an inappropriate treatment decision may lead to severe ADEs and even death. Therefore, the safety of high-alert medications is still a challenge all over the world.

The objective of this study was to predict the high risk patients of high-alert medication treatment. Six machine-learning techniques, including kNN, C4.5, SVM, RF, ANN and LGR, were adopted to construct the prediction models. In this study, the medical records of 513 inpatients were employed to obtain the experimental results and confirm the prediction efficiency of all adopted techniques. Finally, among all classification techniques, the RF exhibited the best performance. Overall, the decision tree-based methods exhibited an average performance superior to that of other techniques and can support clinicians as aids for making treatment decisions.

Although high-alert medications have a narrow therapeutic range and complex drug properties, this research verified that the properly use of medical records and consideration of drug-related variables can achieve better prediction outcomes. In conjunction with clinical experience, the prediction models can facilitate improving medication safety for patients, decreasing the risk of ADEs and economizing the use of medical resources.

Several limitations of this study should be addressed for further research. First, the data used in this study were collected from a tertiary medical center only. Further evaluation of clinical cases in other medical institutions is essential to confirm the validity of the model. Second, we only considered the concomitant medications with major degree DDIs. To construct a more powerful predictive model, including all drugs having DDI when used in combination with high-alert drugs is indispensable. Finally, the main limitation of the machine learning methods is lack of interpretability. How to build trust between physicians and the prediction models is another critical issue.

Improper use of high-alert medication would increase ADEs and may induce serious morbidity and mortality. This study confirmed that machine-learning techniques can yield favorable prediction effectiveness for high-alert medication treatment, thereby decreasing the risk of ADEs and improving medication safety. Future applications in the research of other medications are expected to enhance the patient safety.

**Author Contributions:** Conceptualization, C.-T.T. and Y.-H.H.; methodology, K.-L.S. and. Y.-H.H.; software, K.-L.S.; validation, K.-L.S. and Y.-H.H.; formal analysis, C.-T.T., K.-L.S., an Y.-H.H.; resources, Y.-H.H.; data curation, Y.-H.H.; writing—original draft preparation, C.-T.T., K.-L.S. and Y.-H.H.; writing—review and editing, C.-T.T., K.-L.S. and Y.-H.H.; visualization, K.-L.S.; supervision, Y.-H.H.; project administration, C.-T.T.; funding acquisition, C.-T.T. All authors have read and agreed to the published version of the manuscript.

**Acknowledgments:** The work was supported by the Ministry of Science and Technology of Taiwan under Grant MOST 107-2410-H-194 -054-MY2.

## References

1. Mitchell, I.; Schuster, A.; Smith, K.; Pronovost, P.; Wu, A. Patient safety incident reporting: A qualitative study of thoughts and perceptions of experts 15 years after 'To Err is Human'. *BMJ Qual. Saf.* **2016**, *25*, 92–99. [CrossRef] [PubMed]
2. Landrigan, C.P.; Parry, G.J.; Bones, C.B.; Hackbarth, A.D.; Goldmann, D.A.; Sharek, P.J. Temporal trends in rates of patient harm resulting from medical care. *N. Engl. J. Med.* **2010**, *363*, 2124–2134. [CrossRef]

3. Dixon-Woods, M.; Pronovost, P.J. Patient safety and the problem of many hands. *BMJ Qual. Saf.* **2016**, *25*, 485–488. [CrossRef]
4. World Health Organization. WHO Launches Global Effort to Halve Medication-Related Errors in 5 Years. Available online: http://www.who.int/mediacentre/news/releases/2017/medication-related-errors/en/ (accessed on 20 August 2017).
5. Donaldson, L.J.; Kelley, E.T.; Dhingra-Kumar, N.; Kieny, M.P.; Sheikh, A. Medication without harm: WHO's third global patient safety challenge. *Lancet* **2017**, *389*, 1680–1681. [CrossRef]
6. Salman, M.; Mustafa, Z.U.; Rao, A.Z.; Khan, Q.U.A.; Asif, N.; Hussain, K.; Rashid, A. Serious Inadequacies in High Alert Medication-Related Knowledge Among Pakistani Nurses: Findings of a Large, Multicenter, Cross-sectional Survey. *Front. Pharmacol.* **2020**, *11*, 1026. [CrossRef]
7. Institute for Safe Medication Practices. ISMP List of High-Alert Medications in Acute Care Settings. Available online: https://www.ismp.org/recommendations/high-alert-medications-acute-list (accessed on 23 August 2018).
8. Lee, J.; Han, H.; Ock, M.; Lee, S.I.; Lee, S.; Jo, M.W. Impact of a clinical decision support system for high-alert medications on the prevention of prescription errors. *Int. J. Med. Inform.* **2014**, *83*, 929–940. [CrossRef]
9. Sharabiani, A.; Bress, A.; Douzali, E.; Darabi, H. Revisiting warfarin dosing using machine learning techniques. *Comput. Math. Methods Med.* **2015**. [CrossRef]
10. Ma, Z.; Wang, P.; Gao, Z.; Wang, R.; Khalighi, K. Ensemble of machine learning algorithms using the stacked generalization approach to estimate the warfarin dose. *PLoS ONE* **2018**, *13*, e0205872. [CrossRef]
11. Mc Namara, K.; Alzubaidi, H.; Jackson, J.K. Cardiovascular disease as a leading cause of death: How are pharmacists getting involved? *Integr. Pharm. Res. Pract.* **2019**, *8*, 1–11. [CrossRef] [PubMed]
12. Naghavi, M.; Wang, H.; Lozano, R.; Davis, A.; Liang, X.; Zhou, M. GBD 2013 Mortality and Causes of Death Collaborators. Global, regional, and national age-sex specific all-cause and cause-specific mortality for 240 causes of death, 1990–2013: A systematic analysis for the Global Burden of Disease Study 2013. *Lancet* **2015**, *385*, 117–171.
13. Levy, M.; Kewitz, H.; Altwein, W.; Hillebrand, J.; Eliakim, M. Hospital admissions due to adverse drug reactions: A comparative study from Jerusalem and Berlin. *Eur. J. Clin. Pharmacol.* **1980**, *17*, 25–31. [CrossRef] [PubMed]
14. Rodgers, A.D.; Zhu, H.; Fourches, D.; Rusyn, I.; Tropsha, A. Modeling liver-related adverse effects of drugs using k nearest neighbor quantitative structure-activity relationship method. *Chem. Res. Toxicol.* **2010**, *23*, 724–732. [CrossRef] [PubMed]
15. Zhang, W.; Liu, F.; Luo, L.; Zhang, J. Predicting drug side effects by multi-label learning and ensemble learning. *BMC Bioinform.* **2015**, *16*, 365. [CrossRef] [PubMed]
16. Shakeel, D.; Mir, S.A. Personalized drug concentration predictions with machine learning: An exploratory study. *Int. J. Basic Clin. Pharmacol.* **2020**, *9*, 980. [CrossRef]
17. Glasgow, J.M.; Kaboli, P.J. Detecting adverse drug events through data mining. *Am. J. Health-Syst. Pharm.* **2010**, *67*, 317–320. [CrossRef] [PubMed]
18. Imai, S.; Yamada, T.; Kasashi, K.; Kobayashi, M.; Iseki, K. Usefulness of a decision tree model for the analysis of adverse drug reactions: Evaluation of a risk prediction model of vancomycin–associated nephrotoxicity constructed using a data mining procedure. *J. Evaluat. Clin. Pract.* **2017**, *23*, 1240–1246. [CrossRef] [PubMed]
19. Mansour, A.M. Decision tree-based expert system for adverse drug reaction detection using fuzzy logic and genetic algorithm. *Int. J. Adv. Comp. Res.* **2018**, *8*, 110–128. [CrossRef]
20. Kang, S.; Kang, P.; Ko, T.; Cho, S.; Rhee, S.J.; Yu, K.S. An efficient and effective ensemble of support vector machines for anti-diabetic drug failure prediction. *Exp. Syst. Appl.* **2015**, *42*, 4265–4273. [CrossRef]
21. Kim, E.; Nam, H. Prediction models for drug-induced hepatotoxicity by using weighted molecular fingerprints. *BMC Bioinform.* **2017**, *18*, 227. [CrossRef]
22. Zhang, H.; Yu, P.; Xiang, M.L.; Li, X.B.; Kong, W.B.; Ma, J.Y.; Zhang, J. Prediction of drug-induced eosinophilia adverse effect by using SVM and naïve Bayesian approaches. *Med. Biol. Eng. Comp.* **2016**, *54*, 361–369. [CrossRef]
23. Chen, T.; Brewster, P.; Tuttle, K.R.; Dworkin, L.D.; Henrich, W.; Greco, B.A.; Massaro, J.M. Prediction of cardiovascular outcomes with machine learning techniques: Application to the Cardiovascular Outcomes in Renal Atherosclerotic Lesions (CORAL) study. *Int. J. Nephrol. Renovasc. Dis.* **2019**, *12*, 49. [CrossRef] [PubMed]

24. Su, R.; Li, Y.; Zink, D.; Loo, L.H. Supervised prediction of drug-induced nephrotoxicity based on interleukin-6 and-8 expression levels. *BMC Bioinform.* **2014**, *15*, S16. [CrossRef] [PubMed]
25. Yao, S.H.; Tsai, H.T.; Lin, W.L.; Chen, Y.C.; Chou, C.; Lin, H.W. Predicting the serum digoxin concentrations of infants in the neonatal intensive care unit through an artificial neural network. *BMC Pediatr.* **2019**, *19*, 517. [CrossRef] [PubMed]
26. Yen, P.F.; Mital, D.P.; Srinivasan, S. Prediction of the serious adverse drug reactions using an artificial neural network model. *Int. J. Med. Eng. Inform.* **2011**, *3*, 53–59. [CrossRef]
27. Albert, A.; Serrano, A.J.; Soria, E.; Jiménez, N.V. Clinical decision support system to prevent toxicity in patients treated with digoxin. In *Intelligent Medical Technologies and Biomedical Engineering: Tools and Applications*; IGI Global: Hershey, PA, USA, 2010; pp. 1–21.
28. Kockova, R.; Skvaril, J.; Cernohous, M.; Maly, M.; Kocka, V. Five year two center retrospective analysis of patients with toxic digoxin serum concentration. *Int. J. Cardiol.* **2011**, *146*, 447–448. [CrossRef]
29. Gheorghiade, M.; Adams, K.F., Jr.; Colucci, W.S. Digoxin in the management of cardiovascular disorders. *Circulation* **2004**, *109*, 2959–2964. [CrossRef]
30. Thomson Reuters. *Thomson Micromedex Database*; Thomson Reuters: New York, NY, USA, 2013.
31. Bauman, J.L.; DiDomenico, R.J.; Viana, M.; Fitch, M. A method of determining the dose of digoxin for heart failure in the modern era. *Arch. Intern. Med.* **2006**, *166*, 2539–2545. [CrossRef]
32. Aha, D.W.; Kibler, D.; Albert, M.K. Instance-based learning algorithms. *Mach. Learn.* **1991**, *6*, 37–66. [CrossRef]
33. Quinlan, J.R. *C4. 5: Programs for Machine Learning*; Elsevier: Amsterdam, The Netherlands, 2014.
34. Karegowda, A.G.; Manjunath, A.S.; Jayaram, M.A. Comparative study of attribute selection using gain ratio and correlation based feature selection. *Int. J. Inf. Tech. Knowl. Manag.* **2010**, *2*, 271–277.
35. Vapnik, V. *The Nature of Statistical Learning Theory*; Springer Science & Business Media: Berlin, Germany, 2013.
36. Breiman, L. Random forests. *Mach. Learn.* **2001**, *45*, 5–32. [CrossRef]
37. Rumelhart, D.E.; Hinton, G.E.; Williams, R.J. Learning representations by back-propagating errors. *Nature* **1986**, *323*, 533–536. [CrossRef]
38. Hosmer, D.W., Jr.; Lemeshow, S.; Sturdivant, R.X. *Applied Logistic Regression*; John Wiley & Sons: Hoboken, NJ, USA, 2013; Volume 398.
39. Tan, P.N.; Steinbach, M.; Kumar, V. *Introduction to Data Mining*; Pearson Education India: Bengaluru, India, 2016.
40. Lin, H.J.; Chao, C.L.; Chien, K.L.; Ho, Y.L.; Lee, C.M.; Lin, Y.H.; Chen, C.Y. Elevated blood urea nitrogen-to-creatinine ratio increased the risk of hospitalization and all-cause death in patients with chronic heart failure. *Clin. Res. Cardiol.* **2009**, *98*, 487. [CrossRef] [PubMed]
41. Doherty, J.E.; Flanigan, W.J.; Perkins, W.H.; Ackerman, G.L.; Gammill, J.; Sherwood, J. Studies with tritiated digoxin in anephric human subjects. *Circulation* **1967**, *35*, 298–303. [CrossRef] [PubMed]
42. Pawlosky, N.; MacDonald, E.; Patel, R.; Kanji, S. Evaluation of digoxin concentration after loading dose in patients with renal dysfunction. *Can. J. Hosp. Pharm.* **2013**, *66*, 104. [CrossRef]
43. Bajraktarević, A. Safety and efficacy of digoxin therapy—Where are we now? *J. Pharm. Pharmacol.* **2016**, *4*, 128–134. [CrossRef]
44. Chen, R.; Zou, S.L.; Wang, M.L.; Jiang, Y.; Xue, H.; Qian, C.Y.; Xia, Z.L. Population pharmacokinetics of digoxin in elderly patients. *Eur. J. Drug Metab. Pharmacokinet.* **2013**, *38*, 115–121. [CrossRef]
45. Kroese, W.L.G.; Avery, A.J.; Savelyich, B.S.P.; Brown, N.S.; Schers, H.; Howard, R.; Horsfield, P. Assessing the accuracy of a computerized decision support system for digoxin dosing in primary care: An observational study. *J. Clin. Pharm. Ther.* **2005**, *30*, 279–283. [CrossRef]
46. Muzzarelli, S.; Stricker, H.; Pfister, O.; Foglia, P.; Moschovitis, G.; Mombelli, G.; Brunner-La Rocca, H. Individual dosage of digoxin in patients with heart failure. *QJM-Int. J. Med.* **2011**, *104*, 309–317. [CrossRef]
47. Suematsu, F.; Yukawa, E.; Yukawa, M.; Minemoto, M.; Ohdo, S.; Higuchi, S.; Goto, Y. Population-based investigation of relative clearance of digoxin in Japanese neonates and infants by multiple-trough screen analysis. *Eur. J. Clin. Pharmacol.* **2001**, *57*, 19–24. [CrossRef]
48. Yukawa, M.; Yukawa, E.; Suematsu, F.; Takiguchi, T.; Ikeda, H.; Aki, H.; Mimemoto, M. Determination of Digoxin Clearance in Japanese Elderly Patients for Optimization of Drug Therapy. *Drugs Aging* **2011**, *28*, 831–841. [CrossRef]

49. Zhou, X.D.; Gao, Y.; Guan, Z.; Li, Z.D.; Li, J. Population pharmacokinetic model of digoxin in older Chinese patients and its application in clinical practice. *Acta Pharmacol. Sin.* **2010**, *31*, 753–758. [CrossRef] [PubMed]
50. Vamos, M.; Erath, J.W.; Hohnloser, S.H. Digoxin-associated mortality: A systematic review and meta-analysis of the literature. *Eur. Heart J.* **2015**, *36*, 1831–1838. [CrossRef] [PubMed]
51. Hu, Y.H.; Tai, C.T.; Tsai, C.F.; Huang, M.W. Improvement of Adequate Digoxin Dosage: An Application of Machine Learning Approach. *J. Healthcare Eng.* 2018. [CrossRef] [PubMed]

# 4

# Developing a Novel Machine Learning-Based Classification Scheme for Predicting SPCs in Colorectal Cancer Survivors

**Wen-Chien Ting [1,2], Horng-Rong Chang [3,4,*], Chi-Chang Chang [5,*] and Chi-Jie Lu [6,7,*]**

1 Division of Colorectal Surgery, Department of Surgery, Chung Shan Medical University Hospital, Taichung 40201, Taiwan; tingwenchien@gmail.com
2 Institute of Medicine, Chung Shan Medical University, Taichung 40201, Taiwan
3 Division of Nephrology, Department of Internal Medicine, Chung Shan Medical University Hospital, Taichung 40201, Taiwan
4 School of Medicine, Chung Shan Medical University, Taichung 40201, Taiwan
5 School of Medical Informatics, Chung Shan Medical University & IT office, Chung Shan Medical University Hospital, Taichung 40201, Taiwan
6 Graduate Institute of Business Administration, Fu Jen Catholic University, Taipei 24205, Taiwan
7 Artificial Intelligence Development Center, Fu Jen Catholic University, Taipei 24205, Taiwan
* Correspondence: chrcsmu@gmail.com (H.-R.C.); threec@csmu.edu.tw (C.-C.C.); 055099@mail.fju.edu.tw (C.-J.L.)(ext. 34711) (H.-R.C.);

**Abstract:** Colorectal cancer is ranked third and fourth in terms of mortality and cancer incidence in the world. While advances in treatment strategies have provided cancer patients with longer survival, potentially harmful second primary cancers can occur. Therefore, second primary colorectal cancer analysis is an important issue with regard to clinical management. In this study, a novel predictive scheme was developed for predicting the risk factors associated with second colorectal cancer in patients with colorectal cancer by integrating five machine learning classification techniques, including support vector machine, random forest, multivariate adaptive regression splines, extreme learning machine, and extreme gradient boosting. A total of 4287 patients in the datasets provided by three hospital tumor registries were used. Our empirical results revealed that this proposed predictive scheme provided promising classification results and the identification of important risk factors for predicting second colorectal cancer based on accuracy, sensitivity, specificity, and area under the curve metrics. Collectively, our clinical findings suggested that the most important risk factors were the combined stage, age at diagnosis, BMI, surgical margins of the primary site, tumor size, sex, regional lymph nodes positive, grade/differentiation, primary site, and drinking behavior. Accordingly, these risk factors should be monitored for the early detection of second primary tumors in order to improve treatment and intervention strategies.

**Keywords:** risk factors; second primary cancer (SPC), colorectal cancer; machine learning; classification techniques; extreme gradient boosting

---

## 1. Introduction

Worldwide, colorectal cancer is considered one of the top three causes of cancer-related deaths in developed countries [1]. Due to the success of cancer screening, the early detection and diagnosis of malignant tumors have become feasible. In addition, due to advances in therapeutic instruments and techniques, such as three-dimensional spatial conformal radiation therapy, intensity-modulated radiation therapy, and proximity radiation therapy, cancer patients have longer survival. However, there is a risk of the occurrence of potentially harmful second primary cancers (SPCs) [2–4].

Five-year cancer survival rates have historically been an important indicator of clinical treatment. One of the most difficult clinical issues for cancer survivors is the occurrence of multiple primary malignant neoplasms (MPMNs). Multiple malignancies are characterized by two or more independent primary malignancies diagnosed in different tissues/organs in the same individual [5]. In general, MPMNs are most present in double cancers. According to the literature, the incidence of second primary malignant tumors in patients with malignant tumors is six times higher than that in healthy people. Second primary malignant tumors occur most often within 3 years of the first tumor treatment; the shorter the interval between the first cancer and the SPC, the worse the prognosis [6]. The prevention of MPMNs has always been a significant problem faced by both doctors and patients. The high prevalence age range for MPMNs is 50–59, with most patients being over 50 years old [2].

The first research report on MPMNs was published by Warren and Gates in 1932. According to their definition, MPMNs should have first and second malignant tumors; there should be at least 2 cm between the two tumors; they should exclude metastatic tumors occurring within 5 years; and occurring at a time more than 3 years after the primary tumor [7]. The definition of SPC (synchronous vs, metachronous) is based on the diagnosed time of the first primary cancer. Accordingly, primary cancers found within 6 months of the first diagnosis are considered to be synchronous, whereas metachronous cancers refer to primary cancers discovered 6 months after the first diagnosis [8]. In general, cancer treatment is characterized followed by the targeted therapy and palliative treatment. The treatment target can be divided into cancer-free survival and chronic comorbid management. The latter can result in treatment failure, leading to palliative treatment, and in more severe cases, to an SPC [9].

According to the guidelines of the Institute of Medicine's prevention and treatment recommendations for multiple malignancies, "Based on the cancer-registered population, it is imperative to use the empirical medical perspective and systematic analysis of therapeutic techniques to further develop clinical treatment guidelines for multiple malignancies (MPMNs)" [10].

With recent developments in information technology, data classification methods represent an important research field and have also become useful tools to support clinical diagnostic guidelines. Machine learning is one of the most used data mining methods, and has been applied to analyze important information hidden in the vast amount of data stored in medical databases. There are many different kinds of machine learning methods used for building predictive models for cancer classification/prediction. For example, Tseng et al. [11] used a support vector machine (SVM) and extreme learning machine (ELM) to predict the recurrence-proneness of cervical cancer. Tseng et al. [12] utilized SVM, ELM, multivariate adaptive regression splines (MARS), and random forest (RF) to identify risk factors and diagnose ovarian cancer recurrence. Ting et al. [13] also applied SVM, ELM, MARS, and the RF method to detect recurrence in patients diagnosed with colorectal cancer. Chang and Chen [14] proposed a classification model using extreme gradient boosting (XGBoost) as the classifier for predicting second primary cancers in women with breast cancer. MARS, SVM, ELM, RF, and XGBoost methods have achieved good performances for constructing effective predictive models of cancer. In addition, gene expression classifiers are currently being used in therapeutic intervention. Kopetz et al. [15] developed ColoPrint prediction method for improving prognostic accuracy independent of microsatellite status. Gao et al. [16] developed cancer hallmark-based gene signature sets (CSS sets) for prognostic predictions and for facilitating the identification of patients with stage II colorectal cancer. Since they are based on different concepts, involving nonparametric statistics, statistical learning, a neural network, and a decision tree, to make effective algorithms with different characteristics for cancer data analysis, they are used in this study for analyzing SPCs in colorectal cancer.

Over the last two decades, cancer registration databases have been used to store records related to the treatment of colorectal cancer patients. Indeed, a vast network of useful information is hidden in these collected datasets. Although traditional data query and statistical functions can be utilized, such as prediction of primary colorectal cancer by National Cancer Institute's Surveillance, Epidemiology, and End Results (SEER) data [17]. Statistic methods such as the chi-square test and Student's t-test were used in univariate statistical analysis, and the Kaplan-Meier method and log-rank test are used for continued variables in traditional medical articles [18,19]. It is not easy to find unknown information features in practice, and information about their potential value cannot be directly observed from the dataset. As such, how to explore hidden, unknown, and valuable information from SPC databases through specific procedures and methods is an important research topic that aims to improve prevention and treatment strategies for colorectal cancer survivors.

In this study, we used five machine learning techniques to develop a predictive model for the SPC among colorectal cancer patients. The model can be used to identify various analyzable risk factors and clinical features within primary tumors, providing decision support for intensive treatments such as adjuvant chemotherapy, or aggressive following up procedures, such as positron emission tomography (PET).

## 2. Methods

### 2.1. MARS

Multivariate adaptive regression splines (MARS) is a flexible procedure used to find optimal variable transformations and interactions. It can be used to identify model relationships that are nearly additive or that involve interactions with fewer variables. MARS is a nonparametric statistical method based on a divide-and-conquer strategy for partitioning training datasets into separate groups, each of which gets its own regression equation. The non-linearity of the MARS model is approximated via the use of separate linear regression slopes in distinct intervals of the independent variable space.

The MARS function is a weighted sum of the basis functions (BFs), which are splines piecewise polynomial functions. It can be represented using the following equation [20]:

$$f(x) = \alpha_0 + \sum_{m=1}^{M} \alpha_m \mathrm{B}_m(x) \tag{1}$$

where $\alpha_0$ and $\alpha_m$ are constant coefficients that can be estimated using the least-squares method. $M$ is the number of basis functions. $\mathrm{B}_m(x)$ represents the basis functions. The hinge functions, $max(0, x-k)$ or $max(0, k-x)$, with a knot defined at value $t$, are used in MARS modeling. In addition, MARS automatically selects the variables and values of those variables for knots of the hinge functions based on generalized cross-validation criterion [21].

### 2.2. RF

Random forest (RF) is an ensemble classification method that combines several individual classification trees [22,23]. RF is a supervised machine learning algorithm that considers the unweighted majority of the class votes. First, various random samples of variables are selected as the training dataset using the bagging procedure, which is a meta-algorithm that uses random sampling with replacement to synchronously reduce variance and elude over-fitting. Classification trees using selected samples are then built into the training process. A large number of classification trees are then used to form a RF from the selected samples. Classification and regression tree (CART) is typically the classification method used for RF modeling. Finally, all classification trees are combined and the final classification results are obtained by voting on each class and then choosing the winner class in terms of the number of votes. RF performance is measured by a metric called "out of bag" error, which is calculated as the average of the rate of error for each weak learner. In RF, each individual tree is explored in a particular way. The most important variable randomly chosen is used as a node and each tree is developed to its maximum expansion [22].

### 2.3. SVM

Support vector machine (SVM) is a machine learning algorithm based on the structural risk minimization principle for estimating a function by minimizing the upper bound of the generalization error [24]. In modeling an SVM model, one can initially use the kernel function to, either linearly or non-linearly, map the input vectors into one feature space. Then, within the feature space, the SVM attempts to seek an optimized linear division to construct a hyperplane that separates the classes. In order to optimize the hyperplane, SVM solves the optimization problem using the following equation [24]:

$$\begin{gathered} Min\ \phi(x) = \tfrac{1}{2}\|w\|^2 \\ Subject\ to\ y_i\left(w^T x_i + b\right) \geq 1,\ i = 1, 2, \ldots, N \end{gathered} \tag{2}$$

where $x_i \in R^d$ is the input variable, $y_i \in \{-1, 1\}$ is the known target variable, $N$ is the number of sample observations, $d$ is the dimension of each observation, $w$ is the vector of the hyperplane, and $b$ is a bias term.

In order to solve Equation (2), the Lagrange method is used to transform the optimization problem into a dual problem. The penalty factor is used as a tuning parameter in the transformed dual problem to control the trade-off between maximizing the margin and the classification error. In general, SVM does not find the linear separate hyperplane for all application data. For non-linear data, it must transform the original data to a higher dimension of linearity separately as the best solution. The higher dimension is called the feature space and it improves the data separated by classification. The common kernel functions are linear, polynomial, radial basis function, and sigmoid. Although several choices for the kernel function are available, the most widely used is the radial basis function kernel [25].

### 2.4. ELM

Extreme learning machine (ELM) is a single hidden layer feed-forward neural-network (SLFN) that randomly selects the input weights and analytically determines the output weights of the SLFN [26]. The modeling time of ELM is faster than traditional feedforward network learning algorithms such as the back-propagation (BP) algorithm. It also avoids many difficulties present in gradient-based methods, such as the stopping criteria, learning rate, learning epochs, local minimal, and over tuning issues.

In SLFNs, $N$ represents the arbitrary distinct samples $(x_i,\ y_i)$, using $\rho$ hidden neurons and the activation function vector $\theta(x)$, and approximates $N$ samples with zero error, written as:

$$\boldsymbol{HA} = \boldsymbol{Y} \tag{3}$$

where $\boldsymbol{H}_{N\times\rho} = \left[\theta\left(w_i x_j + b_i\right)\right]$ is the hidden layer output matrix of the neural network and the i-th column of $\boldsymbol{H}$; $\boldsymbol{A}$ is the matrix of the output weights; $w_i$ is the weight vector connecting the i-th hidden node and the input nodes; $b_i$ is the threshold (bias) of the i-th hidden node; and $\boldsymbol{Y}$ is the matrix of the targets.

Huang et al. [26] demonstrated that the input weights and hidden layer biases can be randomly generated in the ELM algorithm, and the output weights can be determined as simply as finding the least-square solution to a given linear system. Accordingly, the minimum norm least-square solution to the linear system is $\hat{\boldsymbol{A}} = \widetilde{\boldsymbol{H}}\boldsymbol{Y}$, where $\widetilde{\boldsymbol{H}}$ is the Moore-Penrose generalized inverse of the matrix $\boldsymbol{H}$. The minimum norm least-square solution is unique and has the smallest norm among all least-square solutions [26].

### 2.5. XGboost

XGBoost belongs to the group of widely used tree learning algorithms. It is a supervised learning algorithm based on a scalable end-to-end gradient tree boosting system [27]. Boosting refers to the ensemble learning technique of building many models sequentially, with each new model attempting to correct for the imperfections or inadequacies in the previous model. In other words, in gradient boosting, a new weak learner is constructed to be maximally correlated with the negative gradient of the loss function associated with the whole assembly for each iteration [28].

XGBoost is the implementation of a generalized gradient boosting decision tree that uses a new distributed algorithm for tree searching, which speeds up tree construction. XGBoost includes a regularization term that is used to alleviate overfitting, and as support for arbitrary differentiable loss functions [29]. The objective function of Xgboost consists of two parts; namely, a loss function over the training set and a regularization term that penalizes the complexity of the model as follows [30]:

$$\text{Objective} = \sum_i \boldsymbol{L}(y_i, \hat{y}_i) + \sum_k \boldsymbol{\Omega}(t_k) \tag{4}$$

where $\boldsymbol{L}(y_i, \hat{y}_i)$ can be any convex differentiable loss function that measures the difference between the prediction and the true label for a given training instance. $\boldsymbol{\Omega}(t_k)$ describes the complexity of the tree $f_k$ and is defined in the XGBoost algorithm as:

$$\boldsymbol{\Omega}(t_k) = \gamma \boldsymbol{T} + \frac{1}{2}\lambda\omega^2 \tag{5}$$

where $\boldsymbol{T}$ is the number of leaves on tree $t_k$ and $\omega$ is the weight of the leaves. When $\boldsymbol{\Omega}(t_k)$ is included in the objective function, it is forced to optimize for a less complex tree, which simultaneously minimizes $\boldsymbol{L}(y_i, \hat{y}_i)$. This helps to alleviate any overfitting issues. $\gamma\boldsymbol{T}$ provides a constant penalty for each additional tree leaf, and $\lambda\omega^2$ penalizes for extreme weights. $\gamma$ and $\lambda$ are user configurable parameters [30].

### *2.6. Model Implementation*

The five machine learning methods have been implemented in the R of version 3.6.1 (R core team, Vienna, Austria). The algorithm used for each method is based on that applied in the corresponding R package. In the first method, MARS was implemented using *earth* R package of version 5.1.2 [31]. The default setting of this package was used; all variables were included to build an additive MARS model. Second, the *randomForest* R package of version 4.6.14 was used for constructing RF classification models [32]. Using the default setting, each forest was built with 500 trees. The best value of the minimum number of variables randomly sampled as candidates at each split is searched from the square root of total number of predictors to the number of predictors. Third, SVM classification models were built by using *e1071* R package of version 1.7-1 [33]. The radial basis kernel function with the gamma parameter at its default setting was used this study. In order to find the best parameter set of cost and gamma parameters for building effective SVM models, the tune function of *e1071* R package was applied. Fourth, for building ELM models, the *elmNN* R package of version 1.0 was used [34]. The default used activation function in this package is radial basis. To search the best number of hidden neurons which can generate promising ELM models, *caret* R package of version 6.0-84 was implemented [35]. For the fifth method, XGBoost model was constructed by implementing *xgboost* R package of version 0.90.0.2 [36]. To estimate the best parameter set for building effective XGBoost models, *caret* R package of version 6.0-84 was also used for tuning the six important hyper-parameters: the maximum number of boosting iterations, learning rate, minimum loss reduction, maximum depth of a tree, subsample ratio of the training instances, and subsample ratio of features.

## 3. Proposed Prediction Scheme

In this study, the five machine learning classification techniques described above were integrated to propose a scheme for predicting SPC in colorectal cancer patients. The flowchart of the proposed scheme is shown in Figure 1.

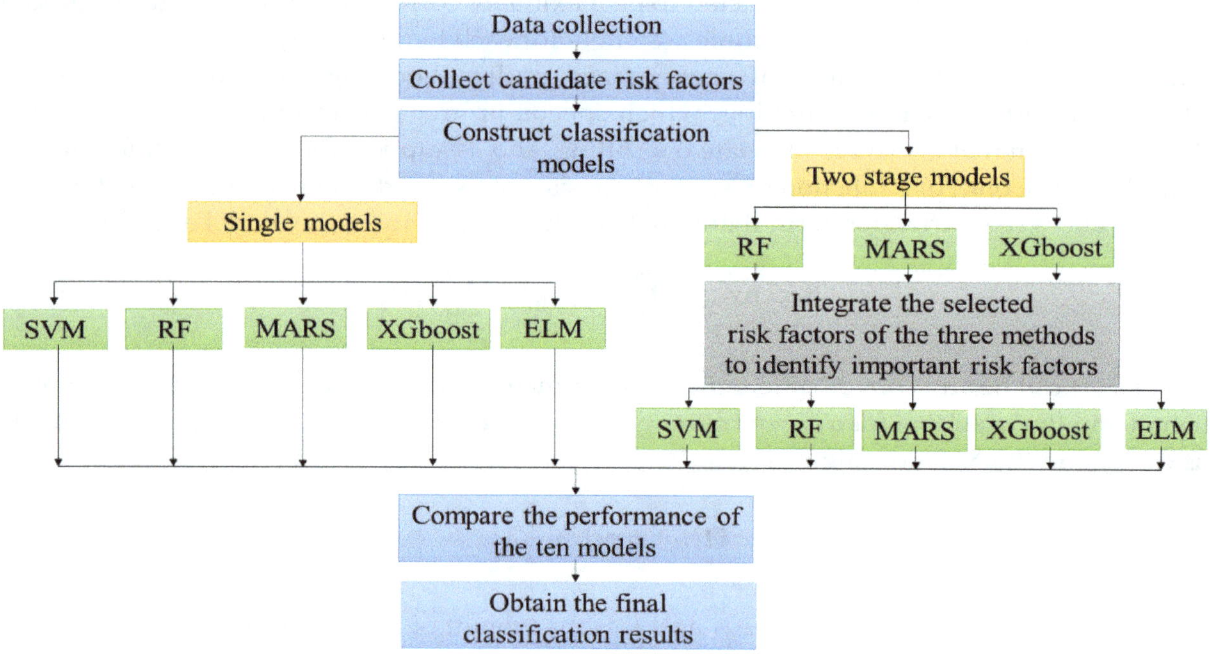


**Figure 1.** The flowchart of the proposed second primary cancer (SPC) prediction scheme in colorectal cancer patients.

The first step of the proposed scheme was to collect the data. The second step was to collect candidate risk factors as predictor variables. In addition, this paper reviews the available literature on what variables are associated with the risk factors for the recurrence of ovarian cancer [13]. As shown in Table 1, the 14 risk factors for SPC in colorectal cancer patients are represented as X1 to X14. The target variable is SPC or not (Y).

**Table 1.** The fourteen candidate risk factors for SPC in colorectal cancer patients.

| Variables | Description |
|---|---|
| X1. Sex | Male/female |
| X2. Age at diagnosis | Age at diagnosis |
| X3. Primary site | Colon/rectal |
| X4. Grade/differentiation | Grade of tumor differentiation |
| X5. Tumor size | Distinguish by unit size (in center meter) |
| X6. Regional lymph nodes positive | Regional lymphoid node involved by tumor |
| X7. Combined stage | Combined pathological and clinical stage as mixed stages |
| X8. Surgical margins of the primary site | Residual/no residual |
| X9. Radiation therapy/no radiation therapy | Radiation therapy/no radiation therapy |
| X10. Chemotherapy/no chemotherapy | Chemotherapy/no chemotherapy |
| X11. BMI | BMI (Body Mass Index) |
| X12. Smoking behavior | Smoking behavior/no smoking behavior |
| X13. Betel nut chewing | Betel nut chewing/no betel nut chewing |
| X14. Drinking | Drinking/no drinking |
| Y: SPC | 1: No, 2: yes |

In the third step, we constructed classification models for predicting SPC in colorectal cancer patients. In building the classification models, we used two types of modeling processes. One was a single model and the other was a two-stage model. In modeling the single models, all 14 risk factors were directly used as predictors for SVM, RF, MARS, ELM, and XGboost for constructing five single classification models. These were termed single SVM (S-SVM), single RF (S-RF), single MARS (S-MARS), single ELM (S-ELM), and single XGboost (S-XGboost) models.

The two-stage model integrating the feature selection method and classifier were used in the third step of the proposed scheme, as important disease risk factors are often fundamental indicators that provide useful information for modeling effective disease predictions. In modeling the two-stage model, a feature selection method was first used to select the important risk factors. Among the five machine learning methods, only RF, MARS, and XGboost can be used to select important risk factors based on their fundamental algorithms; thus, these were used as the three feature selection methods to identify and rank important risk factors for predicting SPC in colorectal cancer patients. Each feature selection method generated one set of important risk factors. Using only one feature selection technique may not provide stable and effective selection results. A simple average rank method was used to combine the risk factor selection results of the three methods.

Table 2 shows the selected and ranked risk factors using the RF, MARS, and XGboost methods. Note that a risk factor with a rank of 1 indicates that it is the most important risk factor, while one with a rank of 14 indicates that it is a risk factor not selected by the method. For each risk factor, the average rank was obtained by calculating the average value of its rankings in the RF, MARS, and XGboost methods. Table 2 shows, also, the average rank of every risk factor. The ranked overall variable importance of all the risk factors is shown in Figure 2. It can be observed that X7, with an average rank of 1, is the most important risk factor, followed by X2 and X11.

**Table 2.** The selected and ranked risk factors using the RF, MARS, and XGboost methods.

| Risk factors | RF | MARS | XGboost | Average Rank |
|---|---|---|---|---|
| X1 | 10 | 2 | 4 | 5.3 |
| X2 | 2 | 3 | 2 | 2.3 |
| X3 | 11 | 5 | 11 | 9.0 |
| X4 | 6 | 14 | 5 | 8.3 |
| X5 | 5 | 8 | 3 | 5.3 |
| X6 | 7 | 9 | 9 | 8.3 |
| X7 | 1 | 1 | 1 | 1.0 |
| X8 | 4 | 4 | 8 | 5.3 |
| X9 | 14 | 9 | 14 | 12.3 |
| X10 | 13 | 14 | 13 | 13.3 |
| X11 | 3 | 6 | 6 | 5.0 |
| X12 | 12 | 7 | 12 | 10.3 |
| X13 | 9 | 14 | 10 | 11.0 |
| X14 | 8 | 14 | 7 | 9.7 |

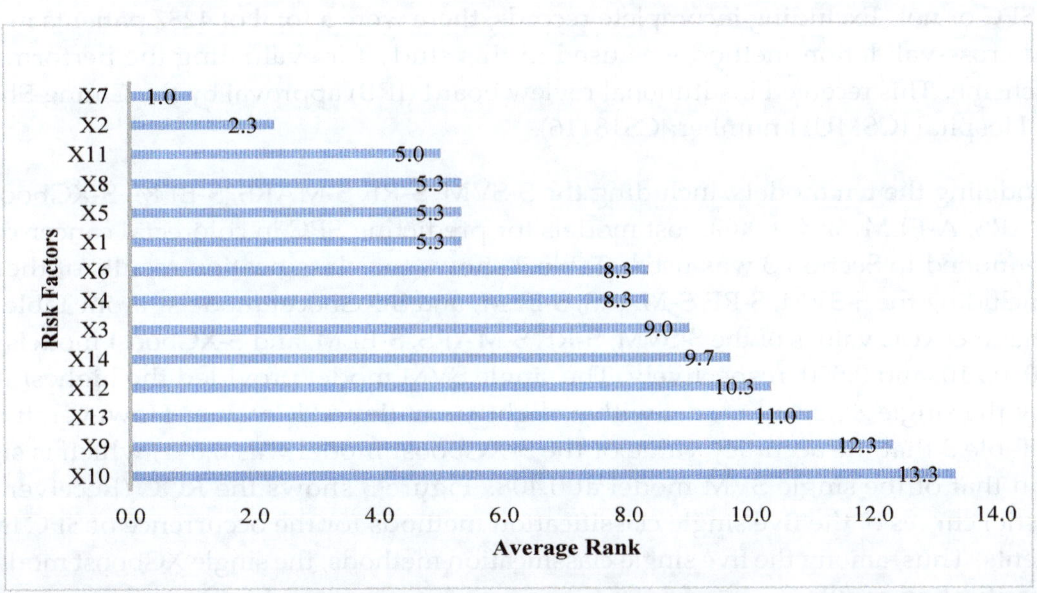


**Figure 2.** The ranking of all risk factors.

In the modeling process of the two-stage method, after obtaining the average rank of each risk factor, the overall important risk factors should be identified before constructing a classification model. In this study, an average rank value less than 10 was used as the criterion for selecting the overall important risk factors. This criterion was determined by the suggestion of clinical physicians. Based on this criterion, it can be observed from Figure 2 that the 10 risk factors including X7 (combined stage), X2 (age at diagnosis), X11 (BMI), X8 (surgical margins of the primary site), X5 (tumor size), X1 (sex), X6 (regional lymph nodes positive), X4 (grade/differentiation), X3 (primary site), and X14 (drinking), were selected as the important risk factors.

In the final stage of the two-stage method, the identified 10 overall important risk factors served as the input variables for the SVM, RF, MARS, ELM, and XGboost methods in order to predict SPC in colorectal cancer patients. The five two-stage methods were termed A-SVM, A-RF, A-MARS, A-ELM, and A-XGboost, respectively.

In the fourth step of the proposed scheme, after obtaining the classification results from the five single methods and the five two-stage methods, we used accuracy, sensitivity, specificity, and area under the curve (AUC) parameters as classification accuracy metrics to compare the performances of the ten models.

In the final step, after comparing the classification performances of the ten models, including S-SVM, S-RF, S-MARS, S-ELM, S-XGboost, A-SVM, A-RF, A-MARS, A-ELM, and A-XGboost models, we obtained the final diagnosis results and identified the important risk factors for predicting SPC in colorectal cancer patients.

This study used 10-fold cross validation methods to estimate the performances of the proposed ten models. First, we randomly split the whole dataset into 10 equal sized parts, with nine folds as the training data set and one fold as the testing data set. That was repeated 10 times, with each of the 10 folds used exactly once as the testing data set. The ten results of classification accuracy metrics could then be averaged to produce the final performances of the methods.

## 4. Empirical Results

In this study, colorectal cancer datasets provided by three hospital cancer registries were used to verify the proposed medical diagnostic scheme for predicting the occurrence of SPC in colorectal cancer patients. Each patient in the dataset had 14 predictor variables, with one response variable indicating SPC or not. Excluding incomplete records, there were a total of 4287 patients in the dataset. The 10-fold cross-validation method was used in this study for evaluating the performance of the proposed scheme. This received institutional review board (IRB) approval by the Chung-Shan Medical University Hospital (CSMUH number: CS18116).

For modeling the ten models, including the S-SVM, S-RF, S-MARS, S-ELM, S-XGboost, A-SVM, A-RF, A-MARS, A-ELM, and A-XGboost models for predicting SPC in colorectal cancer patients, the process mentioned in Section 3 was used. Table 3 shows the classification results of the five single methods, including the S-SVM, S-RF, S-MARS, S-ELM, and S-XGboost models. From Table 3, it can be observed that the AUC values of the S-SVM, S-RF, S-MARS, S-ELM, and S-XGboost models were 0.711, 0.618, 0.640, 0.710, and 0.550, respectively. The single SVM model provided the highest AUC value, followed by the single XGboost model with a slightly smaller AUC value. However, it also can be seen from Table 3 that the accuracy value of the S-XGboost model was 0.641, which is significantly greater than that of the single SVM model at 0.408. Figure 3 shows the ROC (Receiver Operating Characteristic) curves of the five single classification methods for the occurrence of SPC in colorectal cancer patients. Thus, among the five single classification methods, the single XGboost model provided the best classification results.

**Table 3.** Classification results of the five single methods.

| Methods | Accuracy | Sensitivity | Specificity | AUC |
|---|---|---|---|---|
| S-SVM | 0.408 | 0.233 | 0.428 | 0.711 |
| S-RF | 0.819 | 0.384 | 0.868 | 0.618 |
| S-MARS | 0.727 | 0.488 | 0.754 | 0.640 |
| S-XGboost | 0.641 | 0.709 | 0.633 | 0.710 |
| S-ELM | 0.483 | 0.361 | 0.496 | 0.550 |

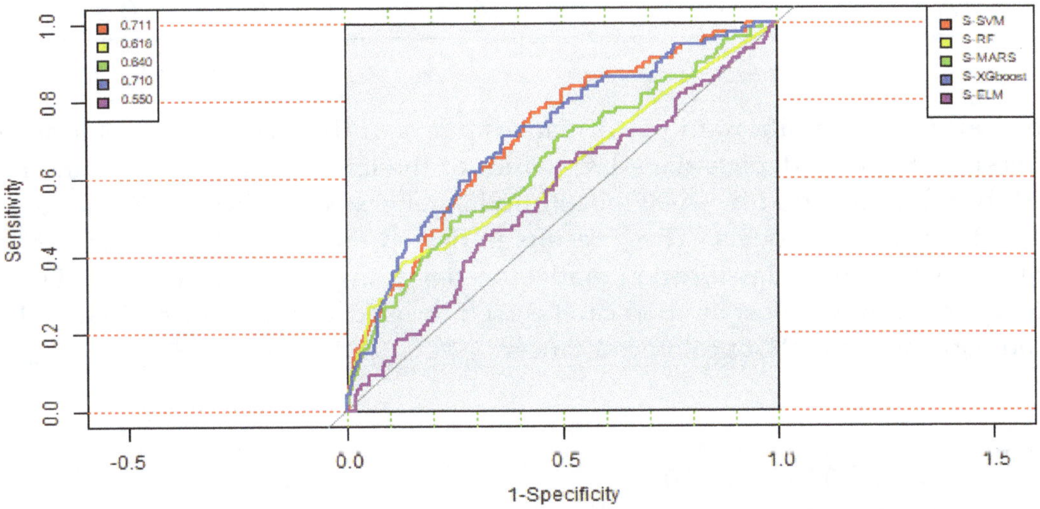


**Figure 3.** ROC (Receiver Operating Characteristic) curves of the five single methods.

As aforementioned, the 10 risk factors, including X7, X2, X11, X8, X5, X1, X6, X4, X3, and X14, were selected as the important risk factors and then served as the critical predictor variables for constructing the five two-stage methods, including the A-SVM, A-RF, A-MARS, A-ELM, and A-XGboost models.

Table 4 shows the classification accuracy matrices of the five two-stage methods. As depicted in Table 4, it can be observed that the A-XGboost method generated the highest AUC value at 0.714, with a sensitivity value of 0.767, compared with the competing models. Figure 4 displays the ROC curves of the five two-stage methods. From Table 4 and Figure 4, it can be observed that the A-XGboost method generated the best performance for predicting the occurrence of SPC in colorectal cancer patients and is the best method among the five two-stage models.

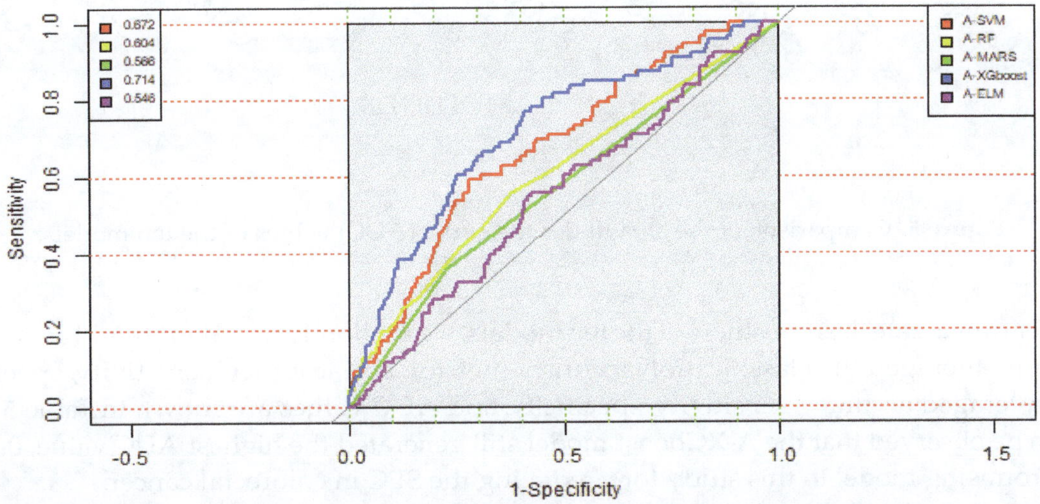


**Figure 4.** ROC curves of the five two-stage methods.

**Table 4.** Classification results of the five two-stage methods.

| Methods | Accuracy | Sensitivity | Specificity | AUC |
|---|---|---|---|---|
| A-SVM | 0.294 | 0.407 | 0.281 | 0.672 |
| A-RF | 0.615 | 0.558 | 0.622 | 0.604 |
| A-MARS | 0.731 | 0.361 | 0.772 | 0.566 |
| A-XGboost | 0.611 | 0.767 | 0.593 | 0.714 |
| A-ELM | 0.425 | 0.442 | 0.424 | 0.546 |

For comparing the classification performances between the five single methods and the five two-stage models, Figure 5 depicts the AUC values of the ten models in decreasing order. It can be observed from Figure 5 that the A-XGboost model generated the best AUC value, followed by the S-SVM and S-XGboost models. These results indicated that the A-XGboost method is a good alternative for constructing a classification model for diagnosing the occurrence of SPC in colorectal cancer. Moreover, the A-XGboost method can be used to select important risk factors that are more influential on patients with SPC of colorectal cancer.

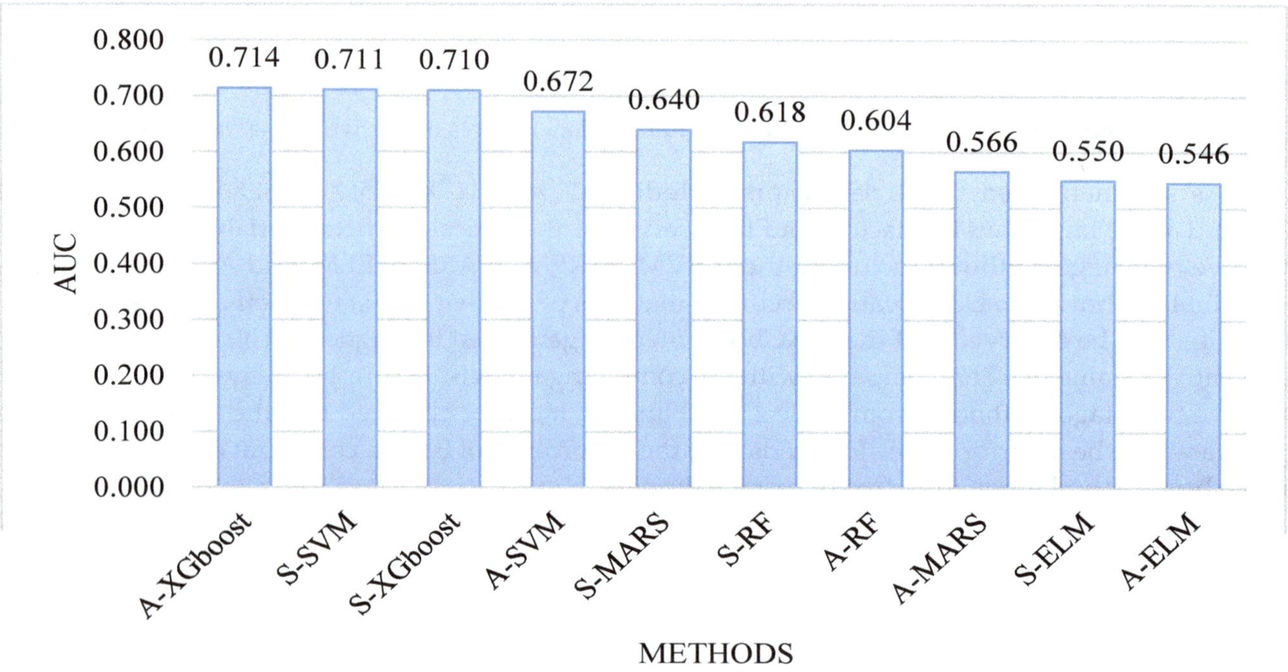


**Figure 5.** Comparison of the area under the curve (AUC) values of the ten models.

In order to evaluate the robustness of the ten models, we randomly repeated 10-fold cross-validation 100 times and averaged the classification accuracy metrics; i.e., accuracy, sensitivity, specificity, and AUC. The averaged accuracy, sensitivity, specificity, and AUC values are shown in Table 5. From the Table, it can be observed that the A-XGboost model still generated the highest AUC value, 0.723, and is the most promising model in this study for predicting the SPC in colorectal cancer.

**Table 5.** Evaluation of the ten models based on the averaged classification results.

| Methods | Accuracy | Sensitivity | Specificity | AUC |
|---|---|---|---|---|
| S-SVM | 0.625 | 0.647 | 0.623 | 0.666 |
| S-RF | 0.691 | 0.539 | 0.709 | 0.637 |
| S-MARS | 0.741 | 0.486 | 0.771 | 0.636 |
| S-XGboost | 0.675 | 0.671 | 0.675 | 0.706 |
| S-ELM | 0.482 | 0.649 | 0.455 | 0.535 |
| A-SVM | 0.609 | 0.642 | 0.605 | 0.641 |
| A-RF | 0.732 | 0.455 | 0.763 | 0.616 |
| A-MARS | 0.696 | 0.553 | 0.713 | 0.652 |
| A-XGboost | **0.695** | **0.672** | **0.697** | **0.723** |
| A-ELM | 0.503 | 0.632 | 0.479 | 0.539 |

## 5. Discussion and Conclusions

In this study, 10 important risk factors, including the combined stage, age at diagnosis, BMI, surgical margins of the primary site, tumor size, sex, regional lymph nodes positive, grade/differentiation, primary site, and drinking behavior, were selected by the A-XGboost model, which provided the best classification performance among the ten models constructed in this study.

Colorectal cancer ranks second and third in terms of mortality and incidence, respectively, in Taiwan. It is also the third highest cancer in terms of medical expenditure. While patient survival has improved, the occurrence of second primary cancers in colorectal cancer patients has become an important issue for clinical management. A variety of different ML techniques have been used in the medical study over the last two decades. To address this issue, data from the cancer registry can be used to better understand the disease and maximize the prevention of SPC. Important issues for future research include predictive models (radiotherapy and chemotherapy) and their association with SPC, as well as a better understanding of the interactions with other genetic factors. Besides, the hospital based cancer registry can be easily extended to the national cancer registry easily. Further discussion with patients after diagnosis should help determine the optimal duration of monitoring and follow-up in early detecting the second primary cancer.

**Author Contributions:** W.-C.T. compiled the data set and drafted the manuscript; H.-R.C. participated in the experimental design and drafted the manuscript; C.-C.C. edited the manuscript and conceived the study; C.-J.L. wrote the experimental programs and conceived the study. All authors have read and agreed to the published version of the manuscript.

## References

1. Zinatizadeh, N.; Khalili, F.; Fallah, P.; Farid, M.; Geravand, M.; Yaslianifard, S. Potential preventive effect of lactobacillus acidophilus and lactobacillus plantarum in patients with polyps or colorectal cancer. *Arq. Gastroenterol.* **2018**, *55*, 407–411. [CrossRef] [PubMed]
2. Sakellakis, M. Multiple primary malignancies: A report of two cases. *Chin. J. Cancer Res.* **2014**, *26*, 215–218. [PubMed]
3. Santangelo, M.L. Immunosuppression and multiple primary malignancies in kidney-transplanted patients: A single-institute study. *BioMed Res. Int.* **2015**, *2015*, 183–523. [CrossRef]
4. Xu, W. Multiple primary malignancies in patients with hepatocellular carcinoma: A largest series with 26-year follow-up. *Medicine* **2016**, *95*, e3491. [CrossRef] [PubMed]
5. Li, F. Multiple primary malignancies involving lung cancer. *BMC Cancer* **2015**, *15*, 696. [CrossRef] [PubMed]
6. Wu, L.L.; Gu, K.S. Clinical retrospective analysis of cases with multiple primary malignant neoplasms. *Genet. Mol. Res.* **2014**, *13*, 9271–9284.

7. Meng, L.V.; Zhang, X.; Shen, Y.; Wang, F.; Yang, J.; Wang, B.; Chen, Z.; Li, P.; Zhang, X.; Li, S.; et al. Clinical analysis and prognosis of synchronous and metachronous multiple primary malignant tumors. *Medicine* **2017**, *96*, e6799.
8. Huang, C.S.; Yang, S.H.; Lin, C.C.; Lan, Y.T.; Chang, S.C.; Wang, H.S.; Chen, W.S.; Lin, T.C.; Lin, J.K.; Jiang, J.K. Synchronous and metachronous colorectal cancers: Distinct disease entities or different disease courses? *Hepato Gastroenterol.* **2015**, *62*, 838–842.
9. Patricia, A.G.; Jacqueline, C.; Erin, E.H. Ensuring quality care for cancer survivors: Implementing the survivorship care plan. *Semin. Oncol. Nurs.* **2015**, *24*, 208–217.
10. Vogt, A.; Schmid, S.; Heinimann, K.; Frick, H.; Herrmann, C.; Cerny, T.; Omlin, A. Multiple primary tumours: Challenges and approaches, a review. *ESMO Open* **2017**, *2*, e000172. [CrossRef]
11. Tseng, C.J.; Chang, C.C.; Lu, C.J.; Chen, G.D. Application of machine learning to predict the recurrence-proneness for cervical cancer. *Neural Comput. Appl.* **2014**, *24*, 1311–1316. [CrossRef]
12. Tseng, C.J.; Lu, C.J.; Chang, C.C.; Chen, G.D.; Cheewakriangkrai, C. Integration of data mining classification techniques and ensemble learning to identify risk factors and diagnose ovarian cancer recurrence. *Artif. Intell. Med.* **2017**, *78*, 47–54. [CrossRef] [PubMed]
13. Ting, W.C.; Lu, Y.C.; Lu, C.J.; Cheewakriangkrai, C.; Chang, C.C. Recurrence impact of primary site and pathologic stage in patients diagnosed with colorectal cancer. *J. Qual.* **2018**, *25*, 166–184.
14. Chang, C.C.; Chen, S.H. Developing a novel machine learning-based classification scheme for predicting SPCs in breast cancer survivors. *Front. Genet.* **2019**, *10*, 848. [CrossRef] [PubMed]
15. Kopetz, S.; Tabernero, J.; Rosenberg, R.; Jiang, Z.Q.; Moreno, V.; Bachleitner-Hofmann, T.; Lanza, G.; Stork-Sloots, L.; Maru, D.; Simon, I.; et al. Genomic classifier ColoPrint predicts recurrence in stage II colorectal cancer patients more accurately than clinical factors. *Oncologist* **2015**, *20*, 127–133. [CrossRef] [PubMed]
16. Gao, S.; Tibiche, C.; Zou, J.; Zaman, N.; Trifiro, M.; O'Connormccourt, M.; Wang, E. Identification and construction of combinatory cancer hallmark-based gene signature sets to predict recurrence and chemotherapy benefit in stage II colorectal cancer. *JAMA Oncol.* **2016**, *2*, 37–45. [CrossRef] [PubMed]
17. Yang, L.; Xiong, Z.; Xie, Q.K.; He, W.; Liu, S.; Kong, P. Second primary colorectal cancer after the initial primary colorectal cancer. *BMC Cancer* **2018**, *18*, 931. [CrossRef]
18. Sun, L.C.; Tai, Y.Y.; Liao, S.M.; Lin, T.Y.; Shih, Y.L.; Chang, S.F. Clinical characteristics of second primary cancer in colorectal cancer patients: The impact of colorectal cancer or other second cancer occurring first. *World J. Surg. Oncol.* **2014**, *12*, 73. [CrossRef]
19. Ringland, C.L.; Arkenau, H.T.; O'Connell, D.L.; Ward, R.L. Second primary colorectal cancers (SPCRCs): Experiences from a large Australian Cancer Registry. *Ann. Oncol.* **2010**, *21*, 92–97. [CrossRef]
20. Friedman, J.H. Multivariate adaptive regression splines. *Ann. Stat.* **1991**, *19*, 1–141. [CrossRef]
21. Zhang, W.; Goh, A.T. Multivariate adaptive regression splines and neural network models for prediction of pile drivability. *Geosci. Front.* **2016**, *7*, 45–52. [CrossRef]
22. Breiman, L. Random forests. *Mach. Learn.* **2001**, *45*, 5–32. [CrossRef]
23. Yuk, E.; Park, S.; Park, C.S.; Baek, J.G. Feature-learning-based printed circuit board inspection via speeded-up robust features and random forest. *Appl. Sci.* **2018**, *8*, 932. [CrossRef]
24. Vapnik, V.N. *The Nature of Statistical Learning Theory*; Springer: Berlin/Heidelberg, Germany, 2000.
25. Li, T.; Gao, M.; Song, R.; Yin, Q.; Chen, Y. Support vector machine classifier for accurate identification of piRNA. *Appl. Sci.* **2018**, *8*, 2204. [CrossRef]
26. Huang, G.B.; Zhu, Q.Y.; Siew, C.X. Extreme learning machine: Theory and applications. *Neurocomputing* **2006**, *70*, 489–501. [CrossRef]
27. Chen, T.; Guestrin, C. XGBoost: A Scalable Tree Boosting System. In Proceedings of the 22nd ACM SIGKDD International Conference on Knowledge Discovery and Data Mining, San Francisco, CA, USA, 13–17 August 2016; pp. 785–794.
28. Natekin, A.; Knoll, A. Gradient boosting machines, a tutorial. *Front. Neurorobotics* **2013**, *7*, 21. [CrossRef]
29. Torlay, L.; Perrone-Bertolotti, M.; Thomas, E.; Baciu, M. Machine learning–XGBoost analysis of language networks to classify patients with epilepsy. *Brain Inform.* **2017**, *4*, 159. [CrossRef]
30. Mitchell, R.; Frank, E. Accelerating the XGBoost algorithm using GPU computing. *PeerJ Comput. Sci.* **2017**, *3*, e127. [CrossRef]

31. Milborrow, S.; Hastie, T.; Tibshirani, R.; Miller, A.; Lumley, T. Earth: Multivariate Adaptive Regression Splines. R Package Version 5.1.2. Available online: https://www.rdocumentation.org/packages/earth (accessed on 1 October 2019).
32. Liaw, A.; Wiener, M. randomForest: Breiman and Cutler's Random Forests for Classification and Regression. R Package Version, 4.6.14. Available online: https://www.rdocumentation.org/packages/randomForest (accessed on 1 October 2019).
33. Meyer, D.; Dimitriadou, E.; Hornik, K.; Weingessel, A.; Leisch, F. e1071: Misc Functions of the Department of Statistics, Probability Theory Group (Formerly: E1071), TU Wien, 2017. R Package Version, 1.7-1. Available online: https://www.rdocumentation.org/packages/e1071 (accessed on 1 October 2019).
34. Gosso, A.; Martinez-de-Pison, F. elmNN: Implementation of ELM (Extreme Learning Machine) Algorithm for SLFN (Single Hidden Layer Feedforward Neural Networks). R Package Version, 1. Available online: https://www.rdocumentation.org/packages/elmNN (accessed on 1 October 2019).
35. Kuhn, M.; Wing, J.; Weston, S.; Williams, A.; Keefer, C.; Engelhardt, A.; Kenkel, B. Caret: Classification and Regression Training. R Package Version 6.0-84. Available online: https://www.rdocumentation.org/packages/caret (accessed on 1 October 2019).
36. Chen, T.; He, T.; Benesty, M.; Khotilovich, V.; Tang, Y. Xgboost: Extreme Gradient Boosting. R Package Version 0.90.0.2. Available online: https://www.rdocumentation.org/packages/xgboost (accessed on 1 October 2019).

# 5

# Prediction System for Prostate Cancer Recurrence Using Machine Learning

**Sun Jung Lee [1,2], Sung Hye Yu [1], Yejin Kim [3], Jae Kwon Kim [1], Jun Hyuk Hong [4], Choung-Soo Kim [4], Seong Il Seo [5], Seok-Soo Byun [6], Chang Wook Jeong [7], Ji Youl Lee [8] and In Young Choi [1,2,*]**

1 Department of Medical Informatics, College of Medicine, Catholic University of Korea, Seoul 06591, Korea; lsjadd500@gmail.com (S.J.L.); sala5537@naver.com (S.H.Y.); jaekwonkorea@naver.com (J.K.K.)
2 Department of Biomedicine & Health Sciences, College of Medicine, The Catholic University of Korea, Seoul 06591, Korea
3 School of Biomedical Informatics, University of Texas Health Science Center at Houston, Houston, TX 77030, USA; yejin.kim89@gmail.com
4 Department of Urology, University of Ulsan College of Medicine, Seoul 05505, Korea; jhhong@amc.seoul.kr (J.H.H.); cskim@amc.seoul.kr (C.-S.K.)
5 Department of Urology, Sungkyunkwan University School of Medicine, Seoul 06351, Korea; siseo@skku.edu
6 Department of Urology, Seoul National University Bundang Hospital, Seongnam 13620, Korea; seoksoo.byeon@gmail.com
7 Department of Urology, Seoul National University College of Medicine, Seoul 03080, Korea; drboss@gmail.com
8 Department of Urology, Seoul St. Mary's Hospital, College of Medicine, The Catholic University of Korea, Seoul 06591, Korea; uroljy@catholic.ac.kr
* Correspondence: iychoi@catholic.ac.kr

**Abstract:** Prostate cancer is the fourth most common cancer affecting South Korean males, and the biochemical recurrence (BCR) of prostate cancer occurs in approximately 25% of patients five years after radical prostatectomy. The ability to predict BCR would help clinicians and patients to make better treatment decisions. Therefore, in this study, we have proposed a web-based clinical decision support system that predicts the BCR of prostate cancer in Korean patients. The data were obtained from the Korean Prostate Cancer Registry (KPCR) database, which contained information about 7394 patients with prostate cancer who were treated at one of the six major medical institutions in South Korea between May 2001 and December 2014. We tested 13 prediction models and selected the gradient boosting classifier because it demonstrated excellent prediction performance. Using this model, we were able to create a web application and once clinical data from patients were entered, the three- and five-year post-surgery BCR predictions could be extracted. We developed a clinical decision support system to provide a prostate cancer BCR predictive function to facilitate postoperative follow-up and clinical management. This system will help clinicians develop a strategic approach for prostate cancer treatment by predicting the likelihood of prostate cancer recurrence.

**Keywords:** prostate cancer; machine learning; prediction; clinical decision support system; gradient boost

---

## 1. Introduction

According to a 2017 Korean National Cancer Center survey, prostate cancer is the fourth most common cancer affecting South Korean males, with an incidence rate of 29 per 100,000 people in the country's population [1].

Biochemical recurrence (BCR) of prostate cancer occurs in approximately 25% of patients within five years after radical prostatectomy [2]. BCR is accepted as evidence of cancer recurrence if measurable serum prostate-specific antigen (PSA) levels are confirmed after radical prostatectomy, or if PSA levels increase after radiation treatments [3–5]. BCR is also accepted as an indicator of postoperative progress and outcomes [6]. If we could predict prostate cancer BCR by analyzing data on the progress and recurrence patterns of prostate cancers, it would help clinicians to make better decisions with regard to future treatment options. In addition, depending on the predicted BCR probability, the incidence of recurrence could be reduced by providing patients with physical examinations or related medication.

Most medical institutions use computer-based systems to accurately and efficiently manage medical data [7]. In particular, the clinical decision support system (CDSS) is a valuable tool that helps healthcare providers to make decisions and solve complex problems [8,9]. There are few prostate cancer recurrence prediction systems currently in clinical use, so providing this function, through a facility's CDSS, will facilitate postoperative follow up and aid in the clinical management of patients with prostate cancer [10].

The Memorial Sloan Kettering Cancer Center (MSKCC) in the United States provides a function that can be used to predict the probability of 2-, 5-, 7-, 10-, and 15-year BCR-free survival after prostate cancer surgery. It applies statistical techniques such as linear regression, logistical regression, and survival progress models to provide a web-based cancer recurrence prediction system [11]. However, the incidence of prostate cancer varies with country and race [12–15], which means that the predictive system that was designed for MSKCC patients may not be as accurate at predicting prostate cancer recurrence in South Korea.

Therefore, in this study, we have proposed a web-based CDSS that can predict the BCR of Korean patients with prostate cancer to support radical prostatectomy postoperative care. Our study uses data from Korean patients with prostate cancer to predict the recurrence of prostate cancer in this population. We tested several statistical and machine learning techniques that could be used to predict prostate cancer recurrence and then adopted the model that exhibited the best prediction accuracy for use in our prostate cancer recurrence prediction system.

This study aimed to develop a machine learning model that could use the Korean Prostate Cancer Registry (KPCR) database to predict the three- and five-year BCR in Korean patients who previously had prostate cancer and had undergone radical prostatectomies.

## 2. Materials and Methods

### 2.1. BCR Prediction Data

The data used in this study was obtained from the KPCR database which included 7394 patients with prostate cancer. This database included Electronic Medical Records (EMRs) data collected from the six major medical institutions in South Korea between May 2001 and December 2014 (Figure 1). The study protocol was approved by the institutional review board of the Catholic University of Korea (IRB No. MC16RIMI0107).

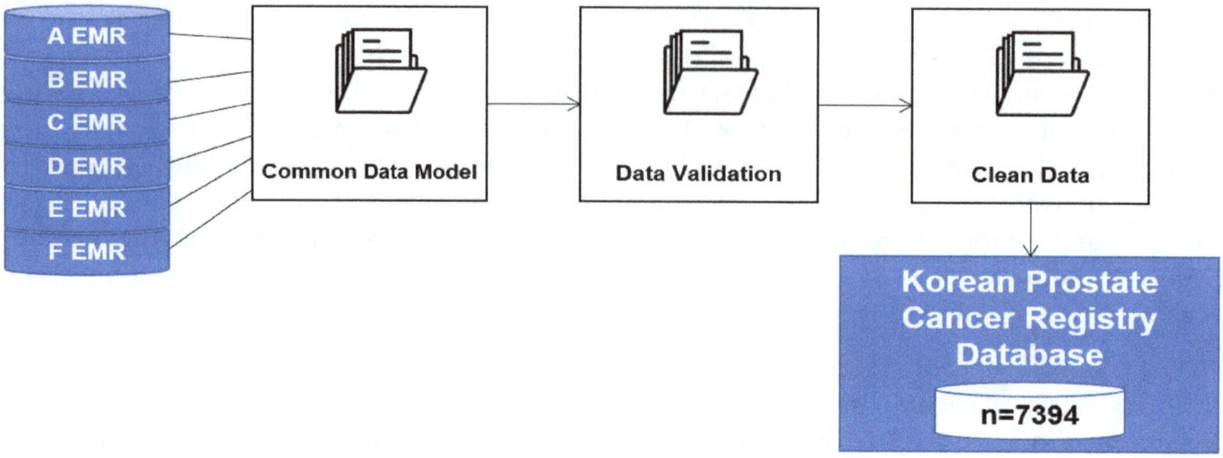


**Figure 1.** The Process of Building a Korean Prostate Cancer Registry (KPCR) Database Based on Electronic Medical Records (EMRs).

Data standardization and quality control were implemented to ensure data integrity, and exclusion criteria were created and applied to the database to refine the data used in the BCR prediction.

Our data subset was created from the main KPCR database using the following processes (Figure 2):

- There were 7394 potentially relevant records in the KPCR database
- 2280 records, including those of non-Koreans (51), those who did not have a full follow-up period of at least one year (633), those who did not have a neoclassical prostatectomy (80), those who performed pre-supplementary therapy (230), and those for whom critical data were missing (1286) were excluded
- We identified 5114 individual records as being statistically usable and relevant
- We classified the 5114 patient data items into BCR (1207) and Non-BCR (3907) groups to identify the characteristics of each group.

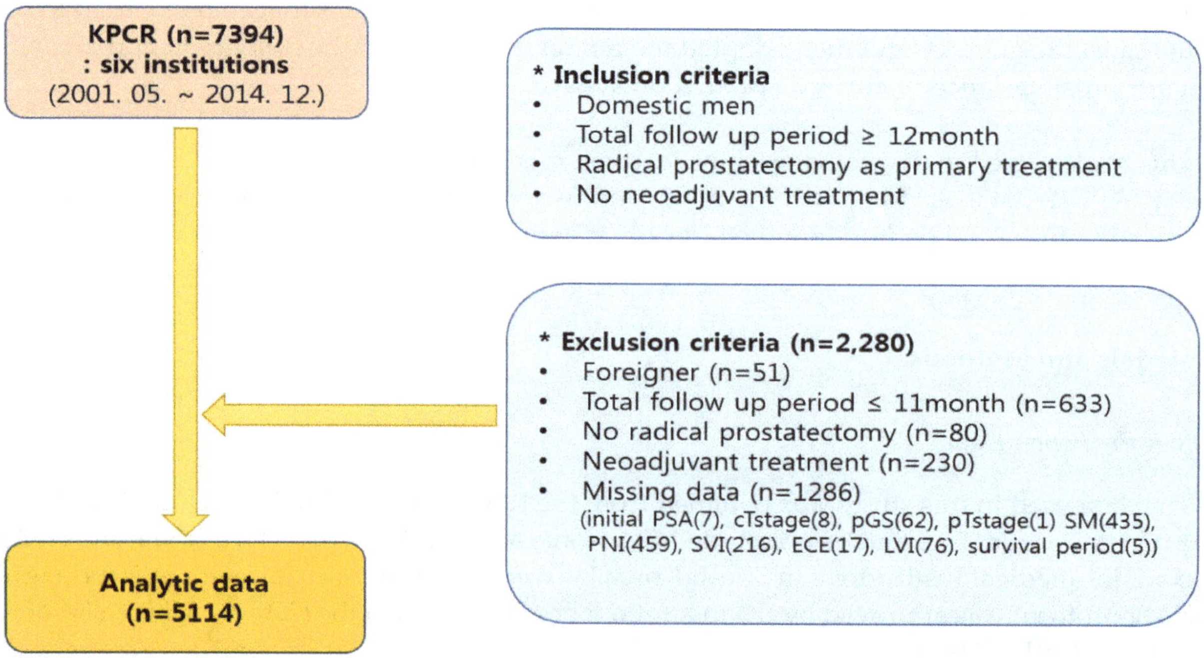


**Figure 2.** Patient Flow Chart.

We found that follow-up periods ranged between 0 and 157 months, and out of the total of 7394 patients, 70% or more had a follow-up period of less than five years. Therefore, we decided to predict BCR likelihood at three and five years after radical prostate cancer surgery.

Factors affecting BCR have been reported to include age, initial PSA, clinical T stage, pathology Gleason score sum, pathology T stage, surgical margin, perineural invasion, seminal vesicles, extracapsular extension, and lymphovascular invasion [16–19]. We extracted these factors from the 5114 analytical data items and generated a training data set for predicting three- and five-year BCR after radical prostate cancer surgery.

### 2.2. *BCR Prediction Statistical Analysis*

In this study, we tested 13 prediction models, including: decision tree [20]; random forest [21] with 20, 50, and 80 trees; a fully-connected feedforward neural network [22]; Cox proportional hazards model [23]; ridge regression [24]; lasso [25]; and gradient boosting classifier (GBC), and analyzed the results produced by each model. GBC iteratively combines weak prediction models to create a more powerful model by allowing optimization of the loss function [26–28].

To select the model with the best BCR prediction performance, we evaluated the area under the receiver operating characteristics curve (AUC), accuracy, sensitivity, specificity, and Matthews correlation coefficient (MCC) for each model. We then selected the analytical model that performed the best and applied it to the BCR prediction system.

### 2.3. *BCR Prediction System*

There was a need for a system that can analyze the database of patients with prostate cancer and review the results to make predictions about prostate cancer recurrence. This system can then be used to analyze data from a new patient and predict the probability of recurrence. Based on the results of the model, clinicians can select treatment options to reduce the incidence of BCR. This system was developed as a web-based application so clinicians could access it easily.

In this study, we proposed a system that used a prediction algorithm to analyze the KPCR database in order to develop a BCR prediction model using data collected from patients with prostate cancer.

## 3. Results

### 3.1. *Patient Characteristics and Distribution*

We analyzed the characteristics and distribution of patients by dividing them into groups with prostate cancer BCR and non-recurrence of prostate cancer (Non-BCR) (Table 1). The average age of the 5114 patients with prostate cancer was 66 years, and the average ages for BCR and Non-BCR were both 65 years, respectively. The oldest and youngest BCR patients were 84 and 38, respectively, while the oldest and youngest Non-BCR patients were 90 and 37, respectively. The average initial PSA value for all patients was 11.59 ng/mL, and the mean PSA values for BCR and Non-BCR patients were 17.58 ng/mL and 9.74 ng/mL, respectively.

**Table 1.** Patient Characteristics and Distribution.

| | | BCR (1207 Patients) | Non-BCR (3907 Patients) |
|---|---|---|---|
| Age | Average | 65 | 65 |
| Initial PSA (ng/mL) | Average | 17.58 | 9.74 |
| Gleason score (sum) | 2–4 | 0 | 5 |
| | 5 | 3 | 19 |
| | 6 | 111 | 994 |
| | 7 | 719 | 2576 |
| | 8–10 | 374 | 313 |
| Clinical T stage | T1 | 399 | 1753 |
| | T2 | 467 | 1416 |
| | T3 | 276 | 677 |
| | T4 | 65 | 61 |

For BCR patients, the initial PSA minimum value was 0.66, and the maximum was 261.77. For Non-BCR patients, the initial PSA minimum was 0.09, while the maximum was 305. Pathological Gleason scores were classified as grade 2–4, 5, 6, 7, and 8–10, and within each grade, 5 (0.09%), 22 (0.43%), 1105 (21%), 3295 (64%), and 687 (13.43%) patients were included, respectively. We classified clinical T stages into four of the existing eight grades [29]: 2152 for T1, 1883 for T2, 953 for T3, and 126 for T4. The BCR patients were widely distributed within T2, and the non-BCR patients were widely distributed within T1.

### *3.2. BCR Prediction Model Analysis*

In order to analyze the statistical performance of the BCR predictions, we evaluated the AUC, accuracy, sensitivity, specificity, and MCC of each analysis method. The analytical data was divided randomly, with 80% of the data allocated to the training dataset and 20% allocated to the test dataset. We trained the model using the training data, and then we evaluated the performance of the model using the test data.

According to the result of analysis (Table 2), the highest AUC value for the three year predictions was 0.8419, which was associated with the GBC model. For the five year predictions, the highest AUC value (0.8071) was associated with the Ridged Regression model. The highest MCC values for the three year and five year predictions were associated with the Random Forest (ntrees = 80) model (0.4621) and the GBC model (0.4836), respectively. The Cox proportional hazard model showed good results in terms of accuracy and specificity but performed poorly in terms of sensitivity, and so was not used as a predictive model. In terms of overall performance across the five analysis criteria (AUC, accuracy, sensitivity, specificity, MCC), the GBC model had the highest average value and showed excellent performance. Therefore, we applied this model to develop the BCR prediction system. To develop prediction models for three and five years after prostate cancer surgery using the GBC model, we developed the BCR prediction system using Python.

**Table 2.** Statistical Method Analysis.

| Analysis | Method | AUC | | Accuracy | | Sensitivity | | Specificity | | MCC | |
|---|---|---|---|---|---|---|---|---|---|---|---|
| | | 3-year | 5-year | 3-year | 5-year | 3-year | 5-year | 3-year | 5-year | 3-year | 5-year |
| Trees | Decision Tree | 0.8186 | 0.7561 | 0.7817 | 0.7033 | 0.4135 | 0.7009 | 0.9447 | 0.7062 | 0.4448 | 0.4055 |
| | Random Forest (ntrees = 20) [1] | 0.8320 | 0.7956 | 0.7817 | 0.7126 | 0.4135 | 0.7308 | 0.9447 | 0.6907 | 0.4448 | 0.4210 |
| | Random Forest (ntrees = 50) | 0.8349 | 0.8047 | 0.7832 | 0.7266 | 0.4279 | 0.7393 | 0.9404 | 0.7113 | 0.4495 | 0.4310 |
| | Random Forest (ntrees = 80) | 0.8362 | 0.8050 | 0.7876 | 0.7196 | 0.4327 | 0.7308 | 0.9447 | 0.7062 | 0.4621 | 0.4360 |
| Neural Networks | 1hidden, dropout = 0.3 at input | 0.7939 | 0.7895 | 0.7611 | 0.7056 | 0.3606 | 0.7821 | 0.9383 | 0.6134 | 0.4385 | 0.4001 |
| | 1hidden dropout = 0.1 at input | 0.8027 | 0.7977 | 0.7699 | 0.6916 | 0.5144 | 0.7393 | 0.8830 | 0.6340 | 0.4089 | −0.0367 |
| | 2hidden, dropout = 0.3 at input | 0.7978 | 0.7941 | 0.6932 | 0.7056 | 0.0000 | 0.7051 | 1.0000 | 0.7062 | 0.3393 | 0.3986 |
| | 2hidden dropout = 0.1 at input | 0.7988 | 0.7967 | 0.7611 | 0.7056 | 0.3702 | 0.8162 | 0.9340 | 0.5722 | 0.3963 | 0.4128 |
| Survival Regression | Cox PH | 0.7944 | 0.7816 | 0.8025 | 0.7830 | 0.2160 | 0.3333 | 0.9568 | 0.9300 | 0.2894 | 0.3159 |
| Logistic Regression | Ridged Regression (L2) | 0.8288 | 0.8071 | 0.7802 | 0.7290 | 0.4279 | 0.7265 | 0.9362 | 0.7320 | 0.4413 | 0.4210 |
| | Lasso (L1) | 0.8319 | 0.7993 | 0.7861 | 0.7243 | 0.4519 | 0.7179 | 0.9340 | 0.7320 | 0.4590 | 0.4481 |
| | GBC | 0.8419 | 0.8031 | 0.7891 | 0.7407 | 0.4567 | 0.7436 | 0.9362 | 0.7371 | 0.4348 | 0.4836 |

[1] "ntrees" means the number of trees in the forest.

### *3.3. Development of BCR Prediction System*

The BCR prediction system used data from Korean patients with prostate cancer to implement a web-based application. The structure of the prediction system was classified into two parts: predictive modeling and web application development (Figure 3). The web application used the predictive model to make predictions.

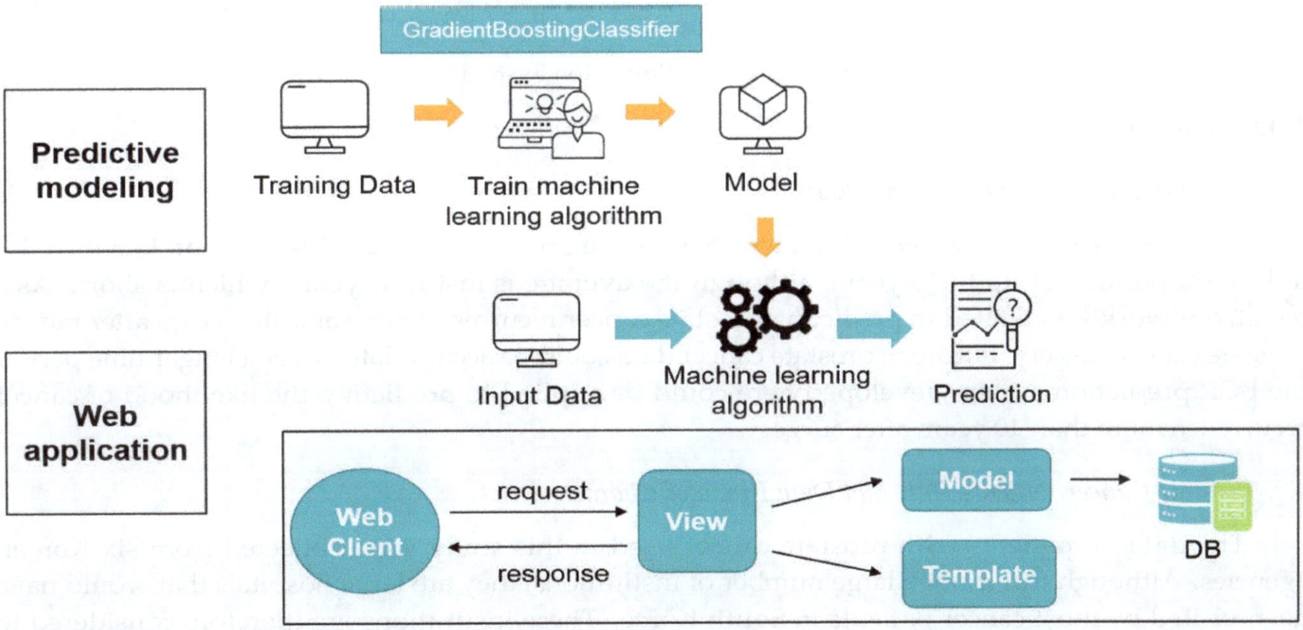


**Figure 3.** System Flow.

The BCR prediction system was set up to perform several functions on one screen, including reading the data list of patients with prostate cancer, inputting the input values, and extracting the prediction results (Figure 4). After the input fields, including age at diagnosis, initial PSA, clinical T stage, pathological Gleason score, and pathological T stage values have been entered and status information such as surgical margin, perineural invasion, seminal vesicle invasion, extracapsular extension, and lymphovascular invasion has been selected, the three and five year post-surgery BCR predictions could be extracted. The prediction results appear as an output item at the bottom of the screen.

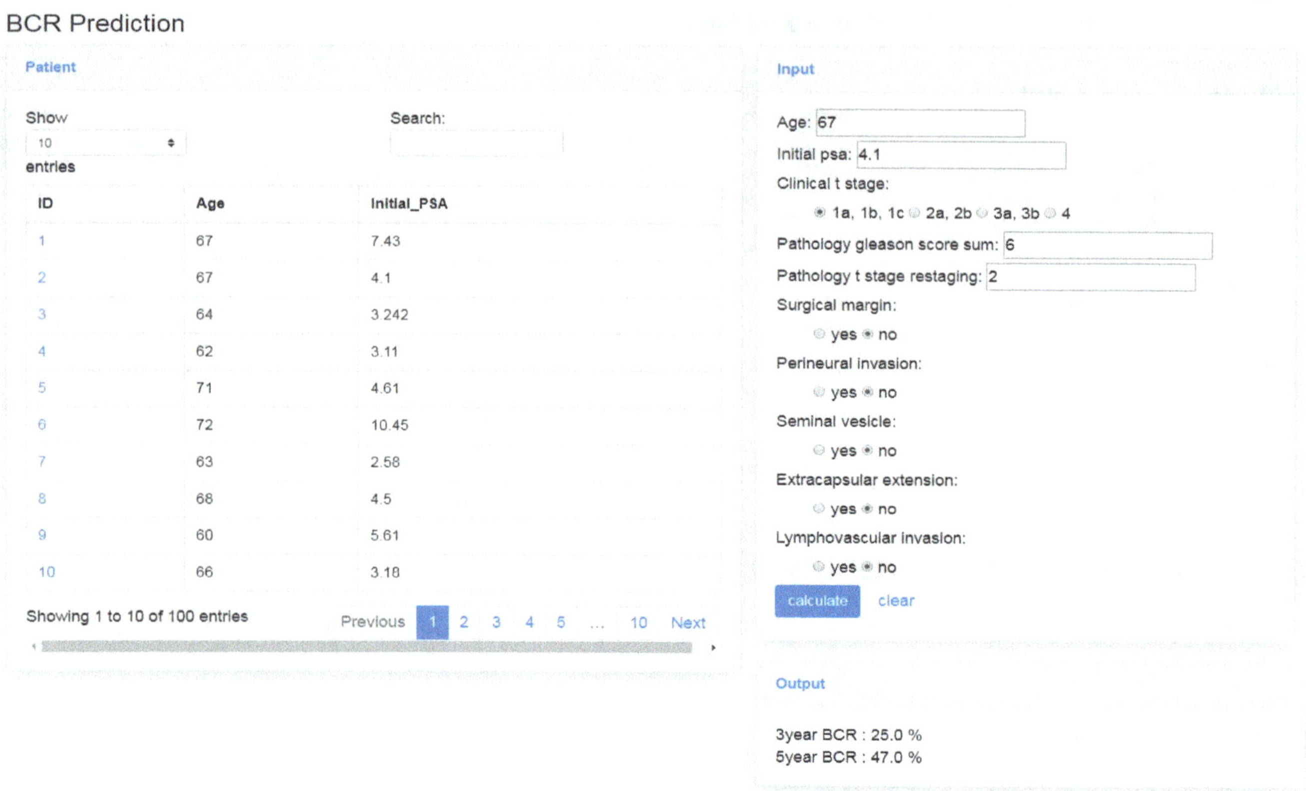


**Figure 4.** BCR Prediction System.

## 4. Discussion

### *4.1. Follow-Up Period for Predicting BCR*

Long-term follow-up is needed to identify prostate cancer recurrence. The current data includes follow-up periods of up to 13 years, although the average is just four years, which is short. As a result, our work was limited to predicting prostate cancer recurrence three and five years after radical prostate cancer surgery. If Korean prostate cancer data could be accumulated over a longer time period, the BCR prediction system developed here could be applied to predicting the likelihood of cancer recurrence more than 10 years after surgery.

### *4.2. Prostate Cancer Patients Data and Data Provider Characteristics*

The data on patients with prostate cancer used in this study were collected from six Korean agencies. Although this is not a large number of institutions, they are large hospitals that would have been visited by most cancer patients in South Korea. These institutions are therefore considered to have provided representative datasets, and it was assumed that institutional dataset characteristics were unlikely to exhibit significant differences.

The analytical classifier used in this study is specific to the Korean prostate cancer dataset. There are racial differences in the recurrence of prostate cancer, and since we currently only have a dataset that represents Korean patients, we can only develop a specific predictive model that applies to that population. We would, therefore, have difficulty predicting recurrence in other races. If we can collect data from other racial populations in the future, we will be able to develop more general models that can predict recurrence in various groups of people.

### *4.3. The Potential of Misdiagnosis*

The CDSS developed in this study can help clinicians determine treatment options by predicting the probability of prostate cancer recurrence. However, there was an error rate of about 20 percent in this study, which means that there is a potential for misdiagnosis. The CDSS should be used as an ancillary tool, and, in the future, measures to improve data quality and the accuracy of predictive models should be investigated to.

## 5. Conclusions

In this study, we designed and developed a CDSS that could predict the likelihood of BCR in Korean patients with prostate cancer. Performance-stable GBC predictive models were used, and the KPCR, a database of Korean patients with prostate cancer, was used for training to develop BCR prediction models that were specialized for use with Korean data. This prediction model was incorporated into a web-based system to allow easy access to data from patients with prostate cancer and facilitate its use for BCR predictions. The BCR prediction could facilitate postoperative follow-up and clinical management of patients with prostate cancer. This system will be able to help clinicians develop a strategic approach by predicting the likelihood that prostate cancer will recur in a particular patient.

**Author Contributions:** Conceptualization, S.J.L., S.H.Y., Y.K., and I.Y.C.; Methodology, S.J.L., Y.K., and I.Y.C.; Software, S.J.L. Formal Analysis, S.J.L.; Investigation, S.J.L, S.H.Y., Y.K., J.H.H., C.-S.K., S.I.S., C.W.J., S.-S.B., J.Y.L., and I.Y.C.; Data Curation, S.H.Y.; Writing—Original Draft Preparation, S.J.L.; Writing—Review & Editing, Y.K., J.K.K., and I.Y.C.; Visualization, S.J.L.; Supervision, I.Y.C. All authors have read and agreed to the published version of the manuscript.

**Acknowledgments:** We thank Hyunmin Kim for reviewing the abstract and providing valuable comments.

## References

1. National Cancer Information Center. 2017 Cancer Statistics; Cancer Incidence Rates. Available online: https://www.cancer.go.kr/lay1/S1T639C641/contents.do (accessed on 6 January 2020).
2. Lee, J.W.; Cho, K.S.; Han, K.S.; Kim, E.K.; Joung, J.Y.; Seo, H.K.; Chung, J.; Park, W.S.; Lee, K.H. Epidermal growth factor receptor as predicting factor on biochemical recurrence after radical prostatectomy: A prospective study. *Korean J. Urol.* **2008**, *49*, 974–980. [CrossRef]
3. Song, S.H.; Kwak, C. Definition of BCR and further evaluation. *Korean J. Urol. Oncol.* **2011**, *9*, 104–111.
4. Cox, J.D.; Grignon, D.J.; Kaplan, R.S.; Parsons, J.T.; Schellhammer, P.F. Consensus statement: Guidelines for PSA following radiation therapy. *Int. J. Radiat. Oncol. Biol. Phys.* **1997**, *37*, 1035–1041.
5. Lange, P.H.; Ercole, C.J.; Lightner, D.J.; Fraley, E.E.; Vessella, R. The value of serum prostate specific antigen determinations before and after radical prostatectomy. *J. Urol.* **1989**, *141*, 873–879. [CrossRef]
6. Hong, J.H.; Lee, H.M.; Choi, H.Y. The predictors of biochemical recurrence and metastasis following radical perineal prostatectomy in clinically localized prostate cancer. *Korean J. Urol.* **2005**, *46*, 1161.
7. Sa, S. Intelligent heart disease prediction system using data mining techniques. *Int. J. Healthc. Biomed. Res.* **2013**, *1*, 94–101.
8. Paydar, K.; Kalhori, S.R.N.; Akbarian, M.; Sheikhtaheri, A. A clinical decision support system for prediction of pregnancy outcome in pregnant women with systemic lupus erythematosus. *Int. J. Med Inform.* **2017**, *97*, 239–246. [CrossRef]
9. Berner, E.S. (Ed.) *Clinical Decision Support Systems*; Springer Science + Business Media, LLC: New York, NY, USA, 2007.
10. Foster, D.; McGregor, C.; El-Masri, S. A survey of agent-based intelligent decision support systems to support clinical management and research. In Proceedings of the Second International Workshop on Multi-Agent Systems for Medicine, Computational Biology, and Bioinformatics, Utrecht, The Netherlands, 25 July 2005; pp. 16–34.
11. Memorial Sloan Kettering Cancer Center. Prostate Cancer Nomograms. Available online: https://www.mskcc.org/nomograms/prostate (accessed on 6 January 2020).
12. National Cancer Information Center. 2017 Cancer Statistics; Global Cancer Incidence. Available online: https://www.cancer.go.kr/lay1/S1T639C644/contents.do (accessed on 6 January 2020).

13. Hoffman, R.M.; Gilliland, F.D.; Eley, J.W.; Harlan, L.C.; Stephenson, R.A.; Stanford, J.L.; Albertson, P.C.; Hamilton, A.S.; Hunt, W.C.; Potosky, A.L. Racial and ethnic differences in advanced-stage prostate cancer: The prostate cancer outcomes study. *J. Natl. Cancer Inst.* **2001**, *93*, 388–395. [CrossRef]
14. Hankey, B.F.; Feuer, E.J.; Clegg, L.X.; Hayes, R.B.; Legler, J.M.; Prorok, P.C.; Ries, L.A.; Merrill, R.M.; Kaplan, R.S. Cancer surveillance series: Interpreting trends in prostate cancer—Part I: Evidence of the effects of screening in recent prostate cancer incidence, mortality, and survival rates. *J. Natl. Cancer Inst.* **1999**, *91*, 1017–1024. [CrossRef]
15. Stanford, J.L.; Stephenson, R.A.; Coyle, L.M.; Cerhan, J.; Correa, R.; Eley, J.W.; Gilliland, F.; Hankey, B.; Kolonel, L.N.; Ross, R. *Prostate Cancer Trends 1973–1995*; NIH Pub. No. 99-4543; Surveillance Research Program, National Cancer Institute: Bethesda, MD, USA, 1999.
16. Ahn, K.I.; Chang, S.G.; Choi, B.K.; Jeon, S.H. The study of biochemical and clinical failure after radical prostatectomy or radiation therapy in localized prostate cancer. *Korean J. Urol. Oncol.* **2004**, *2*, 171–177.
17. De la TaIlle, A.; Rubin, A.A.; Bagiella, E.; Olsson, C.A.; Buttyan, R.; Burchardt, T.; Knight, C.; O'Toole, K.M.; Katz, A.E. Can perineural invasion on prostate needle biopsy predict prostate specific antigen recurrence after radical prostatectomy? *J. Urol.* **1999**, *162*, 103–106. [CrossRef] [PubMed]
18. Blute, M.L.; Bergstralh, E.J.; Iocca, A.; Scherer, B.; Zincke, H. Use of Gleason score, prostate specific antigen, seminal vesicle and margin status to predict biochemical failure after radical prostatectomy. *J. Urol.* **2001**, *165*, 119–125. [CrossRef] [PubMed]
19. Han, M.; Partin, A.W.; Zahurak, M.; Piantadosi, S.; Epstein, J.I.; Walsh, P.C. Biochemical (prostate specific antigen) recurrence probability following radical prostatectomy for clinically localized prostate cancer. *J. Urol.* **2003**, *169*, 517–523. [CrossRef]
20. Pal, M.; Mather, P.M. An assessment of the effectiveness of decision tree methods for land cover classification. *Remote Sens. Environ.* **2003**, *86*, 554–565. [CrossRef]
21. Liaw, A.; Wiener, M. Classification and regression by randomForest. *R News* **2002**, *2*, 18–22.
22. Acion, L.; Kelmansky, D.; van der Laan, M.; Sahker, E.; Jones, D.; Arndt, S. Use of a machine learning framework to predict substance use disorder treatment success. *PLoS ONE* **2017**, *12*, e0175383. [CrossRef]
23. Van Houwelingen, H.; Putter, H. *Dynamic Prediction in Clinical Survival Analysis*, 1st ed.; CRC Press: Boca Raton, FL, USA, 2011.
24. Saunders, C.; Gammerman, A.; Vovk, V. Ridge regression learning algorithm in dual variables. In Proceedings of the Fifteenth International Conference on Machine Learning (ICML 1998), Madison, WI, USA, 24–27 July 1998.
25. Meier, L.; Van De Geer, S.; Bühlmann, P. The group lasso for logistic regression. *J. R. Stat. Soc. Ser. B Stat. Methodol.* **2008**, *70*, 53–71. [CrossRef]
26. Wang, J.; Li, P.; Ran, R.; Che, Y.; Zhou, Y. A short-term photovoltaic power prediction model based on the gradient boost decision tree. *Appl. Sci.* **2018**, *8*, 689. [CrossRef]
27. Friedman, J.H. Stochastic gradient boosting. *Comput. Stat. Data Anal.* **2002**, *38*, 367–378. [CrossRef]
28. Krauss, C.; Do, X.A.; Huck, N. Deep neural networks, gradient-boosted trees, random forests: Statistical arbitrage on the S&P 500. *Eur. J. Oper. Res.* **2017**, *259*, 689–702.
29. Ohori, M.; Wheeler, T.M.; Scardino, P.T. The new American joint committee on cancer and international union against cancer TNM classification of prostate cancer. *Cancer* **1994**, *74*, 104–114. [CrossRef]

# 6

# Taylor Bird Swarm Algorithm Based on Deep Belief Network for Heart Disease Diagnosis

**Afnan M. Alhassan [1,2,*] and Wan Mohd Nazmee Wan Zainon [1]**

1 School of Computer Science, Universiti Sains Malaysia, George Town 11800, Malaysia; nazmee@usm.my
2 College of Computing and Information Technology, Shaqra University, Shaqra 11961, Saudi Arabia
* Correspondence: afnan@student.usm.my

**Abstract:** Contemporary medicine depends on a huge amount of information contained in medical databases. Thus, the extraction of valuable knowledge, and making scientific decisions for the treatment of disease, has progressively become necessary to attain effective diagnosis. The obtainability of a large amount of medical data leads to the requirement of effective data analysis tools for extracting constructive knowledge. This paper proposes a novel method for heart disease diagnosis. Here, the pre-processing of medical data is done using log-transformation that converts the data to its uniform value range. Then, the feature selection process is performed using sparse fuzzy-c-means (FCM) for selecting significant features to classify medical data. Incorporating sparse FCM for the feature selection process provides more benefits for interpreting the models, as this sparse technique provides important features for detection, and can be utilized for handling high dimensional data. Then, the selected features are given to the deep belief network (DBN), which is trained using the proposed Taylor-based bird swarm algorithm (Taylor-BSA) for detection. Here, the proposed Taylor-BSA is designed by combining the Taylor series and bird swarm algorithm (BSA). The proposed Taylor-BSA–DBN outperformed other methods, with maximal accuracy of 93.4%, maximal sensitivity of 95%, and maximal specificity of 90.3%, respectively.

**Keywords:** deep belief network; heart disease diagnosis; sparse FCM; bird swarm algorithm

---

## 1. Introduction

Contemporary medicine depends on a large amount of information accumulated in medical datasets. The extraction of such constructive knowledge can help when making scientific decisions to diagnose disease. Medical data can enhance the management of hospital information and endorse the growth of telemedicine. Medical data primarily focuses on patient care first, and research resources second. The main rationalization to collect medical data is to promote patient health conditions [1]. The accessibility of numerous medical data causes redundancy, which requires effectual and significant techniques for processing data to extract beneficial knowledge. However, the diagnostics of various diseases indicate significant issues in data analysis [2]. Quantifiable diagnosis is performed by adoctor's guidance rather than patterns of the medical dataset; thus, there is the possibility of incorrect diagnosis [3]. Cloud-based services can assist with managing medical data, including compliance management, policy integration, access controls, and identity management [4].

Now a day, heart disease is a foremost source of death. We are moving towards a new industrial revolution; thus, lifestyle changes should take place to prevent risk factors of heart disease, such as obesity, diabetes, hypertension, and smoking [5]. The treatment of disease is a complex mission in medical field. The discovery of heart disease, with different risk factors, is considered a multi-layered issue [6]. Thus, patient medical data are collected to simplify the diagnosis process. Offering a valuable service (at less cost) is a major limitation in the healthcare industry. In [7], valuable quality service refers to the precise diagnosis (and effective treatment) in patients. Poor clinical decisions cause disasters, which may affect the health of patients. Automated approaches, such as the machine-learning approach [8,9] and data mining [10] approach, assist with attaining clinical tests, or diagnoses, at reduced risks [11,12]. The classification and pattern recognition by machine learning algorithms are widely included in prognostic and diagnosis monitoring. The machine learning approach supports decision-making, which increases the safety of the patients and avoids medical errors, so that it can be used in clinical decision support systems (CDSS) [13,14].

Several methods are devised for automatic heart disease detection to evaluate the efficiency of the decision tree and Naive Bayes [15]. Moreover, optimization with the genetic algorithm is employed for minimizing the number of attributes without forfeiting accuracy and efficiency to diagnose heart disease [16]. Data mining methods for heart disease diagnosis include the bagging algorithm, neural network, support vector machine, and automatically defined groups [17]. In [18], the study acquired 493 samples from a cerebrovascular disease prevention program, and utilized three classification techniques (the Bayesian classifier, decision tree, and backpropagation neural network) for constructing classification models. In [19], a method is devised for diagnosing coronary artery disease. The method utilized 303 samples by adapting the feature creation technique. In [20], a methodology is devised for automatically detecting the efficiency of features to reveal heart rate signals. In [21], a hybrid algorithm is devised with K-Nearest Neighbour (KNN), and the genetic algorithm for effectual classification. The method utilized a genetic search as a decency measure for ranking attributes. Then, the classification algorithm was devised on evaluated attributes for heart disease diagnosis. The extraction of valuable information from huge data is a time-consuming task [22]. The size of the medical dataset is increasing in a rapid manner and advanced techniques of data mining help physicians make effective decisions. However, the issues of heart disease data involve feature selection, in which the imbalance of samples and the lack of magnitude of features are just some of the issues [23]. Although there are methods for heart disease detection with real-world medical data, these methods are devised to improve accuracy and time for computation in disease detection [24]. In [25], a hybrid model with the cuckoo search (CS)—and a rough set—is adapted for diagnosing heart disease. The drawback is that a rough set produces an unnecessary number of rules. To solve these challenges in heart disease diagnoses; a novel method, named the Taylor-based bird swarm algorithm–deep belief network (Taylor-BSA–DBN), is proposed for medical data classification.

The purpose of the research is to present a heart disease diagnosis strategy, for which the proposed Taylor-BSA–DBN is employed. The major contribution of the research is the detection of heart disease using selected features. Here, the feature selection is performed using sparse FCM for selecting imperative features. In addition, DBN is employed for detecting heart disease data using the features. Here, the DBN is trained by the proposed Taylor-BSA, in such a way that the model parameters are learned optimally. The proposed Taylor-BSA is developed through the inheritance of the high global convergence property of BSA in the Taylor series. Hence, the proposed Taylor-BSA–DBN renders effective accuracy, sensitivity, and specificity while facilitating heart disease diagnosis.

The major portion of the paper focuses on:

- Proposed Taylor-BSA–DBN for heart disease diagnosis:Taylor-BSA–DBN(a classifier) is proposed by modifying the training algorithm of the DBN with the Taylor-BSA algorithm, which is newly derived by combining the Taylor series and BSA algorithm, for the optimal tuning of weights and biases. The proposed Taylor-BSA–DBN is adapted for heart disease diagnosis.

Other sections of the paper are arranged as follows: Section 2 elaborates the descriptions of conventional heart disease detection strategies utilized in the literature, as well as challenges faced, which are considered as the inspiration for developing the proposed technique. The proposed method for heart disease diagnosis using modified DBN is portrayed in Section 3. The outcomes of the proposed strategy with other methods are depicted in Section 4; Section 5 presents the conclusion.

## 2. Motivations

This section illustrates eight strategies employed for heart disease diagnosis, along with its challenges.

*Literature Survey*

Reddy, G.T. et al. [22] devised an adaptive genetic algorithm with fuzzy logic (AGAFL) model for predicting heart disease, which assists clinicians in treating heart disease at earlier phases. The model comprises rough sets with a fuzzy rule-based classification module and heart disease feature selection module. The obtained rules from fuzzy classifiers are optimized by adapting an adaptive genetic algorithm. Initially, the significant features that affect heart disease are chosen using the rough set theory. Then, the second step predicts heart disease with the AGAFL classifier. The method is effective in handling noisy data and works effectively with large attributes. Nourmohammadi-Khiarak et al. [23] devised a method for selecting features and reducing the number of features.

Here, the imperialist competitive algorithm was devised to choose important features from heart disease. This algorithm offers an optimal response in selecting features. Moreover, the k-nearest neighbor algorithm was utilized for classification. The method showed that the accuracy of feature selection was enhanced. However, the method failed to utilize incomplete or missed data. Magesh, G. and Swarnalatha, P. [26] devised a model using Cleveland heart samples for heart disease diagnosis. The method employed cluster-based Decision Tree learning (CDTL) for diagnosing heart disease. Here, the original set was partitioned using target label distribution. From elevated distribution samples, the possible class was derived. For each class set, the features were detected using entropy for diagnosing heart disease. Thiyagaraj, M. and Suseendran, G. [27] developed Particle Swarm Optimization and Rough Sets with Transductive Support Vector Machines (PSO and RS with TSVM) for heart disease diagnosis. This method improved data integrity to minimize data redundancy. The normalization of data was carried out using Zero-Score (Z-Score). Then, the PSO was employed for selecting the optimal subset of attributes, reduce computational overhead, and enhance prediction performance. The Radial Basis Function-Transductive Support Vector Machines (RBF-TSVM) classifier was employed for heart disease prediction. Abdel-Basset, M. et al. [28] devised a model using Internet of Things (IoT) for determining and monitoring heart patients. The goal of the healthcare model was to obtain improved precision for diagnosis. The neutrosophic multi-criteria decision-making (NMCDM) technique was employed for aiding patients (i.e., for observing patients suffering from heart failure). Moreover, the model provided an accurate solution that decreases the rate of death and the cost of treatment. Nilashi, M. et al. [24] devised a predictive technique for heart disease diagnosis with machine learning models. Here, the method adapted unsupervised and supervised learning for diagnosing heart disease. In addition, the method employed Self-Organizing Map, Fuzzy Support Vector Machine (FSVM), and Principal Component Analysis (PCA) for missing value assertion. Moreover, incremental PCA and FSVM are devised for incremental learning of data to minimize the time taken for computation in disease prediction. Shah, S.M.S. et al. [29] devised an automatic diagnostic technique for diagnosing heart disease. The method evaluated the pertinent feature subset by employing the benefits of feature selection and extraction models. For accomplishing the feature selection, two algorithms: accuracy based feature selection algorithm (AFSA) and Mean Fisher based feature selection algorithm (MFFSA) for heart disease diagnosis. However, the method failed to employ PCA for dimension reduction. Acharjya, D.P. [25] devised a hybrid method for diagnosing heart disease. The method combined the cuckoo search (CS) and rough set to infer decision rules. Moreover, the CS was employed for discovering essential features. In addition, three major features were evaluated with rough set rules. The method improved feasibility, but failed to induce an intuitionistic fuzzy rough set and CS for diagnosing heart disease.

## 3. Proposed Taylor-BSA–DBN for Medical Data Classification

The accessibility of a large amount of medical data led to the requirement of strong data analysis tools for extracting valuable knowledge. Researchers are adapting data mining and statistical tools for improving the analysis of data on huge datasets. The diagnosis of a disease is the foremost application in which data mining tools are offering triumphant results. Medical data tend to be rich in information, but poor in knowledge. Thus, there is a deficiency of effectual analysis tools for discovering hidden relation and trends from medical data generated from clinical records. The processing of medical data brings a manifestation if it has some powerful methods. Thus, the proposed Taylor-BSA–DBN is devised to process medical data for attaining effective heart disease diagnosis. Figure 1 portrays the schematic view of the proposed Taylor-BSA–DBN for heart disease diagnosis. The complete process of the proposed model is pre-processing feature selection, and detection. At first, the medical data is fed as an input to the pre-processing phase, wherein log transformation is applied to pre-process the data. Log transformation is applied for minimizing skew, and to normalize the data. Once the pre-processed data are obtained, then it is further subjected to the feature selection phase. In the feature selection phase, the imperative features are selected with Sparse FCM. After obtaining imperative features, the detection is performed with DBN, wherein the training of DBN is carried out using Taylor-BSA. The proposed Taylor-BSA is devised by combining the Taylor series and BSA. The output produced from the classifier is the classified medical data.

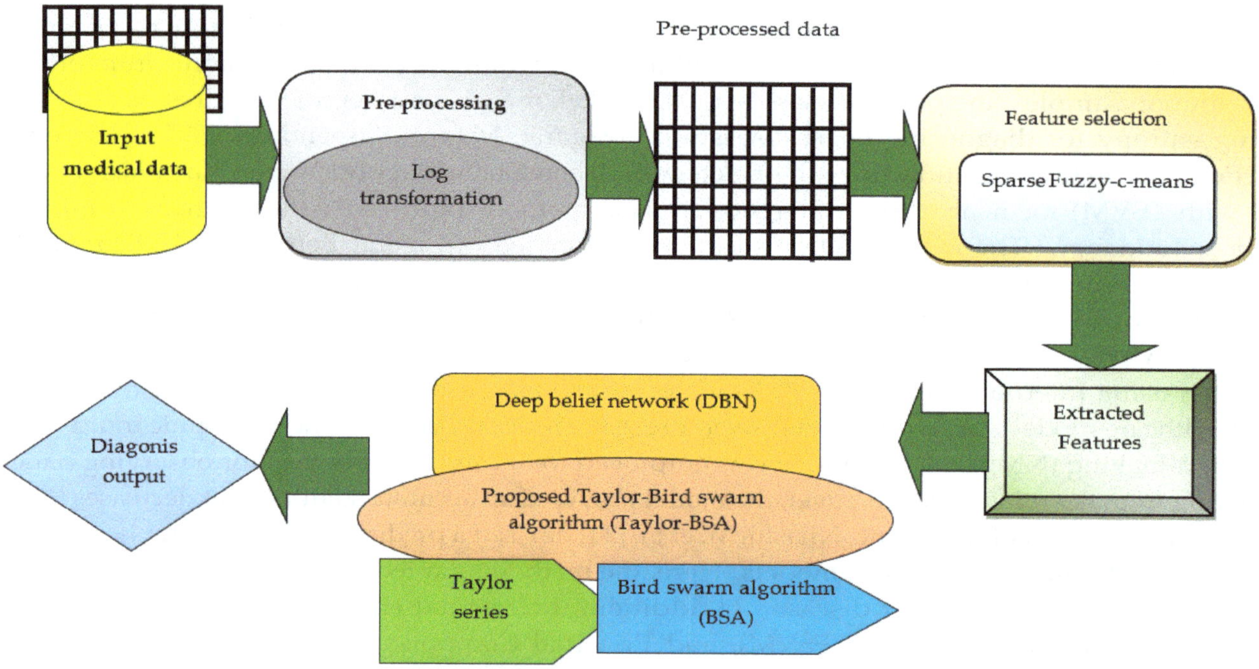


**Figure 1.** Schematic view of the proposed Taylor-based bird swarm algorithm (Taylor-BSA)–deep belief network (DBN) for heart disease diagnosis.

Consider an input medical data be given as $A$, with various attributes, and is expressed as

$$A = \{A_{G,H}\}; (1 \leq G \leq B); (1 \leq H \leq C) \tag{1}$$

where $A_{G,H}$ denotes $H^{th}$ attribute in $G^{th}$ data, $B$ specifies a total number of data, and $C$ specifies total attributes in each data. The dimension of the database is represented as $[B \times C]$.

### *3.1. Pre-Processing*

The importance of pre-processing is to facilitate smoother processing of the input data. Additionally, the pre-processing is carried out for eliminating the noise and artefacts contained in the data.

In this method, the pre-processing is carried out by using log transformation, in which data are replaced with a log function, wherein the base of the log is set by the analyst (maybe 2, or 10). The process is used to compress the massive data. In addition, the log transformation has extensively adapted the method to solve skewed data and assist data normalization. The log transformation is formulated as,

$$D = \log_{10}(A) \tag{2}$$

The dimension of pre-processed dataset $A$ becomes $[B \times C]$.

### 3.2. *Selection of Features with Sparse FCM Clustering*

The pre-processed data are fed to the feature selection module, considering the Sparse FCM algorithm [30], which is the modification of the standard FCM. The benefit of using Sparse FCM is to provide high dimensional data clustering. The pre-processed data contain different types of attributes, each indicating individual value. In the medical data classification strategy, the sparse FCM is applied for determining the features from the data. The sparse FCM clustering algorithm clusters nodes, to attain communication between nodes through the cluster head, and facilitate effective detection of the attacker node. Generally, in sparse FCM, dimensional reduction is effective, poses the ability to handle disease diagnosis without delay, and is easier with optimization techniques.

### 3.3. *Classification of Medical Data with Proposed Taylor-BSA-Based DBN*

In this section, medical data classification using the proposed Taylor-BSA method is presented, and the classification is progressed using the feature vector.

#### 3.3.1. Proposed Taylor-BSA Algorithm

The proposed Taylor-BSA is the combination of the Taylor series and BSA. The Taylor series [31] explains the functions of complex variables, and it is the expansion of a function into an infinite sum of terms. It not only serves as a powerful tool, but also helps in evaluating integrals and infinite sums. Moreover, the Taylor series is aone-step process, and it can deal with higher-order terms. The Taylor series seems to be advantageous for derivations, and can be used to get theoretical error bounds. Above all, the Taylor series ensures the accuracy of classification. Moreover, it is a simple method to solve complex functions. BSA [32] is duly based on the social behaviors of birds that follow some idealistic rules. BSA is more accurate than other standard optimizations with highly efficient, accurate, and robust performances. In addition, there is a perfect balance between exploration and exploitation in BSA. The DBN has recently become a popular approach in machine learning for its promised advantages, such as fast inference and the ability to encode richer and higher order network structures. DBN is used to extract better feature representations, and several related tasks are solved simultaneously by using shared representations. Moreover, it has the advantages of a multi-layer structure, and pre-training with the fine-tuning learning method. The algorithmic steps of the proposed Taylor-BSA are described below:

Step 1. Initialization: the first step is the initialization of population and other algorithmic parameters, including: $F_{i,j}; (1 \le i \le j)$, where, the population size is denoted as $j$, $h_{\max}$ represent maximal iteration, *prob* indicate the probability of foraging food, and the frequency of flight behavior of birds is expressed as $Ft$.

Step 2. Determination of objective function: the selection of the best position of the bird is termed as a minimization issue. The minimal value of error defines the optimal solution.

Step 3. Position update of the birds: for updating the positions, birds have three phases, which are decided using probability. Whenever the random number $Rand(0, 1) < prob$, then the update is based on foraging behavior, or else the vigilance behavior commences. On the other hand, the swarm splits as scroungers and producers, which is modeled as flight behaviors. Finally, the feasibility of the solutions is verified and the best solution is retrieved.

Step 4. Foraging behavior of birds: the individual bird searches for the food based on its own experience, and the behavior of the swarm, which is given below. The standard equation of the foraging behavior of birds [32] is given by,

$$F_{i,j}^{h+1} = F_{i,j}^{h} - F_{i,j}^{h} Rand(0,1)[Z+T] + Rand(0,1)[P_{i,j}Z + Y_j T] \tag{3}$$

where, $F_{i,j}^{h+1}$ and $F_{i,j}^{h}$ denotes the location of $i^{th}$ bird in $j^{th}$ dimension at $(h+1)$ and $h$, $P_{i,j}$ refers to the previous best position of the $i^{th}$ bird, $Rand(0,1)$ is independent uniformly distributed numbers, $Y_j$ indicates the best previous location shared by the birds swarm, $Z$ denotes the cognitive accelerated coefficients, and $T$ denotes the social accelerated coefficients. Here, $Z$ and $T$ are positive numbers.

According to the Taylor series [31], the update equation is expressed as,

$$\begin{array}{c} F_{i,j}^{h+1} = 0.5F_{i,j}^{h} + 1.3591F_{i,j}^{h-1} - 1.359F_{i,j}^{h-2} + 0.6795F_{i,j}^{h-3} \\ -0.2259F_{i,j}^{h-4} + 0.0555F_{i,j}^{h-5} - 0.0104F_{i,j}^{h-6} + 1.38e^{-3}F_{i,j}^{h-7} - 9.92e^{-5}F_{i,j}^{h-8} \end{array} \tag{4}$$

$$F_{i,j}^{h} = \frac{1}{0.5}\left[\begin{array}{c} F_{i,j}^{h+1} - 1.3591F_{i,j}^{h-1} + 1.359F_{i,j}^{h-2} - 0.6795F_{i,j}^{h-3} + 0.2259F_{i,j}^{h-4} \\ -0.0555F_{I,J}^{h-5} + 0.0104F_{i,j}^{h-6} - 1.38e^{-3}F_{i,j}^{h-7} + 9.92e^{-5}F_{i,j}^{h-8} \end{array}\right] \tag{5}$$

Substituting Equation (5) in Equation (3),

$$F_{i,j}^{h+1} = F_{i,j}^{h} - \left[\begin{array}{c} 2F_{i,j}^{h+1} - 2.7182F_{i,j}^{h-1} + 2.718F_{i,j}^{h-2} - 1.359F_{i,j}^{h-3} \\ -0.4518F_{i,j}^{h-4} - 0.111F_{i,j}^{h-5} + 0.0208F_{i,j}^{h-6} - 0.00276F_{i,j}^{h-7} + 0.0001984F_{i,j}^{h-8} \\ Rand(0,1)[Z+T] + Rand(0,1)\left[P_{i,j}Z + Y_j T\right] \end{array}\right] \tag{6}$$

$$F_{i,j}^{h+1} + 2F_{i,j}^{h+1} = F_{i,j}^{h} + \left[\begin{array}{c} 2.7182F_{i,j}^{h-1} - 2.718F_{i,j}^{h-2} + 1.359F_{i,j}^{h-3} \\ +0.4518F_{i,j}^{h-4} + 0.111F_{i,j}^{h-5} - 0.0208F_{i,j}^{h-6} + 0.00276F_{i,j}^{h-7} - 0.0001984F_{i,j}^{h-8} \\ Rand(0,1)[Z+T] + Rand(0,1)\left[P_{i,j}Z + Y_j T\right] \end{array}\right] \tag{7}$$

$$3F_{i,j}^{h+1} = F_{i,j}^{h} + \left[\begin{array}{c} 2.7182F_{i,j}^{h-1} - 2.718F_{i,j}^{h-2} + 1.359F_{i,j}^{h-3} \\ +0.4518F_{i,j}^{h-4} + 0.111F_{i,j}^{h-5} - 0.0208F_{i,j}^{h-6} + 0.00276F_{i,j}^{h-7} - 0.0001984F_{i,j}^{h-8} \\ Rand(0,1)[Z+T] + Rand(0,1)\left[P_{i,j}Z + Y_j T\right] \end{array}\right] \tag{8}$$

$$F_{i,j}^{h+1} = \frac{1}{3}\left[F_{i,j}^{h} + \left[\begin{array}{c} 2.7182F_{i,j}^{h-1} - 2.718F_{i,j}^{h-2} + 1.359F_{i,j}^{h-3} \\ +0.4518F_{i,j}^{h-4} + 0.111F_{i,j}^{h-5} - 0.0208F_{i,j}^{h-6} + 0.00276F_{i,j}^{h-7} - 0.0001984F_{i,j}^{h-8} \\ Rand(0,1)[Z+T] + Rand(0,1)[P_{i,j}Z + Y_j T] \end{array}\right]\right] \tag{9}$$

Step 5. Vigilance Behavior of Birds: the birds move towards the center, during which, the birds compete with each other; the vigilance behavior of birds is modeled as,

$$F_{i,j}^{h+1} = F_{i,j}^{h} + V_1\left(\mu_j - F_{i,j}^{h}\right) \times Rand(0,1) + V_2\left[U_{oj} - F_{i,j}^{h}\right] \times Rand(-1,1) \tag{10}$$

$$V_1 = w_1 \times \exp\left(\frac{-RQ(U)_i}{\sum RQ + \psi} \times v\right) \tag{11}$$

$$V_2 = w_2 \times \exp\left[\left(\frac{RQ(U)_i - RQ(U)_T}{|RQ(U)_T - RQ(U)_i| + \psi}\right)\frac{v \times RQ(U)_T}{\sum RQ + \psi}\right] \tag{12}$$

where, $V$ represents the number of birds, $w_1$ and $w_2$ are the positive constants lying in the range of $[0,2]$, $RQ(U)_i$ denotes the optimal fitness value of $i^{th}$ bird, and $\sum RQ$ corresponds to the addition of the best fitness values of the swarm. $\psi$ be the constant that keeps optimization away from zero-division error. $T$ signifies the positive integer.

Step 6. Flight Behavior: this behavior is of the birds' progress, when the birds fly to another site in case of any threatening events and foraging mechanisms. When the birds reach a new site, they search for food. Some birds in the group act as producers and others as scroungers. The behavior is modeled as,

$$F_{i,j}^{h+1} = F_{i,j}^{h} + Rand\ r(0,1) \times F_{i,j}^{h} \tag{13}$$

$$F_{i,j}^{h+1} = F_{i,j}^{h} + \left(F_{\gamma,j}^{h} - F_{i,j}^{h}\right) \times Fl \times Rand(0,1) \tag{14}$$

where, $Random\ (0,1)$ refer to the Gaussian distributed random number with zero-mean and standard deviation.

Step 7. Determination of best solution:the best solution is evaluated based on error function. If the newly computed solution is better than the previous one, then it is updated by the new solution.

Step 8. Terminate: the optimal solutions are derived in an iterative manner until the maximum number of iterations is reached. The pseudo-code of the proposed Taylor-BSA algorithm is illustrated in Algorithm 1.

**Algorithm 1.** Pseudocode for the proposed Taylor-BSA algorithm

```
Input: Bird swarm population W_{k,l}; (1 ≤ k ≤ b)
Output: Best solution

Procedure:
Begin
  Population initiation: F_{i,j}; (1 ≤ i ≤ p)
  Read the parameters: b – population size; h_max
maximal iteration, prob–probability of foraging food, Fl-frequency of flight behavior of birds
  Determine the fitness of the solutions
  While h < h_max
  For k = 1 : b
    If Rand(0,1) < prob
      Foraging behavior using Equation (3)
    Else
      Vigilance behavior using Equation (12)
    End if
  End for
  Else
  Split the swarm as scroungers and producers
    For k = 1 : b
        If k is a producer
          Update using Equation (13)
        Else
          Update using Equation (14)
        End if
        End for
  Check the feasibility of the solutions
  Return the best solution
  h = h + 1
  End while
  Optimal solution is obtained
End
```

### 3.3.2. Architecture of Deep Belief Network

The DBN [33] is a subset of Deep Neural Network (DNN) and comprises different layers of Multilayer Perceptrons (MLPs) and Restricted Boltzmann Machines (RBMs). RBMs comprise of visible and hidden units that are associated with weights. The basic structural design of the DBN is illustrated in Figure 2.

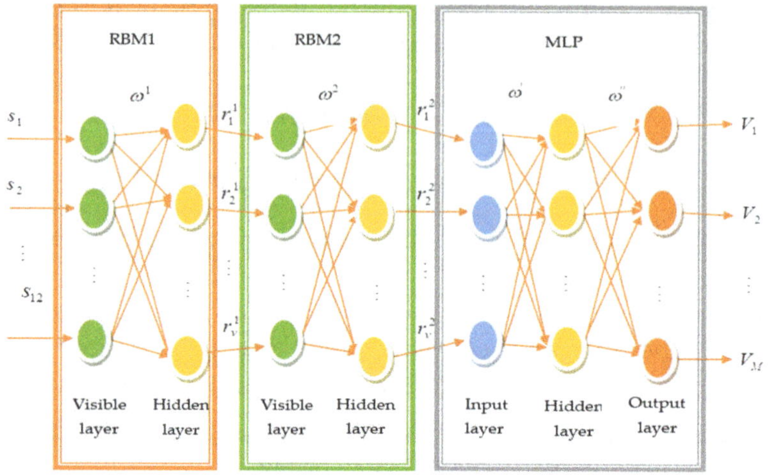


**Figure 2.** Architectural view diagram of DBN classifier.

Training of Deep Belief Network

This section elaborates on the training process of the proposed Taylor-BSA–DBN classifier. A RBM has unsupervised learning based on the gradient descent method, whereas MLP performs a supervised learning method using the standard backpropagation algorithm. Therefore, the training of DBN is based on a gradient descent–backpropagation algorithm. Here, the most appropriate weights are chosen optimally for the update. The training procedure of the proposed DBN classifier is described below,

I. Training of RBM Layers A training sample *N* is given as the input to the first layer of RBM. It computes the probability distribution of the data and encodes it into the weight parameters. The steps involved in the training process of RBM are illustrated below.

  1. The input training sample is read and the weight vector is produced randomly.
  2. The probability function of each hidden neuron in the first RBM is calculated.
  3. The positive gradient is computed using a visible vector and the probability of the hidden layer.
  4. The probability of each visible neuron is obtained by reconstructing the visible layer from the hidden layer.
  5. The probability of reconstruction of hidden neurons is obtained by resampling the hidden states.
  6. The negative gradient is computed.
  7. Weights are updated by subtracting the negative gradient from the positive gradient.
  8. Weights are updated for the next iteration, using the steepest or gradient descent algorithm.
  9. Energy is calculated for a joint configuration of the neurons in the visible and the hidden layers.

II. Training of MLP The training procedure in MLP is based on a backpropagation approach by feeding the training data, which are the hidden output of the second RBM layer through the network. Analyzing the data, the network is adjusted iteratively until the optimal weights are chosen. Moreover, Taylor-BSA is employed to compute the optimal weights, which are determined using the error function. The training procedure is summarized below.

  1. Randomly initialize the weights.

2. Read the input sample from the result of the preceding layer.
3. Obtain the average error, based on the difference between the obtained output and the desired output.
4. Calculate the weight updates in the hidden and the visible layers.
5. Obtain the new weights from the hidden and the visible layers by applying gradient descent.
6. Identify the new weights using the updated equation of Taylor-BSA.
7. Estimate the error function using gradient descent and Taylor-BSA.
8. Choose the minimum error and repeat the steps.

## 4. Results and Discussion

This section elaborates on the assessment of the proposed strategy with classical strategies for medical data classification using accuracy, sensitivity, and specificity. The analysis is done by varying training data. In addition, the effectiveness of the proposed Taylor-BSA–DBN is analyzed.

### 4.1. Experimental Setup

The implementation of the proposed strategy is carried out using Java libraries via Java Archive (JAR) files, utilizing a PC, Windows 10 OS, 2GB RAM, and an Intel i3 core processor. The simulation setup of the proposed system is depicted in Table 1.

**Table 1.** Simulation setup.

| Parameter | Value |
|---|---|
| Number of input layers | 2 |
| Number of hidden layers | 2 |
| Number of output layers | 1 |
| Cluster size | 5 to 9 |
| Number of selected features in Cleveland dataset | 123 |
| Number of selected features in Hungarian dataset | 139 |
| Number of selected features in Switzerland dataset | 139 |
| Learning rate | 0.1 |

### 4.2. Dataset Description

The experimentation is done using Cleveland, Hungarian, and Switzerland datasets taken from healthcare data based on University of California Irvine (UCI) machine learning repository [34], which is commonly used for both detection and classification. The Cleveland database is taken from the Cleveland Clinical Foundation contributed by David W. Aha. The Hungarian dataset is obtained from the Hungarian Institute of Cardiology. The Switzerland dataset is obtained from the University Hospital, Basel, Switzerland. The dataset comprises of 303 number of instances and 75 attributes, ofwhich, 13 attributes are employed for experimentation. Furthermore, the dataset is characterized as multivariate with integer and real attributes. The attributes (features), such asresting blood pressure (trestbps), maximum heart rate achieved (thalach), the slope of the peak exercise ST segment (slope), age (age), sex (sex), fasting blood sugar (fbs), ST depression induced by exercise relative to rest (oldpeak), chest pain (cp), serum cholesterol (chol), exercise-induced angina (exang), resting electrocardiographic results (restecg), number of major vessels (0–3) colored by fluoroscopy (ca), and 3 = normal; 6 = fixed defect; 7 = reversible defect (thal).

### 4.3. Evaluation Metrics

The performance of the proposed Taylor-BSA–DBN is employed for analyzing the methods, including accuracy, sensitivity, and specificity.

4.3.1. Accuracy

The accuracy is described as the degree of closeness of an estimated value with respect to its original value in optimal medical data classification, and it is represented as,

$$Accuracy = \frac{T^p + T^n}{T^p + T^n + F^p + F^n} \tag{15}$$

where, $T^p$ represent true positive, $F^p$ indicate false positive, $T^n$ indicate true negative, and $F^n$ represents false negative, respectively.

4.3.2. Sensitivity

This measure is described as the ratio of positives that are correctly identified by the classifier, and it is represented as,

$$Sensitivity = \frac{T^p}{T^p + F^n} \tag{16}$$

4.3.3. Specificity

This measure is defined as the ratio of negatives that are correctly identified by the classifier, and is formulated as.

$$Specificity = \frac{T^n}{T^n + F^p} \tag{17}$$

*4.4. Comparative Methods*

The methods employed for the analysis include the Support Vector Machine (SVM) [35], Naive Bayes (NB) [36], DBN [33], and the proposed Taylor-BSA–DBN.

*4.5. Comparative Analysis*

The analysis of the proposed Taylor-BSA–DBN, with the conventional methods, with accuracy, sensitivity, and specificity parameters, is evaluated. The analysis is performed by varying the training data using Cleveland, Hungarian, and Switzerland databases.

4.5.1. Analysis with Cluster Size = 5

The analysis of methods, considering cluster size = 5, using Cleveland, Hungarian, and Switzerland databases are specified below:

Analysis Considering Cleveland Database

Table 2 elaborates the analysis of methods using the Cleveland database, considering training data with accuracy, sensitivity, and specificity parameters. The maximum accuracy, sensitivity, and specificity is considered as the best performance. Here, the proposed system offers better performances than the existing methods, such as SVM, NB, and DBN, respectively.

**Table 2.** Analysis of methods with cluster size = 5 using the Cleveland database. Abbreviations: SVM, Support Vector Machine; NB, Naive Bayes; DBN, deep belief network.

| Methods / Training Percentage | SVM | NB | DBN | Proposed Taylor-BSA–DBN |
|---|---|---|---|---|
| | | Accuracy | | |
| 50 | 0.7590 | 0.7603 | 0.7874 | 0.8625 |
| 60 | 0.7143 | 0.7682 | 0.7851 | 0.8632 |
| 70 | 0.7460 | 0.7627 | 0.8122 | 0.8531 |
| 80 | 0.7236 | 0.7619 | 0.7869 | 0.8644 |
| 90 | 0.7538 | 0.7647 | 0.7742 | 0.8710 |
| | | Sensitivity | | |
| 50 | 0.7535 | 0.7613 | 0.7908 | 0.8693 |
| 60 | 0.7120 | 0.7611 | 0.7886 | 0.8699 |
| 70 | 0.7473 | 0.7558 | 0.8172 | 0.8602 |
| 80 | 0.7167 | 0.7656 | 0.7903 | 0.8710 |
| 90 | 0.7576 | 0.7667 | 0.7714 | 0.8788 |
| | | Specificity | | |
| 50 | 0.7566 | 0.7667 | 0.7838 | 0.8551 |
| 60 | 0.7165 | 0.7750 | 0.7815 | 0.8559 |
| 70 | 0.7447 | 0.7692 | 0.8068 | 0.8452 |
| 80 | 0.7302 | 0.7581 | 0.7833 | 0.8571 |
| 90 | 0.7500 | 0.7576 | 0.7813 | 0.8621 |

Analysis Considering Hungarian Database

Table 3 elaborates the analysis of methods using the Hungarian database, considering training data with accuracy, sensitivity, and specificity parameters. The proposed system offers the best performance when considering 90% of training data.

**Table 3.** Analysis of methods with cluster size = 5 using the Hungarian database.

| Methods / Training Percentage | SVM | NB | DBN | Proposed Taylor-BSA–DBN |
|---|---|---|---|---|
| | | Accuracy | | |
| 50 | 0.7810 | 0.8043 | 0.8428 | 0.9200 |
| 60 | 0.7906 | 0.7976 | 0.8595 | 0.8907 |
| 70 | 0.7674 | 0.8143 | 0.8182 | 0.8551 |
| 80 | 0.7576 | 0.8095 | 0.8710 | 0.8710 |
| 90 | 0.6957 | 0.7500 | 0.7647 | 0.9130 |
| | | Sensitivity | | |
| 50 | 0.8160 | 0.8456 | 0.8776 | 0.9388 |
| 60 | 0.8300 | 0.8347 | 0.8908 | 0.9160 |
| 70 | 0.8052 | 0.8539 | 0.8571 | 0.8876 |
| 80 | 0.8065 | 0.8400 | 0.8795 | 0.9000 |
| 90 | 0.7500 | 0.8000 | 0.8125 | 0.9333 |
| | | Specificity | | |
| 50 | 0.7294 | 0.7326 | 0.7805 | 0.8846 |
| 60 | 0.7143 | 0.7500 | 0.8030 | 0.8438 |
| 70 | 0.7115 | 0.7451 | 0.7500 | 0.7959 |
| 80 | 0.6757 | 0.7647 | 0.8182 | 0.8182 |
| 90 | 0.6111 | 0.6667 | 0.6842 | 0.8750 |

Analysis Considering Switzerland Database

Table 4 elaborates the analysis of methods using the Switzerland database considering training data with accuracy, sensitivity, and specificity parameters. The better performances of the proposed system, with values, are 0.8462, 0.8571, and 0.8333 for performance metrics, such as accuracy, sensitivity, and specificity.

**Table 4.** Analysis of methods with cluster size = 5 using the Switzerland database.

| Methods / Training Percentage | SVM | NB | DBN | Proposed Taylor-BSA–DBN |
|---|---|---|---|---|
| | | Accuracy | | |
| 50 | 0.7619 | 0.7710 | 0.7895 | 0.8644 |
| 60 | 0.7009 | 0.7374 | 0.7800 | 0.8557 |
| 70 | 0.7073 | 0.7568 | 0.7895 | 0.8904 |
| 80 | 0.7551 | 0.7647 | 0.7778 | 0.8400 |
| 90 | 0.6774 | 0.7037 | 0.7143 | 0.8462 |
| | | Sensitivity | | |
| 50 | 0.7656 | 0.7742 | 0.7818 | 0.8710 |
| 60 | 0.6981 | 0.7292 | 0.7843 | 0.8627 |
| 70 | 0.7073 | 0.7500 | 0.7948 | 0.8974 |
| 80 | 0.7500 | 0.7692 | 0.7857 | 0.8462 |
| 90 | 0.6875 | 0.6923 | 0.7143 | 0.8571 |
| | | Specificity | | |
| 50 | 0.7581 | 0.7667 | 0.7966 | 0.8571 |
| 60 | 0.7037 | 0.7451 | 0.7755 | 0.8478 |
| 70 | 0.7073 | 0.7632 | 0.7838 | 0.8823 |
| 80 | 0.7600 | 0.7600 | 0.7692 | 0.8333 |
| 90 | 0.6667 | 0.7143 | 0.7143 | 0.8333 |

4.5.2. Analysis with Cluster Size = 9

The analysis of methods considering cluster size = 9, using Cleveland, Hungarian, and Switzerland databases are specified below:

Analysis Considering Cleveland Database

Table 5 depicts the analysis of methods using the Cleveland database, considering training data with accuracy, sensitivity, and specificity parameters. The maximum accuracy, sensitivity, and specificity are considered as the best performances. Here, the proposed system offers better performance than the existing methods, such as SVM, NB, and DBN, respectively.

Analysis Considering Hungarian Database

Table 6 shows the analysis of methods using the Hungarian database, considering training data with accuracy, sensitivity, and specificity parameters. The proposed system offers the best performance when considering 90% of training data.

**Table 5.** Analysis of methods with cluster size = 9 using the Cleveland database.

| Methods / Training Percentage | SVM | NB | DBN | Proposed Taylor-BSA–DBN |
|---|---|---|---|---|
| | | Accuracy | | |
| 50 | 0.7590 | 0.7603 | 0.7993 | 0.8690 |
| 60 | 0.7166 | 0.7430 | 0.7851 | 0.8632 |
| 70 | 0.7354 | 0.7363 | 0.8123 | 0.8857 |
| 80 | 0.7419 | 0.7607 | 0.7619 | 0.8475 |
| 90 | 0.7460 | 0.7910 | 0.8710 | 0.9016 |
| | | Sensitivity | | |
| 50 | 0.7535 | 0.7613 | 0.8039 | 0.8758 |
| 60 | 0.7107 | 0.7440 | 0.7886 | 0.8699 |
| 70 | 0.7303 | 0.7368 | 0.8172 | 0.8925 |
| 80 | 0.7419 | 0.7544 | 0.7656 | 0.8548 |
| 90 | 0.7419 | 0.8000 | 0.8788 | 0.9091 |
| | | Specificity | | |
| 50 | 0.7566 | 0.7667 | 0.7945 | 0.8613 |
| 60 | 0.7222 | 0.7419 | 0.7815 | 0.8559 |
| 70 | 0.7340 | 0.7419 | 0.8068 | 0.8780 |
| 80 | 0.7419 | 0.7581 | 0.7667 | 0.8393 |
| 90 | 0.7500 | 0.7813 | 0.8621 | 0.8929 |

**Table 6.** Analysis of methods with cluster size = 9 using the Hungarian database.

| Methods / Training Percentage | SVM | NB | DBN | Proposed Taylor-BSA–DBN |
|---|---|---|---|---|
| | | Accuracy | | |
| 50 | 0.7500 | 0.7957 | 0.8515 | 0.9200 |
| 60 | 0.7513 | 0.7870 | 0.8075 | 0.8907 |
| 70 | 0.7777 | 0.8273 | 0.8500 | 0.9118 |
| 80 | 0.7755 | 0.8298 | 0.8974 | 0.9341 |
| 90 | 0.7674 | 0.8000 | 0.8298 | 0.8696 |
| | | Sensitivity | | |
| 50 | 0.7907 | 0.8389 | 0.8844 | 0.9388 |
| 60 | 0.8017 | 0.8218 | 0.8487 | 0.9160 |
| 70 | 0.8242 | 0.8652 | 0.8732 | 0.9326 |
| 80 | 0.8226 | 0.8667 | 0.9130 | 0.9500 |
| 90 | 0.8077 | 0.8438 | 0.8667 | 0.9000 |
| | | Specificity | | |
| 50 | 0.6897 | 0.7209 | 0.7927 | 0.8846 |
| 60 | 0.6667 | 0.7353 | 0.7353 | 0.8438 |
| 70 | 0.6981 | 0.7600 | 0.8163 | 0.8723 |
| 80 | 0.6944 | 0.7647 | 0.8750 | 0.9032 |
| 90 | 0.7059 | 0.7222 | 0.7647 | 0.8125 |

Analysis Considering Switzerland Database

Table 7 depicts the analysis of methods using the Switzerland database considering training data with accuracy, sensitivity, and specificity parameters. The better performance of the proposed system with values is 0.7778, 0.7857, and 0.7692, for the performance metrics, such as accuracy, sensitivity, and specificity.

**Table 7.** Analysis of methods with cluster size = 9 using the Switzerland database.

| Methods / Training Percentage | SVM | NB | DBN | Proposed Taylor-BSA–DBN |
|---|---|---|---|---|
| | | Accuracy | | |
| 50 | 0.7460 | 0.7479 | 0.8017 | 0.8644 |
| 60 | 0.7170 | 0.7624 | 0.7684 | 0.8947 |
| 70 | 0.7368 | 0.7500 | 0.7662 | 0.8904 |
| 80 | 0.6786 | 0.7551 | 0.8200 | 0.8400 |
| 90 | 0.7333 | 0.7600 | 0.7679 | 0.7778 |
| | | Sensitivity | | |
| 50 | 0.7414 | 0.7500 | 0.8065 | 0.8710 |
| 60 | 0.7170 | 0.7609 | 0.7647 | 0.9020 |
| 70 | 0.7297 | 0.7561 | 0.7692 | 0.8974 |
| 80 | 0.6786 | 0.7500 | 0.8300 | 0.8462 |
| 90 | 0.7300 | 0.7500 | 0.7667 | 0.7857 |
| | | Specificity | | |
| 50 | 0.7419 | 0.7541 | 0.7966 | 0.8571 |
| 60 | 0.7170 | 0.7600 | 0.7755 | 0.8864 |
| 70 | 0.7436 | 0.7436 | 0.7632 | 0.8824 |
| 80 | 0.6786 | 0.7600 | 0.8200 | 0.8333 |
| 90 | 0.7143 | 0.7300 | 0.7556 | 0.7692 |

#### 4.5.3. Analysis Based on Receiver Operating Characteristic (ROC) Curve

Table 8 depicts the comparative analysis based on ROC curve, using Cleveland, Hungarian, and Switzerland databases. In the Cleveland dataset, when the false positive rate (FPR) is 5, the corresponding true positive rate (TPR) of the methods, such as SVM, NB, DBN, and the proposed Taylor-BSA–DBN is 0.8857, 0.9119, 0.9535, and 0.9684, respectively. By considering the Hungarian dataset, when the FPR is 4, the corresponding TPR of the proposed method is a maximum of 0.9348. For the same FPR, the TPR of the methods, such as SVM, NB, and DBN is 0.9030, 0.9130, and 0.9233, respectively. By considering the Switzerland dataset, when the FPR is 6, the TPR of the methods, such as SVM, NB, DBN, and the proposed Taylor-BSA–DBN is 0.9105, 0.9443, 0.9569, and 0.9794, respectively.

#### 4.5.4. Analysis Based on k-Fold

Table 9 depicts the comparative analysis based on k-fold using the Cleveland, Hungarian, and Switzerland databases, for cluster size = 5. The Hungarian datasets offer the maximum accuracy of 0.9021, when k-fold = 8. By considering k-fold = 7, the specificity offered by the Cleveland datasets for the methods, such as SVM, NB, DBN, and the proposed Taylor-BSA–DBN, is 0.8032, 0.8189, 0.8256, and 0.8321, respectively. The proposed Taylor-BSA–DBN offers maximum accuracy, sensitivity, and specificity, when considering k-fold = 8.

### *4.6. Comparative Discussion*

Table 10 portrays the analysis of methods using accuracy, sensitivity, and specificity parameter with varying training data. The analysis is done with Cleveland, Switzerland, and Hungarian databases. Using cluster size = 5, and considering the Cleveland database, the proposed Taylor-BSA–DBN showed maximal accuracy of 0.871, which is 13.43%, 12.17%, and 11.14%, better than the existing methods, such as SVM, NB, and DBN, respectively. In the existing methods, the DBN offers maximum sensitivity of 0.771, but the proposed method is 12.29% better than the existing DBN. The proposed method has a maximum specificity of 0.862. The percentage of improvement of the proposed method with the existing methods, such as SVM, NB, and DBN, is 12.99%, 12.06%, and 9.40%, respectively. Considering the Hungarian database, the proposed Taylor-BSA–DBN showed maximal accuracy of 0.913, maximal sensitivity of 0.933, and maximal specificity of 0.875. Considering the Switzerland database, the proposed Taylor-BSA–DBN showed maximal accuracy of 0.846, which is 19.98%, 16.78%, and 15.60% better than the existing methods, such as SVM, NB, and DBN, respectively. Similarly, the proposed system has a maximum sensitivity of 0.857. The percentage of improvement of the proposed system sensitivity, with the existing methods, such as SVM, NB, and DBN is 19.72%, 19.25%, and 16.69%, respectively. Likewise, the proposed Taylor-BSA–DBN showed maximal specificity of 0.833.

**Table 8.** Analysis based on ROC.

| Methods | SVM | NB | DBN | Proposed Taylor-BSA–DBN |
|---|---|---|---|---|
| FPR | | | TPR | |
| | | | Cleveland | |
| 1 | 0 | 0 | 0 | 0 |
| 2 | 0.7913 | 0.7949 | 0.8429 | 0.8761 |
| 3 | 0.7961 | 0.8330 | 0.8523 | 0.8798 |
| 4 | 0.8462 | 0.8753 | 0.9149 | 0.9284 |
| 5 | 0.8857 | 0.9119 | 0.9535 | 0.9684 |
| 6 | 0.9153 | 0.9569 | 0.9788 | 0.9847 |
| 7 | 0.9710 | 0.9783 | 0.9895 | 0.9975 |
| 8 | 0.9952 | 0.9989 | 1 | 1 |
| 9 | 1 | 1 | 1 | 1 |
| 10 | 1 | 1 | 1 | 1 |
| | | | Hungarian | |
| 1 | 0 | 0 | 0 | 0 |
| 2 | 0.8233 | 0.8410 | 0.8553 | 0.8941 |
| 3 | 0.8286 | 0.8647 | 0.8734 | 0.8953 |
| 4 | 0.9030 | 0.9130 | 0.9233 | 0.9348 |
| 5 | 0.9246 | 0.9417 | 0.9596 | 0.9789 |
| 6 | 0.9521 | 0.9697 | 0.9803 | 0.9999 |
| 7 | 0.9793 | 0.9800 | 0.9946 | 1 |
| 8 | 0.9981 | 0.9985 | 1 | 1 |
| 9 | 1 | 1 | 1 | 1 |
| 10 | 1 | 1 | 1 | 1 |
| | | | Switzerland | |
| 1 | 0 | 0 | 0 | 0 |
| 2 | 0.7593 | 0.7682 | 0.8024 | 0.8258 |
| 3 | 0.7620 | 0.7923 | 0.8399 | 0.8682 |
| 4 | 0.8452 | 0.8735 | 0.8781 | 0.9101 |
| 5 | 0.8725 | 0.9184 | 0.9194 | 0.9564 |
| 6 | 0.9105 | 0.9443 | 0.9569 | 0.9794 |
| 7 | 0.9701 | 0.9722 | 0.9865 | 0.9924 |
| 8 | 0.9946 | 0.9953 | 0.9994 | 1 |
| 9 | 1 | 1 | 1 | 1 |
| 10 | 1 | 1 | 1 | 1 |

**Table 9.** Analysis based on k-fold.

| Metrics | Methods / k-Fold | SVM | NB | DBN | Proposed Taylor-BSA–DBN |
|---|---|---|---|---|---|
| | | | Cleveland | | |
| Accuracy | 5 | 0.7021 | 0.7088 | 0.7126 | 0.7239 |
| | 6 | 0.7122 | 0.7189 | 0.7245 | 0.7365 |
| | 7 | 0.7345 | 0.7543 | 0.7634 | 0.7843 |
| | 8 | 0.7528 | 0.7843 | 0.7965 | 0.8132 |
| Sensitivity | 5 | 0.7567 | 0.7678 | 0.7898 | 0.7956 |
| | 6 | 0.7834 | 0.8045 | 0.8156 | 0.8232 |
| | 7 | 0.8032 | 0.8189 | 0.8256 | 0.8321 |
| | 8 | 0.8145 | 0.8229 | 0.8365 | 0.8448 |
| Specificity | 5 | 0.7586 | 0.7656 | 0.7699 | 0.7865 |
| | 6 | 0.7854 | 0.7745 | 0.7965 | 0.8043 |
| | 7 | 0.7940 | 0.8088 | 0.8124 | 0.8227 |
| | 8 | 0.8021 | 0.8178 | 0.8249 | 0.8339 |
| | | | Hungarian | | |
| Accuracy | 5 | 0.7960 | 0.8758 | 0.8791 | 0.8822 |
| | 6 | 0.8071 | 0.8413 | 0.8838 | 0.8854 |
| | 7 | 0.7985 | 0.8030 | 0.8324 | 0.8917 |
| | 8 | 0.7982 | 0.8626 | 0.8948 | 0.9021 |
| Sensitivity | 5 | 0.7959 | 0.8027 | 0.8197 | 0.8231 |
| | 6 | 0.7857 | 0.7891 | 0.7925 | 0.8367 |
| | 7 | 0.7891 | 0.7925 | 0.7959 | 0.8393 |
| | 8 | 0.7857 | 0.7925 | 0.8061 | 0.8458 |
| Specificity | 5 | 0.7494 | 0.7513 | 0.7645 | 0.7656 |
| | 6 | 0.7146 | 0.7343 | 0.7645 | 0.7760 |
| | 7 | 0.7433 | 0.7535 | 0.7645 | 0.7719 |
| | 8 | 0.7530 | 0.7645 | 0.7697 | 0.7873 |
| | | | Switzerland | | |
| Accuracy | 5 | 0.7528 | 0.7789 | 0.7799 | 0.7896 |
| | 6 | 0.7658 | 0.7828 | 0.7925 | 0.8012 |
| | 7 | 0.7712 | 0.7958 | 0.8028 | 0.8156 |
| | 8 | 0.7828 | 0.8128 | 0.8159 | 0.8259 |
| Sensitivity | 5 | 0.7428 | 0.7689 | 0.7847 | 0.7956 |
| | 6 | 0.7625 | 0.7758 | 0.7858 | 0.8028 |
| | 7 | 0.7748 | 0.7896 | 0.7952 | 0.8125 |
| | 8 | 0.7828 | 0.7986 | 0.8078 | 0.8225 |
| Specificity | 5 | 0.7658 | 0.7589 | 0.7750 | 0.7896 |
| | 6 | 0.7758 | 0.7832 | 0.7962 | 0.8020 |
| | 7 | 0.7841 | 0.7911 | 0.8025 | 0.8196 |
| | 8 | 0.7958 | 0.8002 | 0.8178 | 0.8219 |

**Table 10.** Comparative analysis.

| Cluster Size | Database | Metrics | SVM | NB | DBN | Proposed Taylor-BSA–DBN |
|---|---|---|---|---|---|---|
| Cluster size = 5 | Cleveland | Accuracy | 0.754 | 0.765 | 0.774 | 0.871 |
| | | Sensitivity | 0.758 | 0.767 | 0.771 | 0.879 |
| | | Specificity | 0.750 | 0.758 | 0.781 | 0.862 |
| | Hungarian | Accuracy | 0.696 | 0.750 | 0.765 | 0.913 |
| | | Sensitivity | 0.750 | 0.800 | 0.813 | 0.933 |
| | | Specificity | 0.611 | 0.667 | 0.684 | 0.875 |
| | Switzerland | Accuracy | 0.677 | 0.704 | 0.714 | 0.846 |
| | | Sensitivity | 0.688 | 0.692 | 0.714 | 0.857 |
| | | Specificity | 0.667 | 0.714 | 0.714 | 0.833 |
| Cluster size = 9 | Cleveland | Accuracy | 0.776 | 0.830 | 0.897 | 0.934 |
| | | Sensitivity | 0.823 | 0.867 | 0.913 | 0.950 |
| | | Specificity | 0.694 | 0.765 | 0.875 | 0.903 |
| | Hungarian | Accuracy | 0.746 | 0.791 | 0.871 | 0.902 |
| | | Sensitivity | 0.742 | 0.800 | 0.879 | 0.909 |
| | | Specificity | 0.750 | 0.781 | 0.862 | 0.893 |
| | Switzerland | Accuracy | 0.679 | 0.755 | 0.820 | 0.840 |
| | | Sensitivity | 0.679 | 0.750 | 0.830 | 0.846 |
| | | Specificity | 0.679 | 0.760 | 0.820 | 0.833 |

Using cluster size = 9, and considering the Cleveland database, the proposed Taylor-BSA–DBN showed maximal accuracy of 0.934, which is 16.92%, 11.13%, and 3.96%, better than the existing methods, such as SVM, NB, and DBN, respectively. In the existing methods, the DBN offers maximum sensitivity of 0.913, but the proposed method is 3.89% better than the existing DBN. The proposed method has a maximum specificity of 0.903. The percentage of improvement of the proposed method with the existing methods, such as SVM, NB, and DBN, is 23.15%, 15.28%, and 3.10%, respectively. Considering the Hungarian database, the proposed Taylor-BSA–DBN showed maximal accuracy of 0.902, maximal sensitivity of 0.909, and maximal specificity of 0.893. Considering the Switzerland database, the proposed Taylor-BSA–DBN showed maximal accuracy of 0.840, which is 19.17%, 10.12%, and 2.38%, better than the existing methods, such as SVM, NB, and DBN, respectively. Similarly, the proposed system has a maximum sensitivity of 0.846. The percentage of improvement of the proposed system sensitivity with the existing methods, such as SVM, NB, and DBN is 19.74%, 11.35%, and 1.89%, respectively. Likewise, the proposed Taylor-BSA–DBN showed maximal specificity of 0.833.

Table 11 shows the computational time of the proposed system and the existing methods, such as SVM, NB, and DBN, in which the proposed Taylor-BSA–DBN has a minimum computation time of 6.31 sec.

**Table 11.** Computational Time.

| Methods | SVM | NB | DBN | Proposed Taylor-BSA–DBN |
|---|---|---|---|---|
| Time (Sec) | 10.08 | 8.79 | 7.56 | 6.31 |

Table 12 shows the statistical analysis of the proposed work and the existing methods based on mean and variance.

**Table 12.** Statistical Analysis.

| Dataset | Methods | Accuracy | Mean | Variance | Sensitivity | Mean | Variance | Specificity | Mean | Variance |
|---|---|---|---|---|---|---|---|---|---|---|
| | | | | Cluster size = 5 | | | | | | |
| Cleveland | SVM | 0.754 | 0.752 | 0.002 | 0.758 | 0.754 | 0.004 | 0.750 | 0.748 | 0.002 |
| | NB | 0.765 | 0.761 | 0.004 | 0.767 | 0.765 | 0.002 | 0.758 | 0.754 | 0.004 |
| | DBN | 0.774 | 0.771 | 0.003 | 0.771 | 0.768 | 0.003 | 0.781 | 0.779 | 0.002 |
| | Proposed Method | 0.871 | 0.869 | 0.002 | 0.879 | 0.878 | 0.001 | 0.862 | 0.860 | 0.002 |
| Hungarian | SVM | 0.696 | 0.693 | 0.003 | 0.750 | 0.748 | 0.002 | 0.611 | 0.608 | 0.003 |
| | NB | 0.750 | 0.746 | 0.004 | 0.800 | 0.799 | 0.001 | 0.667 | 0.665 | 0.002 |
| | DBN | 0.765 | 0.763 | 0.002 | 0.813 | 0.810 | 0.003 | 0.684 | 0.682 | 0.002 |
| | Proposed Method | 0.913 | 0.911 | 0.002 | 0.933 | 0.932 | 0.001 | 0.875 | 0.873 | 0.002 |
| Switzerland | SVM | 0.677 | 0.675 | 0.002 | 0.688 | 0.684 | 0.004 | 0.667 | 0.665 | 0.002 |
| | NB | 0.704 | 0.702 | 0.003 | 0.692 | 0.690 | 0.002 | 0.714 | 0.711 | 0.003 |
| | DBN | 0.714 | 0.711 | 0.003 | 0.714 | 0.713 | 0.001 | 0.714 | 0.712 | 0.002 |
| | Proposed Method | 0.846 | 0.844 | 0.002 | 0.857 | 0.855 | 0.002 | 0.833 | 0.831 | 0.002 |
| | | | | Cluster size = 9 | | | | | | |
| Cleveland | SVM | 0.776 | 0.773 | 0.003 | 0.823 | 0.822 | 0.001 | 0.694 | 0.691 | 0.003 |
| | NB | 0.830 | 0.826 | 0.004 | 0.867 | 0.865 | 0.002 | 0.765 | 0.761 | 0.004 |
| | DBN | 0.897 | 0.895 | 0.002 | 0.913 | 0.911 | 0.002 | 0.875 | 0.873 | 0.002 |
| | Proposed Method | 0.934 | 0.932 | 0.002 | 0.950 | 0.948 | 0.002 | 0.903 | 0.901 | 0.002 |
| Hungarian | SVM | 0.746 | 0.743 | 0.003 | 0.742 | 0.740 | 0.002 | 0.750 | 0.748 | 0.002 |
| | NB | 0.791 | 0.790 | 0.001 | 0.800 | 0.797 | 0.003 | 0.781 | 0.780 | 0.001 |
| | DBN | 0.871 | 0.868 | 0.003 | 0.879 | 0.878 | 0.001 | 0.862 | 0.860 | 0.002 |
| | Proposed Method | 0.902 | 0.900 | 0.002 | 0.909 | 0.907 | 0.002 | 0.893 | 0.891 | 0.002 |
| Switzerland | SVM | 0.679 | 0.677 | 0.002 | 0.679 | 0.675 | 0.004 | 0.679 | 0.677 | 0.002 |
| | NB | 0.755 | 0.752 | 0.003 | 0.750 | 0.748 | 0.002 | 0.760 | 0.758 | 0.002 |
| | DBN | 0.820 | 0.818 | 0.002 | 0.830 | 0.827 | 0.003 | 0.820 | 0.819 | 0.001 |
| | Proposed Method | 0.840 | 0.838 | 0.002 | 0.846 | 0.844 | 0.002 | 0.833 | 0.832 | 0.001 |

## 5. Conclusions

Contemporary medicine depends on a huge amount of information contained in medical databases. The obtainability of large medical data leads to the requirement of effective data analysis tools for extracting constructive knowledge. This paper proposes a novel, fully automated DBN for heart disease diagnosis using medical data. The proposed Taylor-BSA is employed to train DBN. The proposed Taylor-BSA is designed by combining the Taylor series and BSA algorithm, which can be utilized for finding the optimal weights for establishing effective medical data classification. Here, the sparse-FCM is employed for selecting significant features. The incorporation of sparse FCM for the feature selection process provides more benefits for interpreting the models, as this sparse technique provides important features for detection, and can be utilized for handling high dimensional data. The obtained selected features are fed to DBN, which is trained by the proposed Taylor-BSA. The proposed Taylor-BSA is designed by integrating the Taylor series and BSA in order to generate optimal weights for classification. The proposed Taylor-BSA–DBN outperformed other methods with maximal accuracy of 93.4%, maximal sensitivity of 95%, and maximal specificity of 90.3%, respectively. The proposed method does not classify the type of heart disease. In the future, other medical data classification datasets will be employed for computing efficiency of the proposed method. In addition, the proposed system will be further improved to classify heart diseases, such ascongenital heart disease, coronary artery disease, and arrhythmia.

**Author Contributions:** Conceptualization, A.M.A. methodology, A.M.A.; software, A.M.A.; validation, A.M.A.; resources, A.M.A.; data curation, A.M.A.; writing—original draft preparation, A.M.A. and W.M.N.W.Z.;

writing—review and editing, A.M.A. and W.M.N.W.Z.; visualization, A.M.A. and W.M.N.W.Z.; supervision, W.M.N.W.Z. All authors have read and agreed to the published version of the manuscript.

## References


1. Abdel-Basset, M.; Gamal, A.; Manogaran, G.; Long, H.V. A novel group decision making model based on neutrosophic sets for heart disease diagnosis. *Multimed. Tools Appl.* **2019**, *79*, 9977–10002. [CrossRef]
2. Acharjya, D.P. A Hybrid Scheme for Heart Disease Diagnosis Using Rough Set and Cuckoo Search Technique. *J. Med. Syst.* **2020**, *44*, 27.
3. Ahn, G.J.; Hu, H.; Lee, J.; Meng, Y. Representing and Reasoning about Web Access Control Policies. In Proceedings of the IEEE 34th Annual Computer Software and Applications Conference, Seoul, Korea, 19–23 July 2010; pp. 137–146.
4. Alizadehsani, R.; Habibi, J.; Hosseini, M.J.; Mashayekhi, H.; Boghrati, R.; Ghandeharioun, A.; Bahadorian, B.; Sani, Z.A. A data mining approach for diagnosis of coronary artery disease. *Comput. Methods Programs Biomed.* **2013**, *11*, 52–61. [CrossRef] [PubMed]
5. Alzahani, S.M.; Althopity, A.; Alghamdi, A.; Alshehri, B.; Aljuaid, S. An overview of data mining techniques applied for heart disease diagnosis and prediction. *Lect. Notes Inf. Theory* **2014**, *2*, 310–315. [CrossRef]
6. Babič, F.; Olejár, J.; Vantová, Z.; Paralič, J. Predictive and descriptive analysis for heart disease diagnosis. In Proceedings of the Federated Conference on Computer Science and Information Systems (FedCSIS), Prague, Czech Republic, 3–6 September 2017; pp. 155–163.
7. Chang, X.; Wang, Q.; Liu, Y.; Wang, Y. Sparse Regularization in Fuzzy c-Means for High-Dimensional Data Clustering. *IEEE Trans. Cybern.* **2017**, *47*, 2616–2627. [CrossRef]
8. Fatima, M.; Pasha, M. Survey of Machine Learning Algorithms for Disease Diagnostic. *J. Intell. Learn. Syst. Appl.* **2017**, *9*, 1–16. [CrossRef]
9. Ghumbre, S.; Patil, C.; Ghatol, A. Heart disease diagnosis using support vector machine. In Proceedings of the International Conference on Computer Science and Information Technology (ICCSIT), Mumbai, India, 10–12 June 2011.
10. Ghumbre, S.U.; Ghatol, A.A. Heart Disease Diagnosis Using Machine Learning Algorithm. In Proceedings of the International Conference on Information Systems Design and Intelligent Applications, Visakhapatnam, India, 5–7 January 2012; Volume 132, pp. 217–225.
11. Giri, D.; Acharya, U.R. Automated diagnosis of Coronary Artery Disease affected patients usingLDA, PCA, ICA and Discrete WaveletTransform. *Knowl. Based Syst.* **2013**, *37*, 274–282. [CrossRef]
12. Heart Disease Data Set. Available online: http://archive.ics.uci.edu/ml/datasets/Heart+Disease (accessed on 22 April 2020).
13. Jabbar, M.A.; Deekshatulu, B.; LandChandra, P. Classification of Heart Disease Using K- Nearest Neighbor and Genetic Algorithm. *Procedia Technol.* **2013**, *10*, 85–94. [CrossRef]
14. Jabbar, M.A.; Deekshatulu, B.L.; Chandra, P. Heart disease classification using nearest neighbor classifier with feature subset selection. *An. Ser. Inform.* **2013**, *11*, 47–54.
15. Kukar, M.; Kononenko, I.; Groselj, C.; Kralj, K.; Fettich, J. Analysing and Improving the Diagnosis of Ischaemic Heart Disease with Machine Learning. *Artif. Intell. Med.* **1999**, *16*, 25–50. [CrossRef]
16. Magesh, G.; Swarnalatha, P. Optimal feature selection through a cluster-based DT learning (CDTL) in heart disease prediction. *Evol. Intell.* **2020**, 1–11. [CrossRef]
17. Mangai, S.A.; Sankar, B.R.; Alagarsamy, K. Taylor Series Prediction of Time Series Data with Error Propagated by Artificial Neural Network. *Int. J. Comput. Appl.* **2014**, *89*, 41–47.
18. Mannepalli, K.; Sastry, P.N.; Suman, M. A novel Adaptive Fractional Deep Belief Networks for speaker emotion recognition. *Alex. Eng. J.* **2017**, *56*, 485–497. [CrossRef]
19. Medhekar, D.S.; Bote, M.P.; Deshmukh, S.D. Heart disease prediction system using naive Bayes. *Int. J. Enhanc. Res. Sci. Technol. Eng.* **2013**, *2*, 1–5.
20. Meng, X.; Gao, X.Z.; Lu, L.; Liu, Y.; Zhang, H. A new bio-inspired optimisation algorithm: Bird Swarm Algorithm. *J. Exp. Theor. Artif. Intell.* **2016**, *28*, 673–687. [CrossRef]

21. Mohan, S.; Thirumalai, C.; Srivastava, G. Effective Heart Disease Prediction Using Hybrid Machine Learning Techniques. *IEEE Access* **2019**, *7*, 81542–81554. [CrossRef]
22. Nilashi, M.; Ahmadi, H.; Manaf, A.A.; Rashid, T.A.; Samad, S.; Shahmoradi, L.; Aljojo, N.; Akbari, E. Coronary Heart Disease Diagnosis Through Self-Organizing Map and Fuzzy Support Vector Machine with Incremental Updates. *Int. J. Fuzzy Syst.* **2020**, *23*, 1376–1388. [CrossRef]
23. Nourmohammadi-Khiarak, J.; Feizi-Derakhshi, M.R.; Behrouzi, K.; Mazaheri, S.; Zamani-Harghalani, Y.; Tayebi, R.M. New hybrid method for heart disease diagnosis utilizing optimization algorithm in feature selection. *Health Technol.* **2019**, *10*, 667–678. [CrossRef]
24. Oyyathevan, S.; Askarunisa, A. An expert system for heart disease prediction using data mining technique: Neural network. *Int. J. Eng. Res. Sports Sci.* **2014**, *1*, 1–6.
25. Palaniappan, S.; Awang, R. Intelligent heart disease prediction system using data mining techniques. In Proceedings of the International Conference on Computer Systems and Applications, Doha, Qatar, 31 March–4 April 2008.
26. Palaniappan, S.; Awang, R. Intelligent Heart Disease Prediction System Using Data Mining Techniques. *Int. J. Comput. Sci. Netw. Secur.* **2008**, *8*, 343–350.
27. Patil, S.B.; Kumaraswamy, Y.S. Extraction of significant patterns from heart disease warehouses for heart attack prediction. *Int. J. Comput. Sci. Netw. Secur.* **2009**, *9*, 228–235.
28. Pattekari, S.A.; Parveen, A. Prediction system for Heart Disease using Naive Bayes. *Int. J. Adv. Comput. Math. Sci.* **2012**, *3*, 290–294.
29. Ranganatha, S.; Raj, H.P.; Anusha, C.; Vinay, S.K. Medical data mining and analysis for heart disease dataset using classification techniques. In Proceedings of the National Conference on Challenges in Research & Technology in the Coming Decades (CRT), Ujire, India, 27–28 September 2013.
30. Reddy, G.T.; Reddy, M.P.K.; Lakshmanna, K.; Rajput, D.S.; Kaluri, R.; Srivastava, G. Hybrid genetic algorithm and a fuzzy logic classifier for heart disease diagnosis. *Evol. Intell.* **2019**, *13*, 185–196. [CrossRef]
31. Safdar, S.; Zafar, S.; Zafar, N.; Khan, N. Machine learning based decision support systems (DSS) for heart disease diagnosis: A review. *Artif. Intell. Rev.* **2018**, *50*, 597–623. [CrossRef]
32. Shah, S.M.S.; Shah, F.A.; Hussain, S.A.; Batool, S. Support Vector Machines-based Heart Disease Diagnosis using Feature Subset, Wrapping Selection and Extraction Methods. *Comput. Electr. Eng.* **2020**, *84*, 106628. [CrossRef]
33. Shouman, M.; Turner, T.; Stocker, R. Using data mining techniques in heart disease diagnosis and treatment. In Proceedings of the IEEE Japan-Egypt Conference on Electronics, Communications and Computers, Alexandria, Egypt, 6–9 March 2012; pp. 173–177.
34. Subbalakshmi, G. Decision support in heart disease prediction system using naive bayes. *Indian J. Comput. Sci. Eng.* **2011**, *2*, 170–174.
35. Thiyagaraj, M.; Suseendran, G. Enhanced Prediction of Heart Disease Using Particle Swarm Optimization and Rough Sets with Transductive Support Vector Machines Classifier. In *Data Management, Analytics and Innovation*; Springer: Singapore, 2020; Volume 2, pp. 141–152.
36. Yeh, D.Y.; Cheng, C.H.; Chen, Y.W. A predictive model for cerebrovascular disease using data mining. *Expert Syst. Appl.* **2011**, *38*, 8970–8977. [CrossRef]

# 7

# CRISPRLearner: A Deep Learning-Based System to Predict CRISPR/Cas9 sgRNA On-Target Cleavage Efficiency

**Giovanni Dimauro [1,*], Pierpasquale Colagrande [1], Roberto Carlucci [2], Mario Ventura [2], Vitoantonio Bevilacqua [3] and Danilo Caivano [1]**

1 Department of Computer Science, University of Bari, 70125 Bari, Italy; p.colagrande@studenti.uniba.it (P.C.); danilo.caivano@uniba.it (D.C.)
2 Department of Biology, University of Bari, 70125 Bari, Italy; roberto.carlucci@uniba.it (R.C.); mario.ventura@uniba.it (M.V.)
3 Department of Electrical and Information Engineering, Polytechnic University of Bari, 70125 Bari, Italy; vitoantonio.bevilacqua@poliba.it
* Correspondence: giovanni.dimauro@uniba.it

**Abstract:** CRISPRLearner, the system presented in this paper, makes it possible to predict the on-target cleavage efficiency (also called on-target knockout efficiency) of a given sgRNA sequence, specifying the target genome that this sequence is designed for. After efficiency prediction, the researcher can evaluate its sequence and design a new one if the predicted efficiency is low. CRISPRLearner uses a deep convolutional neural network to automatically learn sequence determinants and predict the efficiency, using pre-trained models or using a model trained on a custom dataset. The convolutional neural network uses linear regression to predict efficiency based on efficiencies used to train the model. Ten different models were trained using ten different gene datasets. The efficiency prediction task attained an average Spearman correlation higher than 0.40. This result was obtained using a data augmentation technique that generates mutations of a sgRNA sequence, maintaining the efficiency value. CRISPRLearner supports researchers in sgRNA design task, predicting a sgRNA on-target knockout efficiency.

**Keywords:** convolutional neural network; CRISPR; deep learning

---

## 1. Introduction

### 1.1. Background

Genetic engineering in different living beings has always been used for various tasks, such as treating particular diseases or creating species with particular genetic features. Editing and modifying these features can be accomplished with various biotechnology techniques, which, most of the time, are quite complex.

However, things started to get easier with the discovery of CRISPR, an acronym that stands for Clustered Regularly Interspaced Short Palindromic Repeats. CRISPR was originally discovered in bacteria and archaea in late 1990s and early 2000s as a family of DNA segments containing short repeated sequences. These sequences separate fragments of DNA acquired from viruses that previously attacked the cell, forming an adaptive immunity system. In fact, after a virus attack, new viral DNA is incorporated into the CRISPR locus in form of spacers. Researchers also found that this repeated cluster was accompanied by a set of genes, called CRISPR associated system (Cas) genes, used to generate Cas proteins. Once a virus attacks again, a portion of the CRISPR region is transcribed into CRISPR RNA, or crRNA, that gets joined to a trans-activating crRNA (tracrRNA). These sequences, forming a unique one, are then bound to a Cas9 protein, guiding it to the target site of the virus DNA. The Cas9 protein then unwinds the DNA and performs a double stranded cut, knocking out the virus. The sequence targeted by Cas9 is followed by a 2-6 base pair (bp) sequence called protospacer adjacent motif (PAM), which is part of the invading virus DNA, but not part of the CRISPR region, to prevent Cas9 from cutting the CRISPR locus itself. In fact, Cas9 will not bind to a target sequence if it is not followed by PAM.

Jennifer Doudna and Emmanuelle Charpentier re-engineered the Cas9 endonuclease fusing crRNA and tracrCRNA into a single RNA sequence called sgRNA (single guide RNA). This sequence, when bound with Cas9, can find and cut a target DNA specified by the sequence itself. By manipulating the sgRNA sequence, the artificial Cas9 system can recognize and cut any DNA sequence. CRISPR then becomes a powerful genome editing tool, called CRISPR/Cas9 [1,2]. Recognition and knockout occur via a 23-bp sequence composed by a 20-bp sequence followed by a 3-bp sequence, PAM.

Designing and developing this sequence is an important task because not all the sgRNAs designed to cut a target DNA are equally effective. The efficiency of CRISPR/Cas9 sgRNA depends on the features like the target site, the properties of the endonuclease, and the design of the sequence [3]. Additionally, when DNA gets cut, the cell tends to repair this cut, leading to more or less serious mutations. Predicting efficiency in cutting DNAs (on-target cleavage efficiency or on-target knockout efficiency) and its side effects and mutations (off-target profile or off-target effects) has an important role in sgRNA design task. Also, researchers will be able to obtain these sequence parameters without performing a physical genetic modification, saving time and resources for the actual experimentation. To refine sgRNA design task, various efficiency prediction systems have been developed, using various approaches. For example, locating PAM sequence (CasFinder [4]), scoring efficiencies empirically based on sequence key features (CHOPCHOP [5]), or predicting them with training models (sgRNA designer [6], sgRNA scorer [7,8], SSC [9], CRISPRscan [10]). However, prediction systems based on deep learning principles have surpassed their competitors in both predicting on-target and off-target efficiencies.

The repetitions in a CRISPR locus have variable size: they usually range from 28 to 37 bp. Much shorter repetitions (23 bp) have been discovered and we focused on these ones. Other authors focused on these lengths too, in these preliminary experiments. This paper is presenting CRISPRLearner, a system that uses a deep convolutional neural network (CNN) to extract and automatically learn sequence features and determinants and predict on-target cleavage efficiency of an up to 23-bp sgRNA.

### 1.2. Related Works

Deep learning for sequencing data has been used [11–13]; it has also been used in some works to predict sgRNA on-target and off-target efficiency. For example, a deep learning approach to predict off-target effects is described by Lin in [14]. Another work that used deep learning to predict both off-target and on-target efficiencies is described in [15]. In this system, called DeepCRISPR, the sequence is encoded into a one-hot matrix, composed of 4 rows, one for each nucleobase, and 23 columns, one for each nucleobase in the 23-bp sgRNA sequence. The matrix gets augmented with additional rows corresponding to epigenetic features, to build a generalized model. This matrix then gets passed as input to a CNN, which is able to use both linear regression and classification to predict efficiencies. In the first case, the predicted value is a real value, while in second case a class is predicted (0 low efficiency, 1 high efficiency).

The system developed by Xue [16], called DeepCas9, uses a CNN too. A sequence up to 30-bp is encoded into a one-hot matrix using the same one-hot encoding scheme used in [15], but without adding additional rows for epigenetic features. The obtained matrix gets passed as input to the CNN that uses linear regression to predict efficiency represented by a real value.

All these three studies use similar encoding mechanism to transform each sgRNA sequence into a data format suitable for the CNN. In fact, CNNs take as input a matrix of values, corresponding to the pixel matrix of an image. Each cell of this matrix contains a value representing the color in the corresponding cell of the pixel matrix. For grey-level pictures, matrix cells only contain real values from 0 to 1, where 0 represents white, 1 represents black, and values in between them represent the shades of grey. In [14–16], the sgRNAs get encoded into matrixes where cells assume only 0 and 1 values. Each of them is then served as input to the CNN that makes predictions. Other techniques for comparing images can be found in [17] and an interesting application of NN-based sequencing system is in [18].

The system presented in this paper uses a CNN to predict a score for on-target knockout efficiency: 10 models regarding different type of organisms and cells have been trained using 10 different datasets. The efficiency of a sequence is calculated using one of these 10 models, depending on the organism the sequence has been designed for. In DeepCas9, the efficiency score is calculated with a weighted sum between the scores predicted by three trained models. Moreover, in DeepCas9, the sequence accepted are 30-bp sequence, which we found out was an uncommon type. In DeepCRISPR, different models are used to predict efficiency, some based on a binary classification (1 efficient, 0 not efficient) and some on regression. The system here presented system uses regression, and aims to output a more useful grade of efficiency instead of knowing just if a sequence is efficient or not.

In our work, the sgRNA sequence is encoded into a $4 \times 23$ one-hot matrix that is served as input to the CNN. We also implemented a particular technique to encode sequences with a length less than 23-bp. In addition, datasets are augmented with a particular technique. These details will be described further.

## 2. Materials and Methods

### *2.1. Datasets*

To train and develop the system here presented, the datasets used by Xue in [16] were used, consisting in 10 sgRNA efficiency datasets covering several cell types of five species, which were collected by Haeussler in [19]. These ten datasets were:

- Chari dataset [7], consisting in 1234 guides targeting Human 293T cells
- Wang/Xu dataset [9,20], consisting in 2076 guides targeting 221 genes in Human HL-60 cells
- From Doench dataset [21], 951 guides targeting various mouse-EL4 cells were kept (as said in [16], the sequences that were kept targeted Cd5, Cd28, H2-K, Cd45, Thy1, and Cd43 genes)
- A new version of Doench et al. dataset [6], consisting in 2333 guides targeting CCDC101, MED12, TADA2B, TADA1, HPRT, CUL3, NF1, and NF2 genes from Human A375 cells
- Hart dataset [22], consisting in 4239 guides targeting 829 genes in Human Hct116 cells
- Moreno-Mateos dataset [10], consisting in 1020 guides targeting 128 genes in Zebrafish genome
- Gandhi dataset, consisting in 72 guides targeting different genes in Ciona genome
- Farboud dataset [23], consisting in 50 guides targeting different genes in Caenorhabditis elegans genome
- Varshney dataset [24], consisting in 102 guides targeting different genes in Zebrafish genome
- Gagnon dataset [25], consisting in 111 guides targeting different genes in Zebrafish genome

These datasets were aggregated with others in [19], creating a dataset of 31625 sgRNAs with their relative knockout efficiencies. Unfortunately, we were not able to merge datasets from the same organisms (e.g., Human, Zebrafish datasets). In fact, human datasets were referring to different cell types while for zebrafish dataset were left separated since it was not possible to extract information about cell types or tissues. Each dataset had its own measurement scale for knockout efficiencies, producing a dataset with non-standardized knockout efficiency measurements. Moreover, some datasets presented sequences with a length less than 23-bp, meaning that these sequences were not in form of a 20-bp sequence followed by a 3-bp PAM sequence, leading to non-standardized sequences too. To solve these problems, we adopted some strategies that will be described later.

### 2.2. *Software*

The system was developed using Python language, because of its simplicity and popularity compared to other programming languages. The integrated development environment used to develop CRISPLearner was Pycharm, in combination with VSCode for minor modifications. Also, Git version control system was used, in combination with GitHub.

To develop the core of the system, the convolutional neural network behind the prediction task, Tensorflow has been used, including Keras. Keras uses a data structure called model to represent the way which network layers are organized. In this project, the sequential model has been used. Other libraries used are Scipy, an open library dedicated to scientific computing, NumPy, a library for scientific calculation that provides many functions for operations between matrices, Scikit-learn, a library for machine learning supporting algorithms and Python default libraries, like os, re, and shutil for various purposes.

## 3. System Description

This section will describe the techniques used to extract datasets from Haeussler [19] dataset, the strategies adopted to standardize sequences and efficiencies, along with the sequence representation technique used. In addition, the dataset augmentation technique adopted, the CNN architecture and the CLI (Command-Line Interface) implemented will be described.

### 3.1. *Dataset Creation*

This section will describe the procedure adopted to extract and prepare data.

#### 3.1.1. Data extraction

As said before, the datasets used to train the CNN are ten, which were collected with others in the Haeussler dataset [19]. Each row of this last dataset contained data regarding a single sgRNA sequence. The columns used to extract each dataset were four:

- dataset column, containing the name of the dataset where the sequence was extracted from
- seq column, containing the actual sgRNA sequence
- modFreq column, containing the efficiency value
- longSeq100Bp column, the extended 100-bp sequence

For each of the ten datasets, a file containing only a 23-bp sequence and its efficiency was created. To identify only the sequences from the datasets needed, the dataset column was used, which contained the dataset name. Using these names, ten files corresponding to the ten datasets were created. Each extracted dataset contained only two columns, a column containing the 23-bp sgRNA sequence and a column containing cleavage efficiency.

#### 3.1.2. Standardizing sgRNA Sequences

Some datasets include sequences with a length less than 23-bp. For example, Gandhi dataset had sequences of 22-bp, composed of a 19-bp sequence followed by a 3-bp PAM sequence. Instead, Doench A375 and Hart datasets had sequences of 20-bp not followed by a 3-bp PAM, as it should be.

Therefore, before extracting the datasets, 23-bp sgRNA sequences in form of 20-bp sequences followed by a 3-bp PAM sequence had to be extracted. In fact, in Doench A375 and Hart datasets, the missing PAM sequence was instead in the 3 nucleobases immediately following the seq sequence in longSeq100Bp extended sequence. So, the seq sequence was first found in longSeq100Bp sequence and then extracted along with the 3 immediately following nucleobases (the PAM sequence), obtaining a 23-bp sequence composed of a 20-bp sequence followed the 3-bp PAM sequence.

Instead, for Ghandi dataset, the seq sequence was first found in longSeq100Bp sequence and then extracted along with the first immediately preceding nucleobase.

After this operation, the ten files corresponding to the extracted datasets were created.

#### 3.1.3. Standardizing Efficiency Measurement

Each dataset used a different scale to measure cleavage efficiency, based on the technique used to measure these values. In order to train a regression model, it was necessary to rescale each of these values to a standard measurement scale.

To do this, the same solution described by Xue in [16] was adopted. Each extracted dataset was rescaled using a min–max scaler mapping a value in the range [0, 1]. This function was defined as $f_{nk} = \frac{f_k - f_{min}}{f_{max} - f_{min}}$, where $f_{max}$ and $f_{min}$ are, respectively, the maximum and minimum efficiency value of the dataset, $f_k$ is the original efficiency value to rescale and $f_{nk}$ is the rescaled value. This rescaling function was applied on each sequence of the ten extracted datasets. For each extracted dataset, a rescaled dataset file was created, containing a column with the 23-bp sequence and a column with its rescaled efficiency, rescaled using the minmax function described above. Efficiency was standardized in order to have a general measuring of the it, even if the datasets are not merged, so even if the original efficiency is in a different scale than [0, 1], the system will always output an efficiency included in this interval, no matter what the trained model is.

#### 3.1.4. Data augmentation Technique

During the experimentation, data from different cell types has been used to train the CNN model. Initially, only the rescaled datasets were used, but the results obtained were unsatisfactory, leading to an overfitted and less performing model. Modifying the CNN architecture or changing some of its hyperparameters did not improve model performances.

For this reason, a data augmentation technique was adopted. In particular, the data augmentation technique used by Chuai in [15] was adopted. In fact, it seems that mismatches in the PAM distal region, which is the 5′ end of a 23-bp sgRNA, have no influence on the sequence efficiency [6,15,20], giving us the possibility to generate new sequences, starting from a single sgRNA, with the same efficiency value of the original one. The rescaled sets were then augmented, generating two mismatches in the first two nucleobases of the extracted sequences, obtaining sixteen new sequences for each original sgRNA sequence (one of them was the original sgRNA sequence), each of them having the same identical efficiency value.

Augmenting data has proved to be a key step in improving the CNN performances, as the problem of low performances and high losses seemed to reside in the data itself rather than in the CNN architecture. Table 1 resumes the number of sequences for each dataset before and after augmentation procedure (training on 80% of the sequences, see Section 4).

**Table 1.** Number of sequences in the original and augmented datasets.

| Dataset | Original Sequences | Augmented Sequences |
|---|---|---|
| Chari | 1234 | 19,744 |
| Wang/Xu | 2076 | 33,216 |
| Doench mouse-EL4 | 951 | 15,216 |
| Doench A375 | 2333 | 37,328 |
| Hart | 4239 | 67,824 |
| Moreno-Mateos | 1020 | 16,320 |
| Gandhi | 72 | 1152 |
| Farboud | 50 | 800 |
| Varshney | 102 | 1632 |
| Gagnon | 111 | 1776 |

### *3.2. Data Representation for Training*

To make the sequences usable for the CNN, each sequence was encoded in a one-hot matrix with 23 columns, corresponding to the nucleobases of the sequence, and 4 rows, corresponding to A, C,

G, and T bases channels. CRISPRLearner supports sequence up to a maximum of 23 nucleobases. For sequences with less than 23 nucleobases, a different approach has been adopted. Since an sgRNA gets encoded into a one-hot manner, if a sequence as a length less than 23, some columns of zeros have been added at the beginning of the real one-hot matrix. So, for example, a sequence of 19-bp will be encoded into a $4 \times 19$ one-hot matrix and 4 (23 minus length of sequence) columns of zeros have been added at the start of the matrix, creating a matrix of $4 \times 23$ and making the matrix usable for the CNN. All the dataset that we used for these experiments contains only sequences of 23-bp, so this problem should never appear, since the system is designed to work efficiently with 23-bp sequences. However, we have left the possibility to experiment on shorter sequences if the PAM sequence cannot be extracted, retrieved or is omitted or if a researcher wants to experiment using simply shorter sequences. Figure 1 shows an example of one-hot encoding of a sequence that has a length less than 23-bp.

| | 1 | 2 | 3 | 4 | 5 | 6 | 7 | 8 | 9 | 10 | 11 | 12 | 13 | 14 | 15 | 16 | 17 | 18 | 19 | 20 | 21 | 22 | 23 |
|---|---|---|---|---|---|---|---|---|---|---|---|---|---|---|---|---|---|---|---|---|---|---|---|
| | | | | | G | C | C | C | T | C | A | A | G | T | G | G | C | C | G | T | C | G | G |
| A channel | 0 | 0 | 0 | 0 | 0 | 0 | 0 | 0 | 0 | 0 | 1 | 1 | 0 | 0 | 0 | 0 | 0 | 0 | 0 | 0 | 0 | 0 | 0 |
| C channel | 0 | 0 | 0 | 0 | 0 | 1 | 1 | 1 | 0 | 1 | 0 | 0 | 0 | 0 | 0 | 0 | 1 | 1 | 0 | 0 | 1 | 0 | 0 |
| G channel | 0 | 0 | 0 | 0 | 1 | 0 | 0 | 0 | 0 | 0 | 0 | 0 | 1 | 0 | 1 | 1 | 0 | 0 | 1 | 0 | 0 | 1 | 1 |
| T channel | 0 | 0 | 0 | 0 | 0 | 0 | 0 | 0 | 1 | 0 | 0 | 0 | 0 | 1 | 0 | 0 | 0 | 0 | 0 | 1 | 0 | 0 | 0 |

**Figure 1.** One-hot encoding of a 19-base pair (bp) sequence.

### *3.3. Description of the Convolutional Neural Network Architecture*

The core of the system is a convolutional neural network that performs regression to predict sgRNA cleavage efficiency. Differently from Chuai et al. [15], this model is focused on a regression task instead of a classification task. This system uses only real value labels since it's based on regression instead of using class label. In regression, the labels are real values, indicating precisely the efficiency of the sgRNA on a range of real values between 0 and 1. In classification, labels are class labels, indicating only a binary efficiency, i.e., 0 if a sgRNA is not effective and 1 if it is effective.

The first layer is an input layer that takes as input a $4 \times 23 \times 1$ one-hot matrix. Then, a convolution layer performs 50 convolutions with 4x4 kernel on the input matrix, producing 50 feature maps of size $1 \times 20$. After convolution, a ReLU activation layer removes outputs below 0, transforming them into zeros. After ReLU activation layer, a max pooling layer performs $1 \times 2$ max pooling of the feature maps produced by the convolution layer, producing 50 feature maps of size $1 \times 10$. After pooling, a flatten layer combines the pooling results in a vector with size of 500. Then, two fully connected layers are added, each with 128 nodes. Each fully connected layer is followed by a ReLU activation layer. Between the fully connected layers, a dropout layer is added, with a dropout rate of 0.3, to reduce overfitting. Then, a fully connected (or dense) layer serves as output layer followed by a linear regression activation layer. Table 2 resumes the CNN architecture.

Specifically, after being converted into a one-hot matrix with 4 rows and 23 columns, the sequence is passed to the CNN. The input layer reads the matrix as if it is a $4 \times 23$ black and white image. The first convolutional layer performs 50 convolutions with a $4 \times 4$ filter and a stride of 1, generating 50 feature maps of dimension $1 \times 20$. After convolution, the ReLU layer outputs results above threshold. The next pooling layer performs a $1 \times 2$ max pooling of each feature map using a stride of 1, producing 50 feature maps of size $1 \times 10$. All the pooling results are combined into a single vector by a flatten layer, resulting in a vector of 500 elements. The vector is then passed to two fully connected layers, each composed of 128 nodes, which have a ReLU layer and a dropout layer in between them, with a dropout rate of 0.3, to avoid overfitting. After the fully connected layers, the output layer outputs the prediction for on-target efficiency using linear regression.

**Table 2.** Layers of the convolutional neural network.

| N | Layer |
|---|---|
| 1 | Input: $4 \times 23 \times 1$ |
| 2 | Convolution: $4 \times 4$ size, 50 filters, 1 stride |
| 3 | ReLU |
| 4 | Max pooling: $1 \times 2$ size, 1 stride |
| 5 | Flatten |
| 6 | Fully connected: 128 units |
| 7 | ReLU |
| 8 | Dropout: 0.3 dropout rate |
| 9 | Fully connected: 128 units |
| 10 | ReLU |
| 11 | Fully connected (output): 1 unit |
| 12 | Linear regression |

For each dataset, a model was trained on 250 epochs with a batch size of 32 and a learning rate of 0.001. An early stopping was also added to detect automatically the minimum validation loss, with a patience of 100 epochs. The models were also optimized with Adam algorithm, trained using 80% of each dataset and validated on the remaining 20% [26,27]. Each dataset was also randomly shuffled before training.

To evaluate each model, the loss function used was Mean Squared Error, while the metric used was Spearman correlation coefficient from Scipy library. The Spearman score of each model was calculated between the predicted efficiencies (on the 20% validation set) and the respective real efficiencies from the datasets. After each model training procedure, the model weights were saved.

## 4. Results

The efficiency prediction of the system CRISPRLearner was evaluated using Spearman correlation coefficient and using Mean Squared Error loss. The system was trained on 80% of each dataset and tested on the 20% left, generating ten different models. Few evaluations made before adding the data augmentation technique previously described, pointed out low performances, with an average Spearman correlation coefficient of about 0.2 and a high loss. The models trained also showed overfitting and high validation losses. Adding data augmentation improved both losses and Spearman scores, avoiding overfitting and making the system more effective. In Table 3 it is reported a Spearman score comparison between this system and DeepCas9. The results are interesting, but it is clear that we cannot speak of a decisive improvement in performance in comparison with DeepCas9, which however in some datasets achieves better results. It is also interesting to compare the results with other competitors by analyzing Figure 2 in [16].

**Table 3.** Performance comparison of CRISPRLearner with DeepCas9.

| Dataset | CRISPRLearner | DeepCas9 |
|---|---|---|
| Chari | 0.49 | 0.49 |
| Wang/Xu | 0.69 | 0.61 |
| Doench mouse-EL4 | 0.51 | 0.59 |
| Doench A375 | 0.23 | 0.38 |
| Hart | 0.55 | 0.41 |
| Moreno-Mateos | 0.19 | 0.23 |
| Gandhi | 0.36 | 0.32 |
| Farboud | 0.60 | 0.57 |
| Varshney | 0.35 | 0.3 |
| Gagnon | 0.35 | 0.25 |

## 5. Conclusion and Future Work

As indicated in the Table 3, CNN-based systems perform better that other system on some of the datasets. This means that deep-learning based systems are generally performing better than machine-learning based systems and systems based on other techniques. There are some exceptions, like Doench mEl4, Doench A375, and Ghandi datasets, indicating that some other approaches still may perform better on some kind of data.

The system presented in this paper shows good performances, paying a lower generalization. However, allowing the user to train his own models based on the datasets he provides, leads to a generalization of the system, even if the model itself is not generalized. In fact, a single model was not trained for all the datasets, but for each dataset a model was trained and training more models on new datasets will allow the system to predict more and more sgRNA efficiencies of different genomes, cell types, and genes.

To support multiple cell identification, the user is free to train its own model using a different dataset, expanding the system and allowing it to predict sgRNA efficiencies regarding new cell types, gene, or genome types. This approach will allow researchers to contribute in the overall expansion and improvement of the system, adding new trained models to perform predictions on new types of cells.

A question could be why performance results were not better than the DeepCas9 in some datasets, but the answer could not be definitive. Performances can depend on type of data augmentation, on the number of original sequences, on the similarity between some sequences and obviously on the design details of each system. It is not easy to describe the behavior of the internal layers of the CNN, but we will deepen this argument in a further study.

The system here presented will be expanded, as just said, with more cell and genome types. Also, the ability to predict off-target efficiencies will be added to the system, transforming CRISPRLearner in a complete system for CRISPR/Cas9 sgRNA design. Also, deploying the system online will permit it to be expanded with new trained models more easily.

**Author Contributions:** Conceptualization, G.D. and P.C.; methodology, R.C., M.V. and G.D.; software, P.C. and D.C.; validation, V.B.; formal analysis, V.B.; investigation, P.C. and R.C.; resources, D.C.; data curation, P.C.; writing—original draft preparation, G.D. and P.C.; writing—review and editing, P.C., R.C., and M.V.; project administration, G.D.

## References

1. Jinek, M.; Chylinski, K.; Fonfara, I.; Hauer, M.; Doudna, J.A.; Charpentier, E. A programmable dual-RNA-guided DNA endonuclease in adaptive bacterial immunity. *Science* **2012**, *337*, 816–821. [CrossRef] [PubMed]
2. Doudna, J.A.; Charpentier, E. The new frontier of genome engineering with CRISPR-Cas9. *Science* **2014**, *346*, 1258096. [CrossRef] [PubMed]
3. Zahra, H.; Ali, M.; Hui, W.; Dawei, L.; Yasin, O.; Honghua, R.; Qiang, Z. Strategies to Increase On-Target and Reduce Off-Target Effects of the CRISPR/Cas9 System in Plants. *Int. J. Mol. Sci.* **2019**, *20*, 3718. [CrossRef]
4. Aach, J.; Mali, P.; Church, G.M. CasFinder: Flexible algorithm for identifying specific Cas9 targets in genomes. *bioRxiv* **2014**, 005074. [CrossRef]
5. Labun, K.; Montague, T.G.; Gagnon, J.A.; Thyme, S.B.; Valen, E. CHOPCHOP v2: A web tool for the next generation of CRISPR genome engineering. *Nucleic Acids Res.* **2016**, *44*, W272–W276. [CrossRef]
6. Doench, J.G.; Fusi, N.; Sullender, M.; Hegde, M.; Vaimberg, E.W.; Donovan, K.F.; Smith, I.; Tothova, Z.; Wilen, C.; Orchard, R.; et al. Optimized sgRNA design to maximize activity and minimize off-target effects of CRISPR-Cas9. *Nat. Biotechnol.* **2016**, *34*, 184–191. [CrossRef]
7. Chari, R.; Mali, P.; Moosburner, M.; Church, G.M. Unraveling CRISPR-Cas9 genome engineering parameters via a library-on-library approach. *Nat. Methods* **2015**, *12*, 823–826. [CrossRef]
8. Chari, R.; Yeo, N.C.; Chavez, A.; Church, G.M. sgRNA Scorer 2.0: A Species-Independent Model To Predict CRISPR/Cas9 Activity. *ACS Synth. Biol.* **2017**, *6*, 902–904. [CrossRef]

9. Xu, H.; Xiao, T.; Chen, C.-H.; Li, W.; Meyer, C.A.; Wu, Q.; Wu, D.; Cong, L.; Zhang, F.; Liu, J.S.; et al. Sequence determinants of improved CRISPR sgRNA design. *Genome Res.* **2015**, *25*, 1147–1157. [CrossRef]
10. Moreno-Mateos, M.A.; Vejnar, C.E.; Beaudoin, J.-D.; Fernandez, J.P.; Mis, E.K.; Khokha, M.K.; Giraldez, A.J. CRISPRscan: Designing highly efficient sgRNAs for CRISPR-Cas9 targeting in vivo. *Nat. Methods* **2015**, *12*, 982–988. [CrossRef]
11. Zhang, S.W.; Wang, Y.; Zhang, X.X.; Wang, J.Q. Prediction of the RBP binding sites on lncRNAs using the high-order nucleotide encoding convolutional neural network. *Anal. Biochem.* **2019**, *583*, 113364. [CrossRef] [PubMed]
12. Ding, W.; Mao, W.; Shao, D.; Zhang, W.; Gong, H. DeepConPred2: An Improved Method for the Prediction of Protein Residue Contacts. *Comput. Struct. Biotechnol. J.* **2018**, *16*, 503–510. [CrossRef] [PubMed]
13. Le, N.Q.K.; Ho, Q.T.; Ou, Y.Y. Incorporating deep learning with convolutional neural networks and position specific scoring matrices for identifying electron transport proteins. *Comput. Chem.* **2017**, *38*. [CrossRef] [PubMed]
14. Lin, J.; Wong, K.-C. Off-target predictions in CRISPR-Cas9 gene editing using deep learning. *Oxf. Acad. Bioinform.* **2018**, *34*, i656–i663. [CrossRef] [PubMed]
15. Chuai, G.; Ma, H.; Yan, J.; Chen, M.; Hong, N.; Xue, D.; Zhou, C.; Zhu, C.; Chen, K.; Duan, B.; et al. DeepCRISPR: Optimized CRISPR guide RNA design by deep learning. *Genome Biol.* **2018**, *19*, 80. [CrossRef]
16. Xue, L.; Tang, B.; Chen, W.; Luo, J. Prediction of CRISPR sgRNA activity using a deep convolutional neural network. *J. Chem. Inf. Modeling* **2019**, *59*, 615–624. [CrossRef]
17. Dimauro, G. A new image quality metric based on human visual system. In Proceedings of the 2012 IEEE International Conf. on Virtual Environments Human-Computer Interfaces and Measurement Systems, Tianjin, China, 2–4 July 2012; pp. 69–73. [CrossRef]
18. Casalino, G.; Castellano, G.; Consiglio, A.; Liguori, M.; Nuzziello, N.; Primiceri, e.D. Analysis of microRNA expressions for pediatric multiple sclerosis detection. In *Modeling Decisions for Artificial Intelligence. MDAI2019*; Lecture Notes in Computer Science. LNAI 11676; Springer: Cham, Switzerland, 2019; pp. 177–188. [CrossRef]
19. Haeussler, M.; Schonig, K.; Eckert, H.; Eschstruth, A.; Mianne, J.; Renaud, J.-B.; Schneider-Maunoury, S.; Shkumatava, A.; Teboul, L.; Kent, J.; et al. Evaluation of off- target and on-target scoring algorithms and integration into the guide RNA selection tool CRISPOR. *Genome Biol.* **2016**, *17*, 148. [CrossRef]
20. Wang, T.; Wei, J.J.; Sabatini, D.M.; Lander, E.S. Genetic Screens in Human Cells Using the CRISPR-Cas9 System. *Science* **2014**, *343*, 80–84. [CrossRef]
21. Doench, J.G.; Hartenian, E.; Graham, D.B.; Tothova, Z.; Hegde, M.; Smith, I.; Sullender, M.; Ebert, B.L.; Xavier, R.J.; Root, D.E. Rational design of highly active sgRNAs for CRISPR-Cas9-mediated gene inactivation. *Nat. Biotechnol.* **2014**, *32*, 1262–1267. [CrossRef]
22. Hart, T.; Chandrashekhar, M.; Aregger, M.; Steinhart, Z.; Brown, K.R.; MacLeod, G.; Mis, M.; Zimmermann, M.; Fradet-Turcotte, A.; Sun, S.; et al. High-Resolution CRISPR Screens Reveal Fitness Genes and Genotype-Specific Cancer Liabilities. *Cell* **2015**, *163*, 1515–1526. [CrossRef]
23. Farboud, B.; Meyer, B.J. Dramatic Enhancement of Genome Editing by CRISPR/Cas9 Through Improved Guide RNA Design. *Genetics* **2015**, *199*, 959–971. [CrossRef] [PubMed]
24. Varshney, G.K.; Pei, W.; LaFave, M.C.; Idol, J.; Xu, L.; Gallardo, V.; Carrington, B.; Bishop, K.; Jones, M.; Li, M.; et al. High-throughput gene targeting and phenotyping in zebrafish using CRISPR/Cas9. *Genome Res.* **2015**, *25*, 1030–1042. [CrossRef] [PubMed]
25. Gagnon, J.A.; Valen, E.; Thyme, S.B.; Huang, P.; Ahkmetova, L.; Pauli, A.; Montague, T.G.; Zimmerman, S.; Richter, C.; Schier, A.F. Efficient Mutagenesis by Cas9 Protein-Mediated Oligonucleotide Insertion and Large-Scale Assessment of Single-Guide RNAs. *PLoS ONE* **2014**, *9*, e98186. [CrossRef] [PubMed]
26. Hussain, W.; Khan, Y.D.; Rasool, N.; Khan, S.A.; Chou, K.C. SPalmitoylC-PseAAC: A sequence-based model developed via Chou's 5-steps rule and general PseAAC for identifying S-palmitoylation sites in proteins. *Anal. Biochem.* **2019**, *568*, 14–23. [CrossRef]
27. Le, N.Q.K.; Fertility, G.R.U. Identifying Fertility-Related Proteins by Incorporating Deep-Gated Recurrent Units and Original Position-Specific Scoring Matrix Profiles. *J. Proteome Res.* **2019**, *18*, 3503–3511. [CrossRef]

8

# Applying Machine Learning for Healthcare

**Juan de la Torre [1,*], Javier Marin [1], Sergio Ilarri [2,3] and Jose J. Marin [1,4]**

1 IDERGO-Research and Development in Ergonomics, Biomechanical Laboratory, I3A-University Institute of Research of Engineering of Aragon, University of Zaragoza, 50018 Zaragoza, Spain; 647473@unizar.es (J.M.); jjmarin@unizar.es (J.J.M.)
2 Computer Science for Complex System Modelling (COSMOS), I3A-University Institute of Research of Engineering of Aragon, University of Zaragoza, 50018 Zaragoza, Spain; silarri@unizar.es
3 Department of Computer Science and Systems Engineering, University of Zaragoza, 50018 Zaragoza, Spain
4 Department of Design and Manufacturing Engineering, University of Zaragoza, 50018 Zaragoza, Spain
* Correspondence: 627471@unizar.es

**Abstract:** Given the exponential availability of data in health centers and the massive sensorization that is expected, there is an increasing need to manage and analyze these data in an effective way. For this purpose, data mining (DM) and machine learning (ML) techniques would be helpful. However, due to the specific characteristics of the field of healthcare, a suitable DM and ML methodology adapted to these particularities is required. The applied methodology must structure the different stages needed for data-driven healthcare, from the acquisition of raw data to decision-making by clinicians, considering the specific requirements of this field. In this paper, we focus on a case study of cervical assessment, where the goal is to predict the potential presence of cervical pain in patients affected with whiplash diseases, which is important for example in insurance-related investigations. By analyzing in detail this case study in a real scenario, we show how taking care of those particularities enables the generation of reliable predictive models in the field of healthcare. Using a database of 302 samples, we have generated several predictive models, including logistic regression, support vector machines, k-nearest neighbors, gradient boosting, decision trees, random forest, and neural network algorithms. The results show that it is possible to reliably predict the presence of cervical pain (accuracy, precision, and recall above 90%). We expect that the procedure proposed to apply ML techniques in the field of healthcare will help technologists, researchers, and clinicians to create more objective systems that provide support to objectify the diagnosis, improve test treatment efficacy, and save resources.

**Keywords:** data mining; data anonymization; health; cervical injury; neck pain; inertial sensors

## 1. Introduction

In the field of healthcare, the exponential increase in the data that health centers must produce and manage is significant. The need has arisen to develop procedures that make this process easier and that take advantage of all the data generated [1], detecting unknown and valuable information in health data [2]. Thus, the volume of data generated is such that its processing and analysis by traditional methods is too complex and overwhelming [3]. To tackle this challenge, data mining (DM) can play a key role, as it allows the discovery of patterns and trends in large amounts of complex data and the extraction of hidden information to help in making decisions that can improve the quality of the care processes [4–7]. It is closely linked with the scientific discipline in the field of artificial intelligence called machine learning (ML), which "employs a variety of statistical, probabilistic and optimization techniques that allow computers to learn from past examples and to detect hard-to-discern patterns from large, noisy or complex data sets" [8].

Consequently, ML is generating growing interest in the field of healthcare (e.g., see [9,10]) for relevant special issues related to this topic), mainly derived from its possible applications, such as assessing the effectiveness of treatments, detecting fraud and abuse in health insurance, managing healthcare, making lower-cost medical solutions available to the patients, detecting symptoms and diseases [11], discovering treatment patterns from electronic medical records [12], detecting groups of incidents [13], and identifying medical treatment methods [2,3]. Likewise, ML also presents health benefits: (1) a potential reduction in the time and effort required for diagnosis and treatment, (2) the ability to examine multiple areas simultaneously, (3) a decreased potential for human error, and (4) data that are accessible anytime and anywhere [14]. Besides, DM and ML are key in the path towards personalized medicine, where the goal is to customize treatments to the specifics of each individual [15–18].

However, to take full advantage of the benefits offered by ML in the field of healthcare, several considerations are necessary. Among others, the following aspects can be highlighted:

- The data have to be structured and organized in order to properly process and transform them into suitable variables, which is essential in the development of any pattern recognition software and a highly problem-dependent task [19,20].
- Moreover, the secure treatment and management of data acquires special relevance in the field of healthcare, where the privacy of the patient must be ensured. The management of sensitive data contrasts with other fields of application of ML (fraud detection, stock prediction, etc.), where anonymization treatments may be sometimes not necessary or critical. Therefore, a specific treatment involving the anonymization and categorization of the data must be performed in order to ensure the privacy of the patients [21]. Due to privacy policies, on certain occasions if a suitable anonymization of the data is not performed and/or the required authorizations to access some data are not obtained, the needed health studies cannot be carried out. Therefore, data availability should also be considered as a key factor [21].
- Another difference with other ML applications is the existence of different costs of failures; in the health area, the cost of a false negative (e.g., failing to detect that a patient has a specific disease) is usually much higher than the cost of a false positive (e.g., if a person is initially considered to have a disease that he/she does not really have, additional tests will be performed to rule this out, which may be costly but usually less harmful than failing to diagnose an existing disease).
- It should also be considered that ML hardly ever follows a linear sequence ending at the first attempt; instead, it is rather an iterative feedback process where the stages interact with each other. Furthermore, in the field of healthcare, where the flow of data is continuous and constant, it is reasonable to assume that the model can be designed to be a "learning" model that must be continuously updated to improve its predictions over time. Therefore, the different stages needed to generate a reliable predictive model should be properly structured, from the acquisition of raw data to decision-making, which is essential to achieve the effectiveness of the model [22].

All this motivates the need to define the particularities of the application of ML techniques in the field of healthcare, where different stages in the ML workflow must be correctly defined and structured. The proper application of ML techniques would be beneficial for the clinicians, researchers, developers, and designers involved in the field of health, where the management of information acquires a transcendental role. It would favor the design of new products and services for improving healthcare access [23], creating truly accessible technological solutions [24], and enhance the relationship between health systems and people by providing adequate services at the right time [23].

Based on the above, the aims of this study are the following: (1) to show and develop the particularities of applying ML techniques in the field of healthcare, detailing all the stages that comprise this process, from the acquisition of raw data to the decision-making derived from the predictive model generated; and (2) to demonstrate and show its practical application in a real use case. Specifically, the ML process is applied in a cervical pain assessment study with patients affected by whiplash pathologies derived from traffic accidents or other causes. This case study shows the proposed methodology in action to solve a specific relevant problem. Moreover, the applied procedure can be used as an ML application guide for other similar studies in the field of healthcare. We believe that the combination of the use case study and the machine learning methodology is a relevant contribution of this paper. We do not remain in the theoretical/methodological part only or limit our work to apply different machine learning algorithms and compare the results, as many other works do; instead, we describe the whole machine learning process, highlighting the aspects that are more relevant for our use case but at the same time providing a general framework that could be used in other health-related projects. In this way, we think that the paper could be relevant both as a specific case study and also as a reference and guideline for other similar projects.

The structure of the rest of this paper is as follows. In Section 2, we present the use case scenario studied and the clinical methods used for data collection. In Section 3, we describe the proposed procedure to develop predictive models for healthcare, illustrating each step with our work on the case study. In Section 4, we present an overall discussion of the proposal and the lessons learnt. Finally, in Section 5, we summarize our conclusions, the limitations of the study, and some ideas for future work.

## 2. Use Case Scenario and Clinical Methods

To illustrate the particularities of using ML techniques in the health area, a case study related to the detection of cervical pain is considered. The goal is to try to estimate automatically the presence of cervical pain, which can help to objectify a diagnosis and to clarify issues in case of insurance litigation. The selection of cervical pathology as a case study in this work is motivated by the fact that musculoskeletal disorders of the cervical spine have a high incidence and prevalence and are considered a public health problem, especially in developed countries [25,26]. Likewise, cervical injuries (usually due to whiplash after a traffic accident) are difficult to diagnose [26] because traumatic cervical spine injuries and their associated symptoms are diverse [25].

A real dataset was collected by evaluating the movement of the cervical spine in 151 patients (60 asymptomatic subjects, 42 with cervical pain resulting from a traffic accident, and 49 with neck discomfort due to other causes). Cervical movement assessment tests were performed by using an MH-sensor motion capture system [27,28] (see Figure 1). The participants performed a sequence of functional cervical Range of Motion (ROM) tests of the following movements: flexion-extension, rotation, and lateralization (Figure 2). The patients were collaborating subjects in order to avoid disturbances produced by non-collaborating subjects immersed in a judicial process with an insurance company [29]. The medical test was performed twice with each patient, giving a total of 302 samples.

Moreover, all the participants, who were either asymptomatic or had cervical pain, were also assessed with a clinical examination to verify that they met the inclusion criteria:

- age between 18 and 65 years;
- not immersed in a judicial process;
- no presence of surgery and/or cervical fracture.

The medical inspection, assessment by scales/clinical tests, and development of the clinical profile of the patients were conducted by clinicians. All the participants received information about the experiment and signed a consent agreement prior to the testing. The study received a favorable verdict from the Bioethics Committee of Aragón in Spain (CEICA) on 25 July 2017.

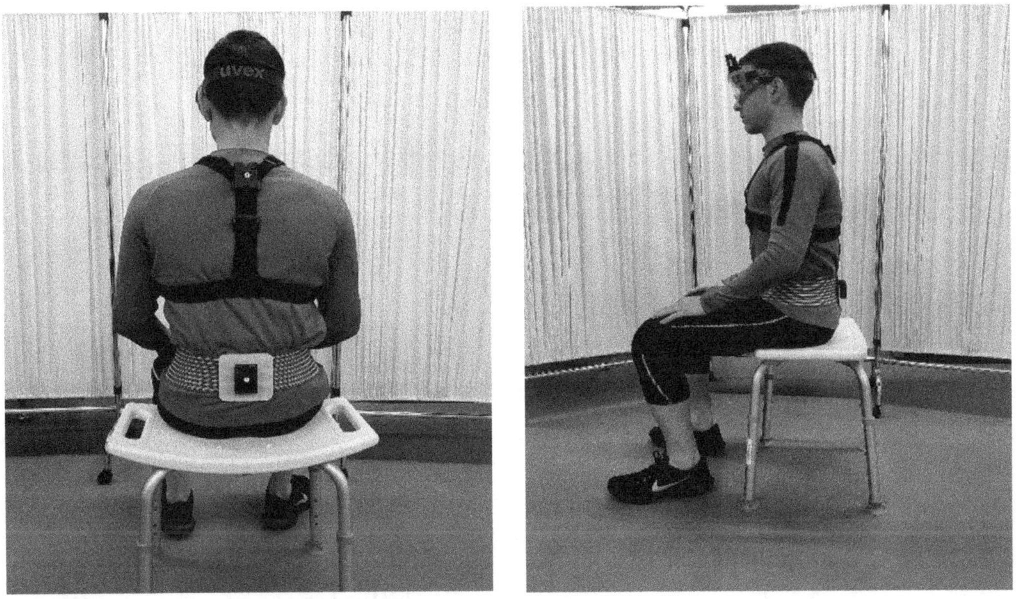


(a) (b)

**Figure 1.** Move Human (MH)-sensor motion capture system, cervical assessment. (**a**) Back view. (**b**) Lateral view.

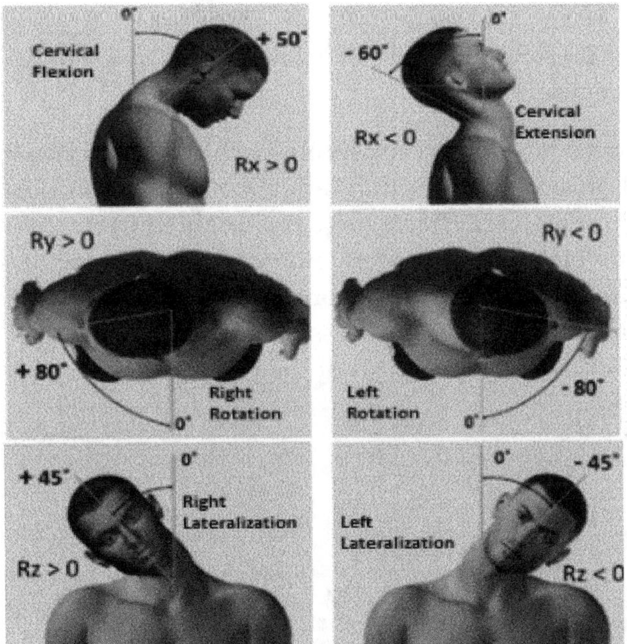


**Figure 2.** Cervical movements evaluated.

## 3. Proposed Procedure to Develop Predictive Models in Healthcare

A predictive model to support decision-making in the field of healthcare should be able to make predictions relative to relevant target clinical variables. The final goal is to deploy a system that can help in clinical decision-making (e.g., objectifying diagnoses, testing the efficacy of treatments, saving resources, providing suitable and customized treatments, etc.). The proposed procedure for continuous use in the field of healthcare is summarized and outlined in Figure 3.

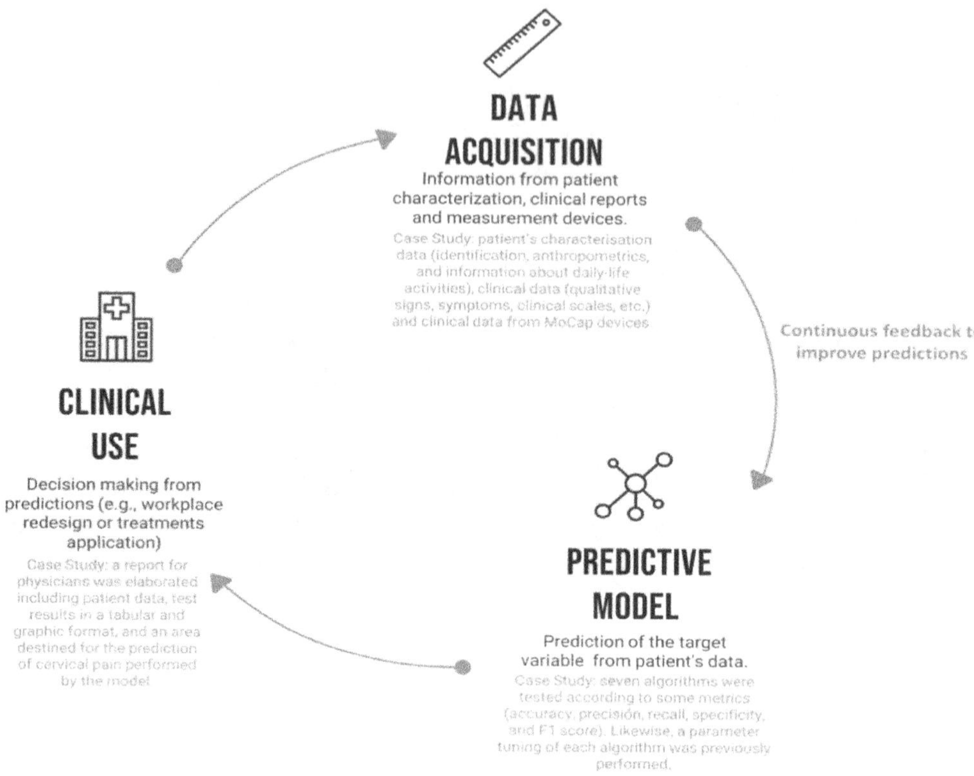


**Figure 3.** Application of predictive models for clinical decision-making. Icons made by monkik, smashicons and mynamepong.

The complete ML process has been considered, with the particularities of its application in the healthcare area. It is based on seven stages that range from the definition of the target to the clinical use of the system, as shown in Figure 4. Each stage is explained in the following subsections. Besides, this paper is accompanied by electronic Supplementary Material to facilitate the understanding of the different stages of application in the case study considered; specifically, we provide sample data files obtained at the end of different stages of the process (anonymized datasets) and an example report that a health professional could obtain as the output of the process.

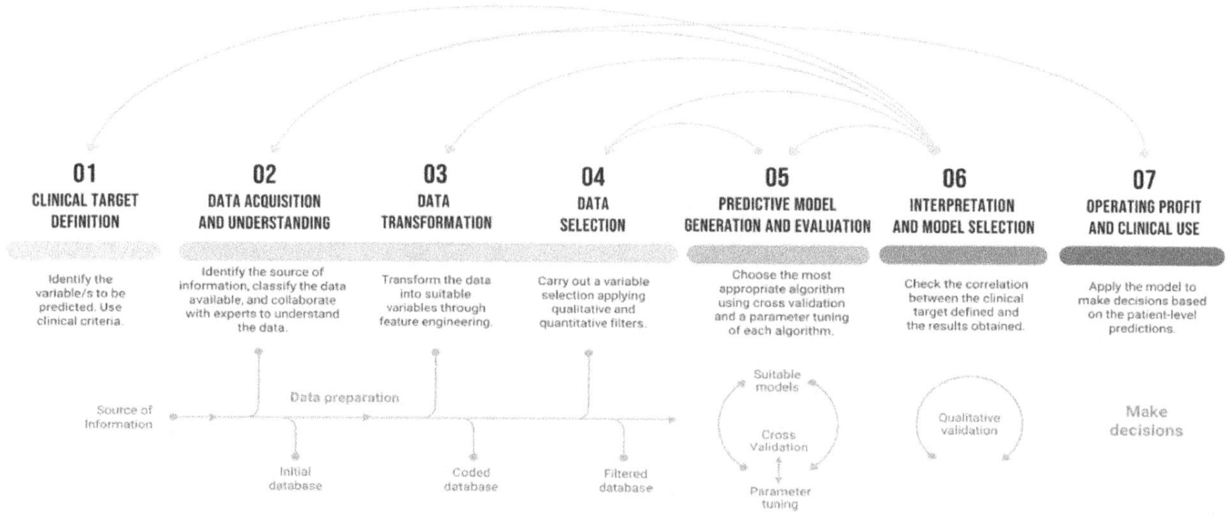


**Figure 4.** Project management procedure proposed for the application of machine learning in healthcare.

In order to adapt and particularize the usual process of applying ML techniques in the healthcare field and develop the project management procedure, some outstanding studies such as [20,30], as well as the most widespread DM processes, such as knowledge discovery in databases (KDD) [31,32]; sample, explore, modify, model, and assess (SEMMA) [14,32]; and the cross-industry standard process for DM (CRISP-DM) [32–35], have been considered as a reference. Likewise, the project management procedure scheme proposed (shown in Figure 4) has been inspired by different outlines of clinical applications proposed by different authors [4,19,36–38] and adapted and extended according to our own experience and the work performed with clinicians in our case study and other related collaborations, such as the project "Mobile units for functional assessment of the musculoskeletal system" (CEICA reference of the project: OTRI-2019/0108) in collaboration with the hospital MAZ (Mutua de Accidentes de Zaragoza, Zaragoza, Spain), whose goal was to predict the degree of collaboration of patients in insurance litigation.

From the related proposals mentioned above, the CRISP-DM process has been our main inspiration to develop the project management procedure proposed in this paper. This is to be expected because CRISP-DM sets a general common framework that can be adapted to different scenarios. Thus, there are similarities between the six stages in CRISP-DM and our seven-stage proposal. For example, the CRISP-DM stage 6 "deployment" is closely related to our last stage, which is "operating profit and clinical use". As another example, stage 6 of CRISP-DM establishes that the creation of the model is not the end of the project and, similarly, in healthcare the knowledge provided to the clinician through the application of the predictive model is not the end of the process, since the system is continuously acquiring new data to improve the clinical performance. As the main difference between both procedures, we put more emphasis on data management aspects, since this is a key point in healthcare, and consider the whole process from the perspective of its application in a healthcare scenario. While only one stage for data management is considered in the CRISP-DM process (stage 3, "data preparation"), data management is the focus of three stages in our proposal (stage 2 "data acquisition and understanding", stage 3 "data transformation", and stage 4 "data selection").

The works mentioned in this section have inspired our proposal, which extends existing models by including a thorough analysis of all the data management challenges, as well as an illustration of each step through a real practical case study. Although the particularities of applying ML techniques in healthcare are exemplified in a specific case study, the procedure presented is flexible enough to adapt to any healthcare case.

### *3.1. Stage 1: Clinical Target Definition*

In the first stage, the aim of the system is established—that is, the variables with clinical significance that the system should be able to predict are identified. Likewise, the final performance of the model and the statistical measures that will define its performance must also be defined. Measures such as the accuracy, precision, or recall are usual metrics used to assess the performance of a classification model, and metrics such as the Mean Absolute Error (MAE) or Root Mean Squared Error (RMSE), to cite two examples can be used to evaluate the accuracy of a numeric prediction.

In predictive classification in a healthcare domain, it is usual that some metric must be highlighted in such a way that the model must always be generated with the aim to minimize it. This metric is usually the number of false negatives (affecting the recall metric). The reason for this is that, in healthcare, false negatives and false positives have no similar costs, which has always been an issue that clinicians have had to deal with [39]. Moreover, the clinical need must be identified (e.g., to classify a certain type of pathology, to predict a pattern or behavior, etc.). In addition, the sample size and viability of the project must be assessed prior to its realization [34].

**Application to our Case Study**

In our case study, the aim of the prediction model is to predict the presence of cervical pain (the target variable) in patients who have suffered whiplash or suffer from chronic cervical pathology. In our collected dataset, the cervical pain is a binary variable (the presence or absence of pain) which has been reported by the collaborating subjects, who were real patients undergoing an assessment process in a hospital.

Predicting the presence of cervical pain is of interest especially in the forensic field, as the incidence and prognosis of whiplash injury from motor vehicles is relevant to insurance litigations for pain and suffering [29]. The aim is to determine the presence or absence of pain with enough confidence to be able to aid clinicians to detect possible magnifications of the injury by the affected individuals and thus establish an unbiased compensation for the cervical pain [40]. It can help to identify and objectify pain in patients with a high degree of anxiety and in hypochondriac patients.

Without a loss of generality, the following target metrics have been determined for the purpose of this study, whose required threshold values have been stablished according to the criteria of clinical experts (for this particular case study, they considered that achieving this quality criteria would be enough for the system to be used as a decision-support system in production):

- Accuracy: greater than 85%.
- Precision: greater than 85%.
- Recall: greater than 90%.

The sample size is 302; although this is not a very large dataset, it contains a lot of variables with relevant information to characterize the presence of cervical pain during insurance litigation, which allows predicting the target variable, thus considering the project viable.

*3.2. Stage 2: Data Acquisition and Understanding*

The second stage implies identifying different sources that will allow access to the data necessary to feed the model, both in the initial phase of model design (initial training), as well as regarding a future continuous feedback when it reaches the operational stage of application in the field of healthcare. Likewise, the typology of these data will also be identified and selected. The level of accuracy that these sources of information can provide and the frequency of data collection (which may be determined by aspects such as the cost of the equipment needed, the availability of collaborating patients, etc.) will be considered in the choice [34].

In the field of healthcare, due to the diverse origins of data, their typology, their consistency, and even their veracity, the process of categorization of the data acquires special relevance for their correct structuring, understanding, and subsequent treatment.

When there are patient's personal data that make the identification of the patient possible, proper anonymization techniques must be applied. Apart from direct identification data (such as the name and last name of the patient, his/her history number, or his/her card ID), other data such as the age, nationality, height, weight, diagnosis, etc., can be used for indirect patient identification. In stage 3 "Data transformation" (see Section 3.3), certain techniques are presented to safeguard the privacy of patients and avoid the loss of useful information for the generation of the model, but these sensitive variables must be identified in this second phase.

Although there are classifications of information and data in the healthcare environment [30], alternative complementary classifications are proposed in this paper for a better understanding and structuring of the data. This has been motivated by the needs of medical staff, as well as by specialists of the medical legal/forensic field collaborating with us in our case study: a greater variety of classifications is of interest in order to include the perspectives of all the parties involved.

**Clinical Data and Patient Data**

Firstly, two types of data related to patients can be identified when we distinguish between clinical data and other data related to the patient:

- Patient characterization data. They are generally static data (although there may be small fluctuations in certain data values over large time intervals, such as in the case of the weight of the patient). They can be grouped in the following categories:

- Identification data: name, age, gender, educational level, nationality, etc.
- Temporary data: dates of control or highlighted clinical evolution, visits to the hospital, start and end of treatments, etc.
- Anthropometric data: measurements of the size and proportions of the human body, such as the height, weight, percentage of fat and muscle, foot length, abdominal perimeter, etc., that usually require instrumentation to be obtained (scale, tape measure, etc.).
- Daily life activities (DLA) data: data usually reported by the patient related to the habits and activities that he/she usually performs on a daily basis. In some cases, some of these data can be measured using wearables sensors or other devices deployed in smart homes.

- Clinical data: data of a medical nature that may require instrumentation and medical tests for their acquisition.

**Data According to the Degree of Objectivity**

Another possible classification is to categorize the data according to the degree of objectivity:

- Measures: objective data that do not require assessment by a clinician. These data are not affected by the reproducibility factor. Examples are test or clinical scales, test results, or data collected by medical instrumentation. Data recorded by sensor devices provide objective data on some measurable dimensions of the patient and can be of different types: motion capture (MoCap) sensors, surface electromyography (EMG), stabilometric platforms, dynamometers, etc.
- Assessed data: information that depends on the assessment of the clinician, such as diagnoses and treatments.
- Reported data: subjective information provided by the patient regarding his/her condition (perceived symptoms).

**Data According to Clinical Considerations**

We also present a classification that groups the collected data according to clinical considerations:

- Clinical profile: data about symptoms and clinical signs of the patient that can lead to a diagnosis by the clinician. We refer to symptoms when they are of subjective nature, reported by the patient, and to signs if they are objective and obtained by the clinician about the pathology. In addition, the signs can be qualitative (binary) or (discrete or continuous) quantitative (e.g., the temperature of a thermometer, image tests, other measurements, etc.).
- Treatment data: data about the treatment that the clinician has prescribed, such as the type of treatment, number of rehabilitation sessions, drugs received, surgery, etc.
- Clinical scales, tests, or surveys: data resulting from scales or validated and protocolized tests whose objective is to obtain objective information about the patient (e.g., the timed up and go test, the Unterberger test, psychological tests, etc.).
- Medical history: data concerning the patient's clinical history, ordered chronologically (e.g., first hospital visit, imaging test for diagnosis, treatment administration after diagnosis, etc.).

**Data According to their Data Types**

Finally, the different data variables can be grouped according to their types, independently of the specifics of the health area. For example, we could consider:

- Qualitative variables: also called categorical variables, they are variables that are not numerical. They describe data that fit into categories (e.g., educational level, the level of development of a disease, the level of invasiveness of a treatment, etc.).
- Quantitative variables: also called measurement or numerical variables, they represent quantities of different nature. They can be divided into discrete variables that can only take a finite number of values (e.g., the number of rehabilitation sessions, score on a clinical scale, age, etc.),

and continuous variables, which can take values in an infinite/continuous range of possible values (e.g., the temperature of a thermometer, weight, Body Mass Index (BMI), etc.).

- Textual data: data that are directly collected in text format, such as handwritten annotations in medical histories.

In this stage, data profiling [41] and cleaning [42] must be applied to detect potential problems and, if possible, fix them. By categorizing the data, using one of the proposed classifications (or another one that could be useful for a specific use case) independently, or several of them at the same time, the process of the understanding and assimilation of the data available and their scope is facilitated. This step must be carried out to obtain a preliminary database, containing the data collected, that will be called the initial database. For this task, having the support of both a clinical expert and a technologist is recommended. In some cases, when the amount of data to handle is large or coming from different data sources, a data warehouse can be created to integrate all the information and allow the easy and efficient analysis of the data stored [43,44].

During data collection for classification tasks, it is also important to collect enough instances/samples to represent in an appropriate way the different classes that must be predicted. In case there is imbalance regarding the number of samples in the different target classes, this should be identified as part of the data profiling, and some strategies could be applied to deal with this issue [45,46] (e.g., to try to prevent the majority class from dominating the predictions in a harmful way).

### Application to Our Case Study

In this case study, the initial database was prepared according to the final goal, which was predicting the presence/absence of cervical pain. The categorization of the data was jointly agreed by physicians and technologists, considering the application of this research in the legal field and the degree of objectivity of the data. According to the four classifications presented, the data from our case study could be classified as shown in Table 1, following the exposed criteria:

**Table 1.** Possible classifications of the case study data.

| 1. Clinical Data and Patient Data | 2. Data According to the Degree of Objectivity | 3. Data According to the Clinical Considerations | 4. Data According to Their Data Types |
|---|---|---|---|
| Patient characterization data:<br>- Identification: name, age, gender, educational level, etc.<br>- Temporary: accident date, visits to the hospital, date of the range of motion (ROM) test, etc.<br>- Anthropometric: weight, height, body mas index, foot length, etc.<br>- Daily life activities: physical activity intensity, workplace, etc. | Measures: all the data from the MoCap sensors or Whiplash scale (WDQ). | Clinical profile:<br>- Symptoms: pain periodicity, feeling of instability, limitation of mobility, etc.<br>- Signs: contracture, limitation of mobility, spinal column alterations, etc. | Qualitative variables: educational level, limitation of mobility, contracture, etc. |
| Clinical data: feeling of instability, surgery, all the data from the MoCap sensors, etc. | Assessed data: contracture, limitation of mobility, Jackson contraction, etc. | Treatment: n/a. | Quantitative variables:<br>- Discrete: WDQ, age, etc.<br>- Continuous: all the data from the MoCap sensors, weight, height, etc. |
| | Reported data: pain periodicity, feeling of instability, etc. | Clinical scales or tests: WDQ. | Textual data: n/a. |
| | | Medical history: accident date, visits to the hospital, etc. | |

The classifications shown in Table 1 illustrate different useful perspectives of the data collected in the case study. Specifically, and considering the final goal of objectively predicting the presence of cervical pain, the classification that best suited the point of view of the health professionals participating in our case study was the following (a combination of the first two classification approaches described):

- Patient characterization data: the data measured and reported, such as the identification information (e.g., ID, age, gender, etc.), anthropometrics (e.g., height, weight, BMI, etc.), and data relative to the activities of daily life (e.g., weekly physical activity and its intensity, workplace, etc.).
- Assessed and reported data: such as the characterization of a cervical accident (e.g., the time since the accident, type of impact of the traffic accident, position of the head, type of effect, etc.), qualitative signs (e.g., column alterations and contractures), clinical scales (e.g., whiplash scale—WDQ), and symptoms (e.g., instability, limitation of mobility, etc.).
- Measured data: such as data from a cervical assessment test with MoCap or from each movement studied, for example the angles reached and the speeds of the movements (e.g., maximum values, minimum values, average values, etc.).

For the purposes of medical legal/forensic assessments, a classification according to the degree of objectivity of the clinical data (assessed and reported) is of interest. Thanks to the understanding of an expert technologist in insurance litigation, it has been possible to identify objective information in the case study, such as the presence of a contracture, column alterations, the WDQ, the characterization of the traffic accident (in case such an event had occurred), etc.

The initial database is presented as Supplementary Material File S1, which collects the dataset that has been considered for the development of the model.

### *3.3. Stage 3: Data Transformation*

Once the data to be considered in the initial database have been selected, certain transformations of the data must be performed in order to handle empty values, perform data transformations to define the required variables and adapt them to the required format, and ensure the anonymization of the data.

The information obtained from the different sources can correspond to variables already defined and structured or to raw data, and it can be presented as numerical, text, curves, images, etc. [47]. Transforming raw data into the format required for the application of specific ML algorithms is a common pre-processing step to be performed, and it could also be useful because the volume of data to be handled could be reduced, and its predictive power could be significantly increased, making it possible to have a significantly lower volume of data to achieve a reliable and stable predictive model [5,19]. To be exploited by traditional DM and ML algorithms, textual data can be transformed into structured variables and different text mining techniques can be applied [48,49]. Besides, depending on the purpose, unsupervised learning approaches can be applied on the texts—for example, for dimensionality reduction (e.g., using the Self-Organizing Map (SOM) method [50]), for clustering documents according to their similarity, or for discovering topics in documents (e.g., probabilistic topic modeling by using Latent Dirichlet allocation) [51].

This stage of transformation of raw data is known as feature engineering and is performed prior to modelling [52]. In some cases, several data mining techniques can be applied to extract features from raw data. For example, Principal Component Analysis (PCA), like the SOM method mentioned above, is a dimensionality reduction method that is often used to reduce the dimensionality of large data sets; it can be used to tackle the problem of high dimensionality that appears in some projects when the number of variables is excessively high compared to the total number of samples (see Section 3.5) [39]. In the field of healthcare, the following types of transformations can be highlighted:

- Texts that become "positive or negative opinions", concepts, dates, values, etc., through the application of text mining techniques [53,54].

- Images of medical tests that are converted into binary variables related to a pathology or other binary representations.
- Curves or other graphical representations from which information can be extracted as statistical variables, such as the mean, standard deviation, skewness, quartiles, etc.
- Different imputation techniques [18,55–57] that can be applied in order to fill empty values, either by means of interpolation or by using other procedures. Alternatively, some records may need to be discarded (e.g., if several key data values are missing).
- The potential addition or creation of variables based on the knowledge of clinical experts and technologists, either as a combination of existing variables or based on experience acquired in similar studies [30].
- Data anonymization, applied in order to preserve the privacy of patients [58]. The trade-off between privacy and information loss should be considered. A detailed analysis of data anonymization techniques for health data is out of the scope of this work but, for illustration purposes, some examples of transformations that can be applied to guarantee the privacy of sensitive information are:

    - Transformation of continuous variables (e.g., age, size, weight, income, etc.) into ordinal variables by defining suitable ranges. Normalization (e.g., min-max normalization) or standardization (z-score scaling) techniques could also be applied to transform the quantitative variables into variables in the range from 0 to 1.
    - Transformation of qualitative variables (e.g., diagnosis, treatment, education level, etc.), that could be classified, according to a scale, into ordinal variables (e.g., severity of diagnosis, treatment risks, range of studies ("high school", "BS", "MS", "PhD"), etc.). In this way, these variables cannot be associated with a specific patient, thus preserving the patient's privacy.
    - Transformation of qualitative variables (e.g., nationality, physical description, address, etc.), that could not be classified according to a scale into groups (e.g., by continents or country grouping, by groups according to a general description, by postal code, etc.) so that these variables cannot be associated with a specific patient.
    - The previous anonymization techniques are examples of the generalization of attribute values. Other possible techniques and privacy-preservation methodologies include adding noise [59], k-anonymity [60], differential privacy [61], etc.

Another important aspect to mention here is the need for the normalization of quantitative attributes; if we have quantitative variables with very different scales, the variables that can take larger values could end up dominating others when learning a predictive model. This is unsuitable because it mistakenly attributes more importance to those variables just because their usual values are higher than the values of other variables.

After applying the specified transformations, the initial database is transformed to an encoded (modified) database, which includes all the available information in the format of multiple variables.

**Application to Our Case Study**

In the case of the cervical pain assessment study, this process consisted of transforming the data from the MoCap sensors into variables (i.e., mean, deviation, maximum, minimum, etc., of the range of the movement) and transforming the clinical and characterization data of the patients into variables considering sensitive variables and their anonymization. Some ranges of variables were associated with a numeric coding to improve the anonymization process and the generation of the predictive model. The process was carried out jointly by a clinical expert and a technologist. As in our case study we have transformed all the quantitative variables into discrete variables, no additional normalization was needed. The following are examples of the transformations performed (the numeric coding used is indicated in brackets):

- Age transformation in a three-tier classification: under 30 (0), between 30 and 55 (1), and over 55 (2).
- Transformation of the level of weekly exercise into a classification of three levels as a function of the time required and the intensity of the exercise: slight (0), moderate (1), and intense (2).
- Transformation of the level of studies in a classification of three levels with their assigned numerical coding: basic/high school (0), medium/bachelor (1), and superior/university studies (2).
- Weight transformation in a three-tier classification: less than 60 Kg (0), between 60 and 85 Kg (1), and greater than 85 Kg (2).
- Height transformation in a three-level classification: less than 158 cm (0), between 158 and 185 cm (1), and greater than 185 cm (2).
- Transformation of the body mass index (BMI) into a three-tier classification: under 24 (0), between 24 and 30 (1), and over 30 (2).
- Grouping of the cervical pain periodicity to create a variable of three levels: sporadic (0), discontinuous (1), and frequent (2).

The completeness and quality of the data recorded is also a key aspect in any ML pipeline, and particularly in the health area. In our case study, some variables were initially incomplete, due to the lack of collected data from certain patients (five patients). These incomplete data were related to specific features (e.g., the workplace of the patient, his/her age, the dominant side of his/her body, the date of the traffic accident, etc.), and were later collected by a telephone call.

The encoded database is presented as Supplementary Material File S2, where the variables are obtained after the transformations that are carried out from the initial database are collected and the anonymized variables are highlighted (see Variable_View).

### 3.4. *Stage 4: Data Selection*

The next stage is to filter the encoded database obtained in the previous phase and select the most useful variables, applying different filters in a way that will lead to obtaining a filtered database, which will be the basis of the predictive model. Possible successive filters to be used include the following:

1. Filters due to ethical and legal issues: Discard personal or private variables and those that are unimportant for the purpose of the predictive model, such as names, clinical history numbers, telephone numbers, and addresses. The filtered database must be anonymous with respect to existing regulations on the protection of personal data, so a previous anonymization process becomes essential in order to keep as much important data as possible. Notice that during the previous step (data transformation, see Section 3.3), some data are transformed to increase privacy; in this step, privacy might need to be further increased by not selecting some sensitive data in case those data have not been properly transformed previously or in the case of other sensitive data that are irrelevant for predictions.
2. Manual selection: Screening based on the needs set by the target of the prediction, removing outliers or variables with a lot of missing data [5]. It is highly recommended that this filtering be conducted by an expert in the healthcare field.
3. Automated attribute selection: specific software and algorithms can be used for filtering, calculating the gain ratio for each of the variables and rejecting those with low predictive power—for example, using regression techniques.

#### Application to Our Case Study

In our case study, the encoded database initially included 230 variables in the initial dataset (the "Coded database"), which were reduced to 28 after the following consecutive filtering steps (see Table 2):

1. The removal of variables related to personal and ethical data not anonymized previously and with no predictive power. The variables name, surname, telephone number, address, and email were removed in this filtering.
2. Manual filtering performed by physicians and technologists, corresponding to non-objective or inappropriate variables in the medical legal/forensic field (e.g., the sensation of instability, mobility limitation, pain periodicity, etc.), as well as variables with missing data that could not be completed (e.g., the position of the head and type of effect in case of a traffic accident, intensity of work, etc.). In this filtering, 74 variables were removed according to the criteria indicated.
3. Finally, a filtering was applied based on the gain ratio of the variables. We used the IBM SPSS modeler software [62] (v. 18), discarding 123 variables with low predictive power (we selected those with a gain ratio higher than 0.95 out of 1). Variables such as the average angle, standard deviation, complementary angle, weight, height, etc., were selected. The selection of these 28 variables is consistent with the target variable (the presence or absence of pain) and its associated requirements, since it is a desirable situation for clinicians that these variables are objective, represent the main cervical movements, and correspond to clinical data objectively acquired by the clinicians.

**Table 2.** Final variables considered in the case study after feature selection.

| **Patient Characterization Data** | **Gender** | **Age** | **Educational Level** | |
|---|---|---|---|---|
| **Clinical data: assessed and reported data** | Contracture | Traffic accident | Spinal column alterations | WDQ |
| **Clinical data: data measured with sensors** | Mean Speed [°/s] in: | Flex.-Ext. | Rotation | Lateralization |
| | Max Speed [°/s] in: | Flexion | Right Rotation | Right Lateral |
| | | Extension | Left Rotation | Left Lateral |
| | Max Angle [°] in: | Flexion | Right Rotation | Right Lateral |
| | | Extension | Left Rotation | Left Lateral |
| | Total Range [°] in: | Flex.-Ext. | Rotation | Lateralization |
| | Total Length [°] in: | Flex.-Ext. | Rotation | Lateralization |

Table 2 shows the 28 final variables of the filtered database; the detailed information of each variable, with the different associated values for the different data instances, is included as Supplementary Material File S3.

### *3.5. Stage 5: Predictive Model Generation and Evaluation*

In the next stage, a predictive model according to the established objective is designed based on the filtered database obtained in the previous stage. To do this, we must select those algorithms that are considered viable for the specific clinical project, such as decision trees, neural networks, or support vector machines (SVM), among others [63]. If the volume of data is very high, the use of specific support software can facilitate selecting a suitable algorithm by performing iterations before generating the full predictive model. For example, the IBM SPSS modeler classifier node (v. 18) can create several models and then compare them to select the best approach for a particular analysis.

In this stage, the performance of the selected algorithms should be tested to choose the most convenient one to implement in the predictive model. To evaluate their stability and effectiveness, different cross-validation approaches can be considered [19,30,64–66]. The simplest method consists of separating the sample into two sub-samples: one to train the model and another one to test it (holdout method). Other more advanced methods include dividing the sample into k sub-samples (k-fold cross validation), stratifying the sample with the same percentage of each class (stratified k-fold cross validation), or even making as many combinations as the number of data instances (leave-one-out cross validation). Furthermore, a validation set could be used (besides the "test set" and the "training set"), which is a set of examples used to tune the parameters of a classifier [67]. This is useful because the performance of the selected algorithms can be improved through parameter tuning, which consists of varying values of parameters of the algorithms in order to find the most suitable configuration for each of them. Once the suitable parameter configuration for each algorithm is selected, the performance of the different algorithms can be compared.

It must be stressed that the most appropriate prediction method depends on the data. Besides, overfitting (a phenomenon that occurs when the adjustment of the model to the training data is too strong and, as a consequence, finds difficulties in obtaining suitable conclusions about unobserved data) should be avoided, as this would lead to a model that will only be able to make predictions for the data with which it has been trained [52]. There are several techniques to deal with this, such as regularization (smoothing the models), data augmentation (increasing the training data), early stopping, etc. As an example, early stopping implies that the training process of the model must be stopped before overfitting [30,68,69], that is, before the model adjusts too much to the training data (i.e., before the performance of model gets worse on the validation data).

Over-parametrization is a recurrent problem in the application of ML techniques in healthcare, where there are cases where the ratio between variables and data is very high and overfitting effects can occur. The opposite can also happen when the volume of data is very high, but the number of variables is excessively reduced and/or has little predictive power. Therefore, if needed, depending on the results obtained we could come back to Stage 4 "Data Selection" to reduce the number of variables. As a guideline, to avoid over-parametrization the 1 to 10 ratio between variables (attributes or features) and data (number of instances) should not be exceeded [20,52]. If there was a smaller ratio between the variables and data, a more exhaustive screening of variables would have to be carried or a larger sample would have to be obtained. In terms of classification, having an excessive number of variables will lead to not solving the problem or not achieving the proposed objective because the model will only be able to classify the training data correctly [70].

To select the most suitable algorithm for the project, it is necessary to follow an organization strategy, storing each previous version and modification of the project [52]. In this way, the results are contrasted (training data, validation, errors, etc.). After the selection of the most effective algorithm, we will be able to generate the definitive predictive model that incorporates the already-existing filtered database. If the predictive model were evaluated positively, a continuous learning process could begin by receiving periodic information from the assessment tests performed on future patients, as shown in Figure 3.

### Application to Our Case Study

In view of the target of our clinical study to classify the presence of cervical pain, only supervised learning algorithms must be selected, dismissing unsupervised learning algorithms. The algorithms selected in our study were logistic regression [71], decision trees [72], random forests [73], SVM [73], neural networks (MLP neural networks) [74], k-Nearest Neighbors (KNN) [73], and Gradient Boosting Algorithm (GBA) [75]. All these are popular supervised machine learning approaches. The main parameters selected to perform the parameter tuning of those algorithms are shown in Table 3. In our experimental evaluation, we combined the parameters of each algorithm presented in Table 3 using the software tool Weka [76] (v. 3.8); specifically, for the parameter tuning we used the Weka Experimenter user interface.

**Table 3.** ML approaches considered and their main parameters.

| Approach | Main Parameters |
|---|---|
| **Logistic regression** | Ridge value in the log-likelihood: from $10^{-4}$ to $10^{-12}$ (parameter change every $10^{-2}$). |
| **Decision tree (C4 pruned)** | Number of instances per leaf: 3/5/10/15/20. Confidence factor for pruning (Conf.): 0.15/0.25/0.35. |
| **Random forest** | Maximum depth of the tree: 3/4/5. Number of trees: 25/50/100/200. |
| **Support vector machine (SVM)** | Tolerance: $10^{-3}$. Kernel function: radial basis function (RBF). Epsilon for round-off error: $10^{-12}$. Complexity (C): 0.25/0.5/1/2/4. Gamma (kernel width): 0.01/0.25/0.5/1/2. |
| **Neural Network (MLP neural network)** | Type: multilayer perceptron (MLP). Learning Rate (LR, the amount the weights are updated): 0.2/0.3/0.4/0.5. Momentum (Mom., applied to the weights during updating): 0.1/0.2/0.3. Number of epochs for training: 500. Number of hidden layers: 15. Auto-built option in Weka set to true. |
| **K-Nearest Neighbors (KNN)** | Number of Neighbors (K): 1/3/5/7/9/11/13/15/20. Distance function: Euclidean distance, Manhattan distance. |
| **Gradient Boosting Algorithm (GBA)** | Iterations (Iter.): 10/20/50/100. Weight threshold (W.T.): 50/100/200. AdaBoost implementation provided by Weka. |

In our case study, the predictive models generated by applying the previously selected algorithms are shown in Table 3. As mentioned previously, the DM software used in this study was Weka (v. 3.8). Considering the current availability of data for our case study, the performance of each parameter configuration of each algorithm was tested using a validation set which is the same as the test set; using the same set for validation and testing is not the ideal situation, but we decided not to reserve a part of the available dataset for validation because of the moderate size of our sample. We considered the accuracy metric (i.e., the percentage of instances correctly classified) for determining the most suitable algorithm configuration. Figure 5 shows the performance of the algorithms obtained during parameter tuning using a k-fold cross validation (k = 10).

Consequently, the parameter configuration selected for each algorithm is shown in the first row of Table 4. The effectiveness of the models generated by k-fold cross validation (k = 10) was evaluated. The following metrics were computed in order to determine the most suitable algorithms (see Table 4): the accuracy (the percentage of instances correctly classified), the precision (the percentage of patients with pain correctly classified over all the patients labelled by the algorithms as patients with pain), the recall/sensitivity (the percentage of patients with pain correctly classified over all the patients with real pain), the specificity (the percentage of healthy patients correctly classified over all the patients who are really healthy), and the F1-score (the harmonic average of the precision and recall).

We have noticed using the software Weka, which provides the attribute weights of each model in the results display section, that the variables with greater predictive power in all the predictive models evaluated are the following: maximum speed in all the movements, the existence of a traffic accident, and the presence of a contracture. In our case study, there is no indication of over-parametrization; as described in Section 3.4, we have a sample of 302 instances and 28 selected variables, which complies with the 1 to 10 ratio between the variables and data.

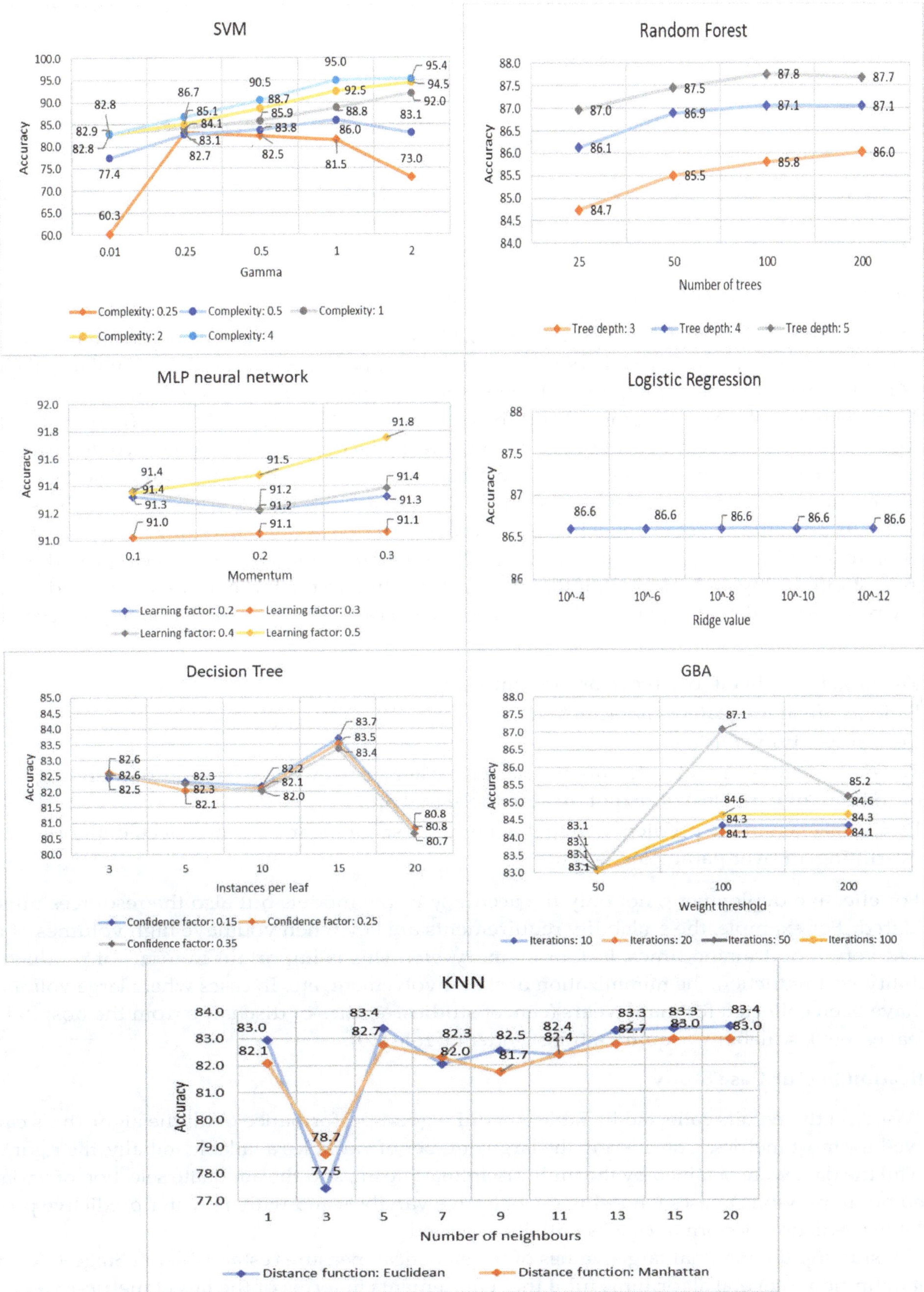


**Figure 5.** Parameter tuning of the seven algorithms selected.

**Table 4.** Metrics considered for algorithm selection and the results obtained for each algorithm.

| | Logistic Regression | SVM | Decision Tree | Random Forest | MLP Neural Network | KNN | GBA |
|---|---|---|---|---|---|---|---|
| **Parameter Selection** | Ridge: $10^{-8}$ | C: 4; Gamma: 2 | Instances per leaf: 15; Conf.: 0.15 | Trees: 200 Depth: 5 | LR: 0.5; Mom.: 0.3 | K: 20; Euclidean | Iterat.: 50 W.T.:100 |
| **Accuracy** | 86.6% | 95.4% | 83.7% | 87.7% | 91.8% | 83.4% | 87.1% |
| **Precision** | 88.6% | 95.4% | 86.9% | 86.1% | 93% | 83.5% | 87.1% |
| **Recall/Sensitivity** | 89.6% | 97.8% | 84.1% | 92.3% | 92.5% | 91.2% | 92.9% |
| **Specificity** | 82.5% | 91.7% | 80.8% | 76.6% | 90.5% | 71.7% | 78.3% |
| **F1 Score** | 89.1% | 95.3% | 85.5% | 88.9% | 92.8% | 83.2% | 86.9% |

### *3.6. Stage 6: Interpretation of Results and Model Selection*

Once a statistically acceptable predictive model has been created, it can be deployed to be used in production, since it can provide predictions with good accuracy to support decision-making (Figure 4, stage 6). However, for the exploitation of the model, it is necessary first to evaluate the degree of correlation between the results obtained and the previously defined clinical target (in our case study, the prediction of cervical pain). Besides, some models (e.g., the tree-based classifiers) could be explored to analyze which particular features are the most decisive factors in the classification model.

If the evaluation of the correlation does not yield satisfactory results—that is, if the consonance of the results with the target is not achieved or the model does not have enough predictive power according to the minimum goals established initially—the previous stages must be repeated with the objective of improving and optimizing the process according to the target initially set, leading to an iterative process (see Figure 4) [20,77]. There can be several causes of low correlation or poor predictive power:

- The target is difficult to achieve or too complex;
- Patients are inadequately characterized;
- The sample is insufficient;
- The data include variables that are not necessary (e.g., irrelevant variables, confounding factors, or redundant variables) or do not include those that are;
- Problems exist in the predictive model generation stage regarding the selected algorithm [78], overfitting, or over-parameterization.

For effective deployment, not only the accuracy of the models but also the resources must be considered. For example, the scalability requirements are key when you have high volumes of data to avoid very long training times, lack of memory, etc. This is important in terms of productivity, portability, cost reduction, the minimization of staff involvement, etc. In cases where large volumes of data have been collected for many years (cancer studies, studies of discharge from the hospital and sick leaves, etc.), scalability acquires a transcendental role [30].

**Application to Our Case Study**

Based on the results collected in Table 4, a quite good performance of all the algorithms can be observed for most metrics. Considering the large number of variables available initially, the rigor with which all the data were obtained by the multidisciplinary team, and the adequate selection of variables carried out in previous phases (choosing the objective variables and with a greater predictive power), a suitable prediction performance was initially expected.

Considering the minimal target values of the statistical measures established in Stage 1 "Clinical target definition", several algorithms fulfil the requirements in terms of the target metrics:

- Accuracy (>85%): logistic regression, SVM, random forest, MLP neural network, and GBA.
- Precision (>85%): logistic regression, SVM, decision tree random forest, MLP neural network, and GBA.

- Recall (>90%): SVM, random forest, MLP neural network, kNN, and GBA.

According to the results, the four algorithms that fulfil the requirements are SVM, random forest, the MLP neural network, and GBA. From all these algorithms, SVM achieves the best results in all the metrics considered, and therefore it could be the model selected for production.

### 3.7. *Stage 7: Operating Profit and Clinical Use*

The last stage (Figure 4, stage 7) concerns the adaptation and organization of the acquired knowledge and the predictive capacity of the system to make it accessible to the physician [47]. At this point, it is important to emphasize the key role played by the expert medical professionals (final decision makers) in interpreting the results, in determining whether certain patterns observed make medical sense and are relevant, or in clearly distinguishing between correlation and causality (as studied for different heath topics [79,80]). The "intelligence" provided is not intended to replace the physician but to advise and guide his/her decisions, which will always prevail [20].

#### Application to Our Case Study

The results obtained directly by the model may involve difficulties when interpreted by the physicians. That is why the information presented to them must be intuitive, simple, and easily interpretable. In this regard, a concise graphic and clear report, where the results of the test and the prediction of the pathology/target variable to be predicted are presented, can help the clinical to more easily interpret the test performed and the results of the predictive model. This paper is accompanied by a report example as Supplementary Material File S4, showing a possible example of a report for our case study that includes patient data, test results in a tabular and graphic format, and an area showing the prediction of cervical pain obtained by the model.

Once the model enters production, it will be possible to add data regarding new patients both with or without cervical pain and verified diagnosis, which would increase the sample and thus the predictive power.

## 4. Discussion and Lessons Learnt

In this paper, the particularities of applying ML techniques in the field of healthcare are shown, developing all the stages that comprise it, to generate reliable and stable models. It has been exemplified through a case study of cervical pain evaluation, where we have been able to predict the presence of cervical pain with accuracy, precision, and recall above 85% with the approaches based on SVM, random forest, MLP neural networks, and GBA.

In order to clarify and structure the knowledge acquired during the development of the current study, a summary of some key aspects and lessons learnt regarding DM and ML in the field of healthcare is shown in Table 5. Every key aspect has been categorized in a general classification, followed by a description, the real situation exemplified in our case study, and some important related references.

**Table 5.** Summary of the key aspects and lessons learnt.

| Category | Key Aspect | Description | Case Study | Sample References |
|---|---|---|---|---|
| **Clinical target** | Proper selection | Clinical target definition according to the aims and clinical needs. This facilitates the subsequent selection of data. | Presence of cervical pain. Only collaborating subjects and objective variables were selected. | [34,40] |
| | Definition of statistical measures | Minimum metrics to be fulfilled by the model according to the clinical target. Metrics are checked in stage 6 (interpretation of results) after the predictive model generation. | Performance required: accuracy: greater than 85%; precision: greater than 85%; recall: greater than 90%. | [39] |

**Table 5.** *Cont.*

| Category | Key Aspect | Description | Case Study | Sample References |
|---|---|---|---|---|
| Data | Identification and understanding | Diversity of the origins of data in healthcare (regarding typology, consistency, and veracity) and need to correctly understand the data. A health expert is required in this stage. | Prior to the field work, relevant clinical information was identified and the tests to perform were determined. | [34] |
| | Clear and concise structure | Categorization of data using appropriate variables/features, applying classifications motivated by medical needs. This is essential to carry out an adequate analysis of the information. | Data classification motivated by clinical staff and forensic experts: patient characterization data, assessed and reported clinical data, measured clinical data. | [30] |
| | Data transformations in healthcare | Feature engineering. Reducing the raw data to be handled and adapting them to the required format in order to increase the predictive power. | Variables such as the age, level of studies, weight, height, etc., were transformed into discrete variables. Ranges of variables were associated with a numeric code. | [5,19,47,52] |
| | Anonymization | Preservation of sensitive patient data by transforming values of data variables into scales or groups, thus avoiding patient identification. This is a key aspect in healthcare data management. | No quantitative variables remained after the anonymization process (through transformation into discrete variables and the removal of identifying attributes) that could be associated with patients. | [58] |
| | Selection | After data transformation, the selection of variables applying a filter according to the target:ethical and legal issues, manual selection, automated attribute selection. | The volume of data in the case study was reduced from 230 variables to 28 after applying the three successive aforementioned filters. | [19,21] |
| | Normalization | Normalization of quantitative attributes avoiding situations where variables that can take larger values could end up dominating others. | No quantitative variables remained after anonymization. | [55–57] |
| | Completeness | Completeness and quality of the data recorded as a key aspect in the health area. | Incomplete data from 5 patients related to specific features were collected through a telephone call. | [81] |
| | Over-parametrisation | Need not to exceed the 1 to 10 ratio between variables and data to avoid overfitting. The dimensionality is an issue in studies with a high number of variables compared to the total number of samples. | This was a real issue in our case study because of the volume of data provided by sensors. A sample of 302 and 28 variables was finally selected, which complies with the 1 to 10 ratio. | [20] |

**Table 5.** *Cont.*

| Category | Key Aspect | Description | Case Study | Sample References |
|---|---|---|---|---|
| | Scalability | Support for handling large amounts of data (efficient and effective collection, storage, management, and exploitation). Depending on the project duration, and especially if it is intended to have an adaptive character (projects with data collected for many years), scalability is a key issue to consider. | The current project is still in an initial stage, with no large-scale deployment. No scalability problems have been detected. | [30] |
| **Predictive model** | High recall and relatively high precision | Minimization of the number of false negatives (increasing recall). This is a key goal in healthcare, since false negatives and false positives have no similar costs in this area. The precision should also be suitable, as a high number of false positives would lead to false alarms, the performance of needless procedures, and increasing costs and discomfort for the patients. | The selected algorithms (SVM, random forest, MLP neural network, and GBA) have recall >90%. | [39] |
| **Project work procedure** | Multidisciplinary work as a key point | Composing teams involving technical people and diverse health professionals. This is required, but not always possible. Insufficient collaboration could be diminished by applying the stages assigned to each of the professionals in a concise and structured way. | There was interaction between professionals in almost all the stages. Nevertheless, more interventions could be encouraged because clinical experts were not present in stage 5. | [34,52] |
| | Continuous data collection | Improvement of the model performance thanks to a continuous learning process. | There is an intention to improve the current system by incorporating data of new collaborating patients. | [30] |
| **MoCap** | Sensors/devices in healthcare | Complementary objective tests to help physicians. | We expect the applicability of the proposal in the forensic field as an objective system of application to aid in judicial processes. | [19,82] |

**Data structuring.** A clear and concise structuring of the data is essential to carry out an adequate analysis of the information as well as to make this information really useful for the purposes of the predictive model. In our case study, and prior to the field work, the relevant clinical information was identified and the tests to perform were determined (cervical ROM in three different planes with a MoCap system of inertial sensors), so that its processing and subsequent structuring were easier. It is essential to accurately structure the available information in a suitable way (using appropriate variables/features) when working with large volumes of data, and to classify the different variables in different groups (using appropriate categories) to facilitate access (for all the parties involved) in a more effective and useful way. Data management is so important that the preparation of the data covers three of the seven stages of the methodology (stages 2, 3, and 4).

**Selection of variables.** Likewise, the selection of the most adequate information to predict a certain characteristic, as well as its transformation in terms of variables, is essential. In relation to this adaptation, sensitive patient data must be anonymized for their use in the generation of a predictive model [19,21]. Although converting continuous predictors to discrete variables (specifically binary variables) is not always recommended [20], the necessary transformation of data for privacy reasons in the field of health conditions the stage of data transformation. The reduction in the volume of data in the case study was from 230 variables to 28 due to the large number of variables provided by the inertial sensors and the clinical data. The variable reduction applied (based on the gain ratio of the variables) after the corresponding selection of the data for ethical and legal issues and the screening made by an expert was necessary to fulfil the 1 to 10 ratio between the variables and data. This key point allowed us to ensure that the predictive models work properly, maximizing the predictive power and avoiding overfitting.

**Selection of the predictive model.** Regarding the selection of the predictive model, after performing a parameter tuning of the seven selected algorithms and comparing the most suitable configuration of each of them (see Figure 5), it was concluded that the models that meet the established requirements regarding accuracy, precision, and recall for the case study were SVM, random forest, MLP neural networks, and GBA. Our results highlight the low number of false negatives achieved (high recall), a fundamental aspect in healthcare studies [39]. These results are in agreement with other investigations of a similar nature, using the same software (Weka), in terms of the accuracy, precision, recall, and F1 score with the SVM and random forest algorithms [36].

**Variability of the measures acquired.** It has been detected that it is possible to assess the measurement capacity of our medical equipment in terms of the variability of the measures that it obtains. A *series* variable identifies whether the data are relative to the first measure of each subject or to the second (which was performed consecutively). The results obtained by the predictive models showed that there were no differences between the two series of cervical ROM (this variable had the lowest predictive power among all the variables introduced in the model). This result indicates that the measure has behaved stably in collaborating subjects. This result is interesting in the forensic field due to the following reason. If repeating the cervical ROM test in a patient results in significant differences, they would not be derived from the variability of the test, but by the type of pathology that prevents the patient from repeating the test normally. Alternatively, the patient may try to simulate or magnify the lesion by not showing consistent results between the first and second series. This aspect would be of relevance to judicial experts [29,83].

**Data collection in production.** Once the system is applied in its context and has been developed, continuous data collection must be planned in production in order to improve the prediction accuracy, resulting in a continuous learning system (Figure 3). In the case study, to increase the sample in the exploitation stage of the model it is possible to include those patients who perform cervical assessment tests in a care or rehabilitation setting; thus, their sincerity can be assumed regarding the degree of cervical pain as well as full collaboration in the performance of the tests. However, for the collection of training data it may be necessary to exclude those patients who are immersed in a judicial and indemnifying process and who report cervical pain because their degree of collaboration or sincerity is unknown. In the future, the system can be used to predict the cervical pain of non-collaborating patients (e.g., patients in a judicial process or patients with a high degree of anxiety or hypochondriacs) from the predictive model previously generated with collaborating patients, serving as objective evidence in judicial proceedings with insurance companies [40].

**Multidisciplinarity.** For a correct interpretation of the results, multidisciplinary work is a key point, since the contribution of each of the branches of knowledge is necessary in this type of project to optimize the possibilities offered by the model. In this way, it will be possible to assess the statistical quality of the results and their medical utility. For example, in our case study questions were raised regarding the way the data and the results should be represented (solved with the databases defined and the design of a report for physicians, presented as Supplementary Material), the possible interpretation and use of the system by the clinician (problems could have arisen if we had not been worked in close collaboration with the clinicians; however, the target variable and how to present the results were clarified from the beginning of the project), and the overlap with other possible decision-support systems (if other systems could also provide in the future a prediction indicating that a patient suffers cervical pain, both results would be presented to the clinician and he/she would take the final decision). Through collaboration with the medical experts, these issues have been solved. However, multidisciplinary work is not always possible, since professionals participate in different stages of the entire process according to their degree of knowledge, experience, and training, so in some cases there may be no direct or sufficient interaction between them [34]. This lack of interaction among professionals could be diminished by following the stages assigned to each of the professionals in a concise and structured way, thus avoiding problems that may lead to project failure [52]. In the case study, the rigor followed by the different professionals involved in the different stages have resulted in adequate results. Nevertheless, although there has been interaction between them, it could have been done in a more collaborative way, since clinical experts were not present in the generation of the predictive model and the interpretation of the results, which could have improved the quality of the study thanks to its specific medical knowledge.

**Exploitation of sensor data.** The use of sensors and devices with the use of ML could be implemented as a complementary objective test to help physicians. This type of test could constitute an aid to the decision-making in the diagnosis or treatment, or if there is doubt about the veracity of the information reported by the patient [19,82]. Although we wanted to show the clinical utility of this type of technology, the lack of studies on the application of ML techniques with motion capture sensors in healthcare, and specifically their applicability in the forensic field as an objective system of application in judicial processes, have further motivated the choice of the case study. Therefore, while our case study focuses on the medical legal/forensic field, the procedure proposed to use ML techniques could be applied in any study of the health field (cancer detection, studies of discharge from the hospital and sick leave, etc.).

**Use of resources.** Regarding the frequency and regularity of data acquisition, it is necessary to previously estimate it to limit the duration of the project [34], as well as to quantify the necessary storage size, which is a factor with high variability between projects. If the project is intended to have an adaptive character that can be applied or expanded for subsequent research, the scalability and magnitude should be considered. If the scalability of the project is not considered, and the intention is to continue acquiring data and adapting the model to the continuous growth of information, there may come a time when the project is no longer viable because it is unable to assimilate the corresponding increase in data size. This situation is common in epidemiological projects of data collection for large periods of time, where the scalability is transcendental for the future of the project [30]. On the other hand, it is important to consider that, in certain projects as in the case study presented in this paper, the ratio between available variables and data can be high. So, not exceeding the 1 to 10 ratio between variables and data is transcendental to avoid overfitting effects [20].

## 5. Conclusions and Future Work

Through a practical guide, the stages and particularities to consider for the application of ML techniques in the field of healthcare have been described, considering all the stages involved in the process. This procedure is shown through objective cervical functional assessment tests that use MoCap technology with inertial sensors and a predictive model whose goal is to estimate the presence of cervical pain from the data collected with the test. Four models (SVM, random forest, MLP neural network, and GBA) from the seven models initially generated obtained an accuracy and precision of more than 85% and a recall of more than 90% (i.e., the percentage of false negatives is smaller than 10%). The approach and the results obtained could help objectify diagnoses, improve test treatment efficacy, and save resources in healthcare systems. The procedure, which has been applied to data derived from a cervical assessment study for verification and evaluation, is also appropriate for any healthcare field regardless of the origin of the data. It can be useful, for example, in gait studies [82], balance studies [84], cardiac failure studies [85], the prediction of events [86], fertility tests [87], etc.

Despite the great usefulness of ML in the field of healthcare, some limitations have been detected in this field. First, a major limitation is how to achieve a suitable flow of data from health centers and hospitals, as well as the accessibility (in relation to privacy policies and authorizations) [21], gathering, and integration of the data [3]. If a global information collaboration policy were established between hospitals [6,69,88], the problem of access to information could be solved, and it would be possible to share more data and feed the predictive models applied to the field of healthcare more efficiently. The explainability of predictions [89,90] is an important issue in a health care domain, as it could increase the trust in the ML systems (for both clinicians and patients) and even lead to the acquisition of new knowledge; however, more research on how to achieve explainability while considering the potential trade-off with accuracy must be performed, especially in the health domain.

Regarding the limitations of the conclusions obtained with this case study, once the model is in the exploitation stage it would be advisable to carry out an external validation to verify the viability of the model in terms of geography, temporality, etc. [30,77]. Regarding the data sample used in our case study, its size has been large enough to obtain good results, but it would be relevant to see the impact of increasing it, as new data about patients becomes available, to enable a continuous learning process that could lead to better results over time. Besides, a study is currently being conducted to check the accuracy of the proposed models with a sample of non-collaborating patients.

Concerning the target variable (presence of cervical pain), which is a binary variable, it could be defined in a more granular way considering not only the presence of pain but also its intensity (as a continuous variable or as a discrete variable with several pain degrees). The problem with pain intensity is that pain scales are highly dependent on the subjectivity of the patient, and this issue could be further exacerbated with non-collaborating subjects. However, as a future goal of our research, it could be useful to tackle this issue and introduce some statistical techniques, such as the numerical measurement z-score, to normalize the subjective values from pain intensity scales (e.g., the Visual Analogue Scale) provided by the patients. The z-score could help to reduce the bias of patients, allowing us to include pain intensity as a target variable in our proposal.

Finally, as future work, it could also be interesting to extend the range of experiments performed and analyze the potential interest of other ML methods; for example, we could consider applying different classifiers applied over different categories of data proposed in the paper and combine them into an ensemble.

**Author Contributions:** Conceptualization, J.d.l.T., J.M., S.I., and J.J.M.; data curation, J.d.l.T., J.M., and J.J.M.; formal analysis, J.d.l.T., J.M., S.I., and J.J.M.; funding acquisition, S.I. and J.J.M.; investigation, J.d.l.T.; methodology, J.d.l.T., J.M., and J.J.M.; project administration, J.J.M.; resources, S.I. and J.J.M.; software, J.d.l.T. and J.J.M.; supervision, S.I. and J.J.M.; validation, J.d.l.T.; visualization, J.d.l.T.; writing—original draft preparation, J.d.l.T., J.M., and J.J.M.; writing—review and editing, J.d.l.T., J.M., S.I., and J.J.M. All authors have read and agreed to the published version of the manuscript.

**Acknowledgments:** We thank Mapfre insurance company (Zaragoza, Spain) for allowing us to use their facilities. We also thank the I3A—University Institute of Research of Engineering of Aragon, University of Zaragoza, Zaragoza, Spain—for the materials and support they provided.

## Abbreviations

The following abbreviations are used in this manuscript:

| | |
|---|---|
| BMI | Body Mass Index |
| CEICA | Bioethics Committee of Aragón |
| CRISP-DM | CRoss-Industry Standard Process for Data Mining |
| DLA | Daily life activities |
| DM | Data Mining |
| EMG | Surface Electromyography |
| GBA | Gradient Boosting Algorithm |
| KDD | Knowledge Discovery in Databases |
| KNN | K-Nearest Neighbors |
| MAE | Mean Absolute Error |
| ML | Machine Learning |
| MLP | MultiLayer Perceptron |
| MoCap | Motion Capture |
| PCA | Principal component analysis |
| RMSE | Root Mean Squared Error |
| ROM | Range of Movement |
| SEMMA | Sample, Explore, Modify, Model, and Assess |
| SVM | Support Vector Machine |
| WDQ | Whiplash Scale |

## References


1. Kayyali, B.; Knott, D.; Van Kuiken, S. *The Big-Data Revolution in US Health Care: Accelerating Value and Innovation*; Mc Kinsey Co.: New York, NY, USA, 2013; Volume 2, pp. 1–13.
2. Tomar, D.; Agarwal, S. A survey on Data Mining approaches for Healthcare. *Int. J. Bio-Sci. Bio-Technol.* **2013**, *5*, 241–266. [CrossRef]
3. Koh, H.C.; Tan, G. Data mining applications in healthcare. *J. Healthc. Inf. Manag.* **2011**, *19*, 65.
4. Maity, N.G.; Das, S. Machine learning for improved diagnosis and prognosis in healthcare. In Proceedings of the 2017 IEEE Aerospace Conference, Big Sky, MT, USA, 4–11 March 2017; pp. 1–9.
5. Yoo, I.; Alafaireet, P.; Marinov, M.; Pena-Hernandez, K.; Gopidi, R.; Chang, J.-F.; Hua, L. Data Mining in Healthcare and Biomedicine: A Survey of the Literature. *J. Med. Syst.* **2012**, *36*, 2431–2448. [CrossRef]
6. Sen, I.; Khandelwal, K. Data Mining in Healthcare. 2018. Available online: https://www.researchgate.net/publication/322754945_DATA_MINING_IN_HEALTHCARE (accessed on 26 August 2020).
7. Clavel, D.; Mahulea, C.; Albareda, J.; Silva, M. A Decision Support System for Elective Surgery Scheduling under Uncertain Durations. *Appl. Sci.* **2020**, *10*, 1937. [CrossRef]
8. Cruz, J.A.; Wishart, D.S. Applications of Machine Learning in Cancer Prediction and Prognosis. *Cancer Inform.* **2006**, *2*, 59–77. [CrossRef]
9. Wang, F.; Stiglic, G.; Obradovic, Z.; Davidson, I. Guest editorial: Special issue on data mining for medicine and healthcare. *Data Min. Knowl. Discov.* **2015**, *29*, 867–870. [CrossRef]
10. Rosales, R.E.; Rao, R.B. Guest Editorial: Special Issue on impacting patient care by mining medical data. *Data Min. Knowl. Discov.* **2010**, *20*, 325–327. [CrossRef]
11. Alotaibi, S.; Mehmood, R.; Katib, I.; Rana, O.; Albeshri, A. Sehaa: A Big Data Analytics Tool for Healthcare Symptoms and Diseases Detection Using Twitter, Apache Spark, and Machine Learning. *Appl. Sci.* **2020**, *10*, 1398. [CrossRef]
12. Huang, Z.; Dong, W.; Bath, P.; Ji, L.; Duan, H. On mining latent treatment patterns from electronic medical records. *Data Min. Knowl. Discov.* **2015**, *29*, 914–949. [CrossRef]
13. Bentham, J.; Hand, D.J. Data mining from a patient safety database: The lessons learned. *Data Min. Knowl. Discov.* **2012**, *24*, 195–217. [CrossRef]
14. Obenshain, M.K. Application of Data Mining Techniques to Healthcare Data. *Infect. Control. Hosp. Epidemiol.* **2004**, *25*, 690–695. [CrossRef] [PubMed]
15. Zhang, P.; Wang, F.; Hu, J.; Sorrentino, R. Towards Personalized Medicine: Leveraging Patient Similarity and Drug Similarity Analytics. *AMIA Summits Transl. Sci. Proc.* **2014**, *2014*, 132. [PubMed]
16. Hamet, P.; Tremblay, J. Artificial intelligence in medicine. *Metab. Clin. Exp.* **2017**, *69*, S36–S40. [CrossRef] [PubMed]

17. Joyner, M.J.; Paneth, N. Seven Questions for Personalized Medicine. *JAMA* **2015**, *314*, 999–1000. [CrossRef]
18. Weiss, J.C.; Natarajan, S.; Peissig, P.L.; McCarty, C.A.; Page, D. Machine Learning for Personalized Medicine: Predicting Primary Myocardial Infarction from Electronic Health Records. *AI Mag.* **2012**, *33*, 33–45. [CrossRef]
19. Mannini, A.; Sabatini, A.M. Machine Learning Methods for Classifying Human Physical Activity from On-Body Accelerometers. *Sensors* **2010**, *10*, 1154–1175. [CrossRef]
20. Moons, K.; Kengne, A.P.; Woodward, M.; Royston, P.; Vergouwe, Y.; Altman, U.G.; Grobbee, D.E. Risk prediction models: I. Development, internal validation, and assessing the incremental value of a new (bio)marker. *Heart* **2012**, *98*, 683–690. [CrossRef]
21. Wilkowska, W.; Ziefle, M. Privacy and data security in E-health: Requirements from the user's perspective. *Heal. Inform. J.* **2012**, *18*, 191–201. [CrossRef]
22. Dolley, S. Big Data Solution to Harnessing Unstructured Data in Healthcare. IBM Report. 2015. Available online: https://assets.sourcemedia.com/31/a6/cb1b019c4d6cb338fab539eea360/ims14428usen.pdf. (accessed on 26 August 2020).
23. Andersen, R.M.; Davidson, P.L.; Baumeister, S.E. Improving access to care. In *Changing the US Health Care System: Key Issues in Health Services Policy and Management*; John Wiley & Sons: Hoboken, NJ, USA, 2013; pp. 33–70.
24. Marin, J.; Blanco, T.; Marin, J.J. Research Lines to Improve Access to Health Instrumentation Design. *Procedia Comput. Sci.* **2017**, *113*, 641–646. [CrossRef]
25. Cassidy, J.D.; Carroll, L.; Côté, P.; Lemstra, M.; Berglund, A.; Nygren, Å. Effect of Eliminating Compensation for Pain and Suffering on the Outcome of Insurance Claims for Whiplash Injury. *N. Engl. J. Med.* **2000**, *342*, 1179–1186. [CrossRef]
26. Moreno, A.J.; Utrilla, G.; Marin, J.; Marin, J.J.; Sanchez-Valverde, M.B.; Royo, A.C. Cervical Spine Assessment with Motion Capture and Passive Mobilization. *J. Chiropr. Med.* **2018**, *17*, 167–181. [CrossRef] [PubMed]
27. Utrilla, G.; Marín, J.J.; Sanchez-Valverde, B.; Gomez, V.; JAuria, J.M.; Marin, J.; Royo, C. *Cervical Mobility Testing in Flexion-Extension and Protraction-Retraction to Evaluate Whiplash Syndrome Through Motion Capture*; Universidad de Zaragoza: Zaragoza, Spain, 2017.
28. Marín, J.J.; Pina, M.J.B.; Gil, C.B. Evaluación de Riesgos de Manipulación Repetitiva a Alta Frecuencia Basada en Análisis de Esfuerzos Dinámicos en las Articulaciones sobre Modelos Humanos Digitales. *Cienc. Trab.* **2013**, *15*, 86–93. [CrossRef]
29. Marín, J.; Boné, M.; Ros, R.; Martínez, M. Move-Human Sensors: Sistema portátil de captura de movimiento humano basado en sensores inerciales, para el análisis de lesiones musculoesqueléticas y utilizable en entornos reales. In Proceedings of the Sixth International Conference on Occupational Risk Prevention, Galicia, Spain, 14–16 May 2008.
30. Steyerberg, E.W. *Clinical Prediction Models: A Practical Approach to Development, Validation, and Updating*; Springer: Berlin, Germany, 2009.
31. Fayyad, U.M.; Piatetsky-Shapiro, G.; Smyth, P.; Uthurusamy, R. *Advances in Knowledge Discovery and Data Mining*; AAAI Press: Menlo Park, CA, USA, 1996.
32. Azevedo, A.I.R.L.; Santos, M.F. KDD, SEMMA and CRISP-DM: A Parallel Overview. ISCAP—Informática—Comunicações em Eventos Científicos. 2008. Available online: https://recipp.ipp.pt/handle/10400.22/136 (accessed on 26 August 2020).
33. Chapman, P.; Clinton, J.; Kerber, R.; Khabaza, T.; Reinartz, T.; Shearer, C.; Wirth, R. *CRISP-DM 1.0 Step-by-Step Data Mining Guide*; SPSS Inc.: Chicago, IL, USA, 2000.
34. McGregor, C.; Catley, C.; James, A. A process mining driven framework for clinical guideline improvement in critical care. In Proceedings of the Learning from Medical Data Streams Workshop, Bled, Slovenia, 6 July 2011.
35. Catley, C.; Smith, K.; McGregor, C.; Tracy, M. Extending CRISP-DM to incorporate temporal data mining of multidimensional medical data streams: A neonatal intensive care unit case study. In Proceedings of the 2009 22nd IEEE International Symposium on Computer-Based Medical Systems, Albuquerque, NM, USA, 3–4 August 2009; pp. 1–5.
36. Araujo, F.H.; Santana, A.M.; Neto, P.S. Using machine learning to support healthcare professionals in making preauthorisation decisions. *Int. J. Med. Inform.* **2016**, *94*, 1–7. [CrossRef]
37. Bose, I.; Mahapatra, R.K. Business data mining—A machine learning perspective. *Inf. Manag.* **2001**, *39*, 211–225. [CrossRef]

38. Bhatla, N.; Jyoti, K. An analysis of heart disease prediction using different data mining techniques. *Int. J. Eng.* **2012**, *1*, 1–4.
39. Raschka, S.; Mirjalili, V. *Python Machine Learning*; Packt Publishing Ltd.: Birmingham, UK, 2017.
40. Schuller, E.; Eisenmenger, W.; Beier, G. Whiplash Injury in Low Speed Car Accidents: Assessment of Biomechanical Cervical Spine Loading and Injury Prevention in a Forensic Sample. *J. Musculoskelet. Pain* **2000**, *8*, 55–67. [CrossRef]
41. Naumann, F. Data profiling revisited. *ACM SIGMOD Rec.* **2014**, *42*, 40–49. [CrossRef]
42. Rahm, E.D.H. Data Cleaning: Problems and Current Approaches. *Bull. Tech. Comm. Data Eng.* **2000**, *23*, 3–13.
43. Jannot, A.-S.; Zapletal, E.; Avillach, P.; Mamzer, M.-F.; Burgun, A.; Degoulet, P. The Georges Pompidou University Hospital Clinical Data Warehouse: A 8-years follow-up experience. *Int. J. Med. Inform.* **2017**, *102*, 21–28. [CrossRef]
44. Evans, R.S.; Lloyd, J.F.; Pierce, L.A. Clinical Use of an Enterprise Data Warehouse. *AMIA Annu. Symp. Proc.* **2012**, *2012*, 189–198.
45. Batista, G.E.A.P.A.; Prati, R.C.; Monard, M.C. A study of the behavior of several methods for balancing machine learning training data. *ACM SIGKDD Explor. Newsl.* **2004**, *6*, 20–29. [CrossRef]
46. Batista, G.E.A.P.A.; Prati, R.C.; Monard, M.C. Balancing Strategies and Class Overlapping. *Lect. Notes Comput. Sci.* **2005**, *3646*, 24–35. [CrossRef]
47. Bhardwaj, R.; Nambiar, A.R.; Dutta, D. A Study of Machine Learning in Healthcare. *2017 IEEE 41st Annu. Comput. Softw. Appl. Conf.* **2017**, *2*, 236–241. [CrossRef]
48. Dörre, J.; Gerstl, P.; Seiffert, R. Text mining: Finding nuggets in mountains of textual data. In Proceedings of the Fifth ACM SIGKDD International Conference on Knowledge Discovery and Data Mining (KDD), San Diego, CA, USA, 23–27 August 1999; pp. 398–401.
49. Aggarwal, C.C.; Zhai, C. *Mining Text Data*; Springer Science & Business Media: Berlin, Germany, 2012.
50. Janasik, N.; Honkela, T.; Bruun, H. Text mining in qualitative research: Application of an unsupervised learning method. *Organ. Res. Methods* **2009**, *12*, 436–460. [CrossRef]
51. Blei, D.M. Probabilistic topic models. *Commun. ACM* **2012**, *55*, 77–84. [CrossRef]
52. Henri, L. *Data Scientist y Lenguaje R Guía de Autoformación Para el uso de Big Data*; Francisco, J., Piqueres, J., Eds.; Colecciones Epsilon: Cornellá de Llobregat, Spain, 2017.
53. Stavrianou, A.; Andritsos, P.; Nicoloyannis, N. Overview and semantic issues of text mining. *ACM SIGMOD Rec.* **2007**, *36*, 23–34. [CrossRef]
54. Carlos, T.; Sergio, I.; Carlos, S. Text Mining of Medical Documents in Spanish: Semantic Annotation and Detection of Recommendations. In Proceedings of the 16th International Conference on Web Information Systems and Technologies (WEBIST 2020), Budapest, Hungary, 3–5 November 2020.
55. Donders, A.R.T.; Van Der Heijden, G.J.; Stijnen, T.; Moons, K.G. Review: A gentle introduction to imputation of missing values. *J. Clin. Epidemiol.* **2006**, *59*, 1087–1091. [CrossRef]
56. Farhangfar, A.; Kurgan, L.; Dy, J. Impact of imputation of missing values on classification error for discrete data. *Pattern Recognit.* **2008**, *41*, 3692–3705. [CrossRef]
57. Bennett, D.A. How can I deal with missing data in my study? *Aust. N. Z. J. Public Health* **2001**, *25*, 464–469. [CrossRef]
58. Arbuckle, L.; El Emam, K. *Anonymizing Health Data*; O'Reilly Media, Inc.: Newton, MA, USA, 2013.
59. Kargupta, H.; Datta, S.; Wang, Q.; Sivakumar, K. On the privacy preserving properties of random data perturbation techniques. In Proceedings of the Third IEEE International Conference on Data Mining, Melbourne, FL, USA, 19–22 November 2003; pp. 99–106.
60. El Emam, K.; Dankar, F.; Issa, R.; Jonker, E.; Amyot, D.; Cogo, E.; Corriveau, J.-P.; Walker, M.; Chowdhury, S.; Vaillancourt, R.; et al. A globally optimal k-anonymity method for the de-identification of health data. *J. Am. Med. Inform. Assoc.* **2009**, *16*, 670–682. [CrossRef]
61. Dankar, F.K.; El Emam, K. The application of differential privacy to health data. *Jt. EDBT/ICDT Workshops EDBT-ICDT* **2012**, *2012*, 158–166. [CrossRef]
62. IBM. SPSS Software. Available online: https://www.routledge.com/IBM-SPSS-Statistics-26-Step-by-Step-A-Simple-Guide-and-Reference/George-Mallery/p/book/9780367174354 (accessed on 16 February 2020).
63. Wu, X.; Kumar, V.; Quinlan, J.R.; Ghosh, J.; Yang, Q.; Motoda, H.; McLachlan, G.J.; Ng, A.; Liu, B.; Yu, P.; et al. Top 10 algorithms in data mining. *Knowl. Inf. Syst.* **2007**, *14*, 1–37. [CrossRef]

64. Gupta, P. Cross Validation in Machine Learning. 2020. Available online: https://towardsdatascience.com/cross-validation-in-machine-learning-72924a69872f (accessed on 26 August 2020).
65. Arlot, S.; Celisse, A. A survey of cross-validation procedures for model selection. *Stat. Surv.* **2010**, *4*, 40–79. [CrossRef]
66. Refaeilzadeh, P.; Tang, L.; Liu, H. Cross-Validation. *Encycl. Database Syst.* **2009**, *5*, 532–538.
67. Xu, Y.; Goodacre, R. On Splitting Training and Validation Set: A Comparative Study of Cross-Validation, Bootstrap and Systematic Sampling for Estimating the Generalization Performance of Supervised Learning. *J. Anal. Test.* **2018**, *2*, 249–262. [CrossRef] [PubMed]
68. McCaffrey, J. Neural Network Train-Validate-Test Stopping. 2020. Available online: https://visualstudiomagazine.com/articles/2015/05/01/train-validate-test-stopping.aspx (accessed on 26 August 2020).
69. Ferber, R.; Osis, S.T.; Hicks, J.L.; Delp, S.L. Gait biomechanics in the era of data science. *J. Biomech.* **2016**, *49*, 3759–3761. [CrossRef] [PubMed]
70. Reed, R.; MarksII, R.J. *Neural Smithing: Supervised Learning in Feedforward Artificial Neural Networks*; Mit Press: Cambridge, MA, USA, 1999.
71. Christodoulou, E.; Ma, J.; Collins, G.S.; Steyerberg, E.W.; Verbakel, J.Y.; Van Calster, B.; Evangelia, C.; Jie, M. A systematic review shows no performance benefit of machine learning over logistic regression for clinical prediction models. *J. Clin. Epidemiol.* **2019**, *110*, 12–22. [CrossRef]
72. Bae, J.M. The clinical decision analysis using decision tree. *Epidemiol. Health* **2014**, *36*. [CrossRef] [PubMed]
73. Noi, P.T.; Kappas, M. Comparison of Random Forest, k-Nearest Neighbor, and Support Vector Machine Classifiers for Land Cover Classification Using Sentinel-2 Imagery. *Sensors* **2018**, *18*, 18. [CrossRef]
74. Penny, W.; Frost, D.; Penny, W. Neural Networks in Clinical Medicine. *Med. Decis. Mak.* **1996**, *16*, 386–398. [CrossRef]
75. Zhang, Z.; Zhao, Y.; Canes, A.; Steinberg, D.; Lyashevska, O.; AME Big-Data Clinical Trial Collaborative Group. Predictive analytics with gradient boosting in clinical medicine. *Ann. Transl. Med.* **2019**, *7*. [CrossRef]
76. Witten, I.; Frank, E.; Hall, M.; Pal, C. Appendix B: The WEKA workbench. In *Data Mining: Practical Machine Learning Tools and Techniques*, 4th ed.; Morgan Kaufmann: Burlington, MA, USA, 2016.
77. Moons, K.; Kengne, A.P.; Grobbee, D.E.; Royston, P.; Vergouwe, Y.; Altman, U.G.; Woodward, M. Risk prediction models: II. External validation, model updating, and impact assessment. *Heart* **2012**, *98*, 691–698. [CrossRef] [PubMed]
78. Murphy, C.K. Identifying Diagnostic Errors with Induced Decision Trees. *Med. Decis. Mak.* **2001**, *21*, 368–375. [CrossRef] [PubMed]
79. Zhao, L. The gut microbiota and obesity: From correlation to causality. *Nat. Rev. Genet.* **2013**, *11*, 639–647. [CrossRef] [PubMed]
80. Dab, W.; Ségala, C.; Dor, F.; Festy, B.; Lameloise, P.; Le Moullec, Y.; Le Tertre, A.; Médina, S.; Quenel, P.; Wallaert, B.; et al. Air pollution and health: Correlation or causality? The case of the relationship between exposure to particles and cardiopulmonary mortality. *J. Air Waste Manag. Assoc.* **2001**, *51*, 220–235. [CrossRef] [PubMed]
81. Liu, C.; Talaei-Khoei, A.; Zowghi, D.; Daniel, J. Data completeness in healthcare: A literature survey. *Pac. Asia J. Assoc. Inf. Syst.* **2017**, *9*, 5. [CrossRef]
82. Mannini, A.; Trojaniello, D.; Cereatti, A.; Sabatini, A.M. A Machine Learning Framework for Gait Classification Using Inertial Sensors: Application to Elderly, Post-Stroke and Huntington's Disease Patients. *Sensors* **2016**, *16*, 134. [CrossRef]
83. Ramírez, P.C.; Ordi, H.G.; Fernández, P.S.; Morales, M.I.C. Detección de exageración de síntomas en esguince cervical: Pacientes clínicos versus sujetos análogos. *Trauma* **2014**, *25*, 4–10.
84. De La Torre, J.; Marin, J.; Marin, J.J.; Auria, J.M.; Sanchez-Valverde, M.B. Balance study in asymptomatic subjects: Determination of significant variables and reference patterns to improve clinical application. *J. Biomech.* **2017**, *65*, 161–168. [CrossRef]
85. Austin, P.C.; Tu, J.V.; Ho, J.E.; Levy, D.; Lee, D.S. Using methods from the data-mining and machine-learning literature for disease classification and prediction: A case study examining classification of heart failure subtypes. *J. Clin. Epidemiol.* **2013**, *66*, 398–407. [CrossRef]
86. Choi, E.; Bahadori, M.T.; Schuetz, A.; Stewart, W.F.; Sun, J. Doctor AI: Predicting Clinical Events via Recurrent Neural Networks. *JMLR Work. Conf. Proc.* **2016**, *56*, 301–318.

87. Uyar, A.; Bener, A.; Ciray, H.N. Predictive modeling of implantation outcome in an in vitro fertilization setting: An application of machine learning methods. *Med. Decis. Mak.* **2015**, *35*, 714–725. [CrossRef] [PubMed]
88. Abdelaziz, A.; Elhoseny, M.; Salama, A.S.; Riad, A. A machine learning model for improving healthcare services on cloud computing environment. *Measurement* **2018**, *119*, 117–128. [CrossRef]
89. Hall, P.; Gill, N. *An Introduction to Machine Learning Interpretability*; O'Reilly Media, Inc.: Sebastopol, CA, USA, 2018.
90. Guidotti, R.; Monreale, A.; Ruggieri, S.; Turini, F.; Giannotti, F.; Pedreschi, D. A Survey of Methods for Explaining Black Box Models. *ACM Comput. Surv.* **2018**, *51*, 1–42. [CrossRef]

# 9

# Stretched Exponential Survival Analysis for South Korean Females

**Byung Mook Weon** [1,2,3]

[1] Soft Matter Physics Laboratory, School of Advanced Materials Science and Engineering, SKKU Advanced Institute of Nanotechnology (SAINT), Sungkyunkwan University, Suwon 16419, Korea; bmweon@skku.edu
[2] Research Center for Advanced Materials Technology, Sungkyunkwan University, Suwon 16419, Korea
[3] Department of Biomedical Engineering, Johns Hopkins University, Baltimore, MD 21218, USA

**Featured Application: The stretched exponential survival analysis enables quantitative and comparative study of female lifespan between South Korea and other countries, particularly quantifying the survival rate, the characteristic life, and the maximum lifespan.**

**Abstract:** South Korea has recently exhibited a remarkable rapid increase in female lifespan. Here, a mathematical analysis is suggested for a clear interpretation of current trends in female lifespan in South Korea. To mathematically analyze life tables, a modified stretched exponential function is employed and demonstrated to estimate current trends of female lifespan in South Korea based on reliable life tables from 1987 to 2016 taken from the Korean Statistical Information Service. This methodology enables us to perform quantitative and comparative analyses of female lifespan in South Korea with representative industrialized countries such as Japan, France, Australia, Switzerland, UK, Sweden, and USA. This analysis provides quantitative and comparative evidence that South Korea has the highest increase rate of female lifespan over the past three decades. Further application would be feasible for a better estimation of human aging statistics.

**Keywords:** modified stretched exponential function; age-dependent stretched exponent; characteristic life; maximum lifespan; South Korean female

---

## 1. Introduction

Statistical analysis of human lifespan is a central topic in demography and gerontology. Life expectancy of humans has risen steadily and rapidly over the past 150 years in most countries and keeps increasing in the 21st century [1–3]. A recent study of 35 industrialized countries shows an interesting projection: there is more than 50% probability that by 2030, female life expectancy is likely to break the 90-year barrier [4]. Interestingly, South Korea is predicted to have the highest female life expectancy at birth by 2030 [4]. This prediction is achieved by applying a mathematical ensemble of 21 forecasting models to reliable statistics data about life tables for humans [4]. South Korean females are an important model to understand current trends in human lifespan and a better survival analysis is required for a better understanding of human lifespan.

To achieve a more reliable prediction, a mathematical model of human survival curves is helpful in quantifying current trends in human lifespan for human aging and demography research [5–8]. In fact, many mathematical models for survival curves have been proposed, including the Gompertz, Weibull, Heligman-Pollard, Kannisto, quadratic, and logistic models [5]. In a recent work, a mathematical model has been suggested owing to a usefulness to describe survival curves with complexity in shape by adopting a modified function from the stretched exponential (Weibull or Kohlrausch–Williams–Watts) function [9–14]. Flexibility of a modified stretched exponential function, originating from an age-dependent stretched exponent, enables us to mathematically describe plasticity and rectangularity of survival curves [5,13]. In this work, by incorporating this mathematical model to the reliable life table datasets taken from the Korean Statistical Information Service (KOSIS, http://kosis.kr/eng), a practical application is demonstrated to quantify current trends in female lifespan for South Korea over three recent decades, from 1987 to 2016. This analysis for South Korea is compared with that for Japan, France, Australia, Switzerland, UK, Sweden, and USA, which are the representative leading countries in longevity [4].

In this study, a mathematical analysis with a modified stretched exponential model is demonstrated to interpret the recent survival curves for South Korean female, taken from the Korean Statistical Information Service. The current trends for 1987–2016 are estimated from the female survival curves in South Korea based on the estimates of the characteristic life and the maximum lifespan.

## 2. Methods

The stretched exponential survival analysis is summarized as follows. The methodology is based on the modified stretched exponential function to describe the human survival curves, which has been developed for the past decade [5,12–14]. This section briefly introduces into the mathematical approach. The survival rate, $s(x)$, is a function of age, $x$. Mathematically the mortality rate (equivalently the hazard function or the force of mortality), $\mu(x) = -d\ln(s(x))/dx$, is the derivative of the survival rate with respect to age. As a mathematical constraint, $s(x)$ is a monotonic decrease function with age, starting from 1 and ending to 0. To mathematically describe the survival curves, a modified stretched exponential function is quite flexible by applying a form of $s(x) = \exp(-(x/\alpha)^{\beta(x)})$ where the stretched exponent, $\beta(x)$, is an age-dependent term as $\beta(x) = \ln[-\ln(s(x))]/\ln(x/\alpha)$ and the characteristic life, $\alpha$, is a reference age, determined at $s(\alpha) = \exp(-1)$ that equals to the interception point between $s(x)$ and $s(\alpha) = \exp(-1)$ [5,12–14]. The characteristic life is an alternative to the life expectancy at birth, $\varepsilon$ [14,15]. The age dependence of the stretched exponent is the critical feature of the modified stretched exponential function, which is fundamentally different from the classical stretched exponential function [5,12–14]. The characteristic life and the stretched exponent are useful to respectively describe the scale effect (associated with *living longer*, characterized by $\alpha$) and the shape effect (associated with *growing older*, characterized by $\beta(x)$) of the individual survival curve [14]. For old-age patterns, the quadratic formula of $\beta(x) = \beta_0 + \beta_1 x + \beta_2 x^2$ is applicable [5,12], which leads to the occurrence of the (mathematical) maximum lifespan, $\omega$, which is obtained at the age for $\beta(x) = -x\ln(x/\alpha)\frac{d\beta(x)}{dx}$ by the mathematical constraint of $\frac{ds(x)}{dx} \to 0$ [12]. This methodology is beneficial in modeling the human mortality curves in very old age [5].

## 3. Results and Discussion

### 3.1. Survival Analysis

The survival curves for women were obtained at the complete life tables taken from the Korean Statistical Information Service (http://kosis.kr/eng). Figure 1 shows how we evaluate the survival curves for Korean female in the most recent decades, 1987–2016. The summarized survival curves in Figure 1a show the historic trends in the survival rates for Korean female over three recent decades. The survival curves for Korean female show that $s(x)$ gradually decreases with age and historically shifts rightwards and towards a rectangular shape over three recent decades, as consistent with Swedish female [5,14].

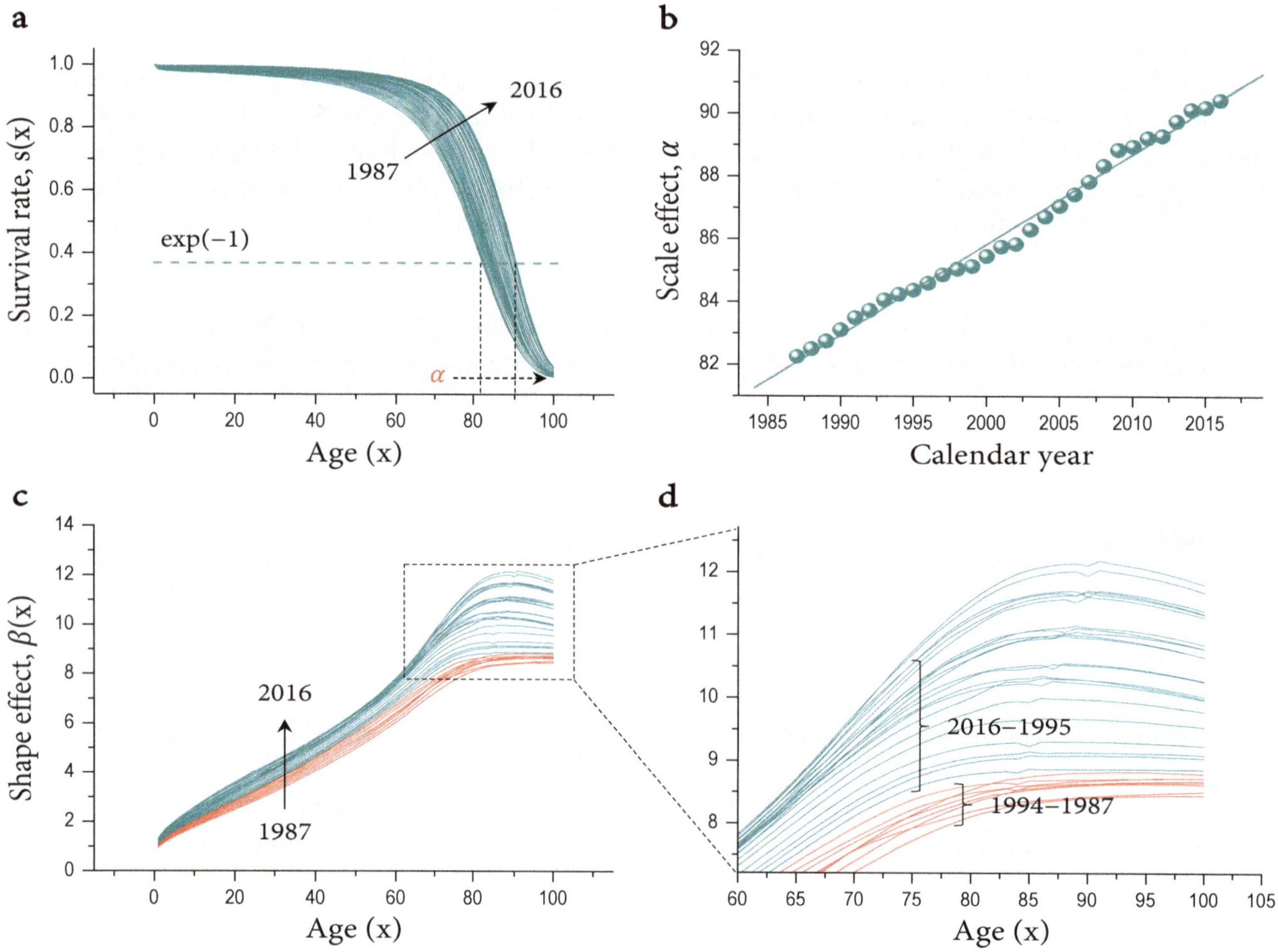


**Figure 1.** Survival analysis. (**a**) The survival curves for Korean female in recent decades, 1987–2016, were obtained at the complete life tables taken from the Korean Statistical Information Service (http://kosis.kr/eng). (**b**) The characteristic life of the given survival curve. (**c**) The age-dependent stretched exponent. (**d**) The old-age patterns of the stretched exponent at ages over 60 years could be fitted with the quadratic formula of age. The phase transition in the stretched exponent with age appears for 1995–2016 but not for 1987–1994.

The characteristic life, $\alpha$, indicating the scale effect of the individual survival curve, was measured for each survival curve through the graphical analysis at $s(\alpha) = \exp(-1) \approx 0.367879$. The recent historic trends in the $\alpha$ values were summarized in Figure 1b. The characteristic life for Korean female was depicted as a function of the calendar year (1987–2016) in Figure 1b. This result shows that the $\alpha$ value linearly increases at a constant rate of $\sim$2.88 years per decade (as marked by the solid line in Figure 1b). This steady increase rate for South Korean female is much higher than the rate of $\sim$1.20 years per decade for Swedish female in the previous analyses (data from the Human Mortality Database, http://www.mortality.org) [5,14]. The historic trends in the characteristic life clearly demonstrate that South Korean women have lived longer in the past three decades.

The $\beta(x)$ value, indicating the shape effect of the individual survival curve, was obtained from $\beta(x) = -x\ln(x/\alpha)\frac{d\beta(x)}{dx}$ as shown in Figure 1c. Particularly as demonstrated in Figure 1d, old-age patterns of $\beta(x)$ at ages over 60 years could be empirically fitted with the quadratic formula as $\beta(x) = \beta_0 + \beta_1 x + \beta_2 x^2$ as suggested previously [5,12,13]. The modified stretched exponential function is successfully applicable to the survival curves and to the age-dependent stretched exponents for all ages (Figure 1c) and for old ages over 60 years (Figure 1d). Most remarkably, the $\beta(x)$ curve smoothly varies with age at old ages over 60 years and old-age $\beta(x)$ patterns over 90 years can be depicted with the quadratic function of age. As found previously, the $\beta(x)$ patterns for old-age populations undergo the phase transition with age: $\beta(x)$ increases with age at $x < \alpha$ and decreases with age at $x > \alpha$ [12]. The phase transition appears in South Korean female datasets after the calendar year of 1995: there are phase transitions for 1995–2016 and no transitions for 1987–1994, as separately marked in Figure 1d. Considering old-age $\beta(x)$ patterns, the female lifespan of South Korea would experience the critical phase change through the calendar year of 1995. The historic trends in age dependence in $\beta(x)$ clearly show how the female lifespan in South Korea has been growing older during 1987–2016.

### 3.2. Characteristic Life Analysis

The comparison in the increase rate of $\alpha$ for South Korea with that for major industrialized countries is shown in Figure 2. The increase rate in $\alpha$ was obtained from Figure 1b for South Korea, 1987–2016 (data from the Korean Statistical Information Service, http://kosis.kr/eng), and from literature [14] for other countries, 1980–2010 (data from the Human Mortality Database, http://www.mortality.org). The error bars were taken from the standard errors by linear fits. The increase rate in $\alpha$ per decade was evaluated as ~2.88 years for South Korea, ~2.71 years for Japan, ~1.96 years for France, ~1.85 years for Australia, ~1.61 years for Switzerland, ~1.49 years for UK, ~1.24 years for Sweden, and ~0.76 years for USA. This analysis result confirms the highest increase rate of the characteristic life for women in South Korea among the representative high-income countries including Japan, France, Australia, Switzerland, UK, Sweden, and USA.

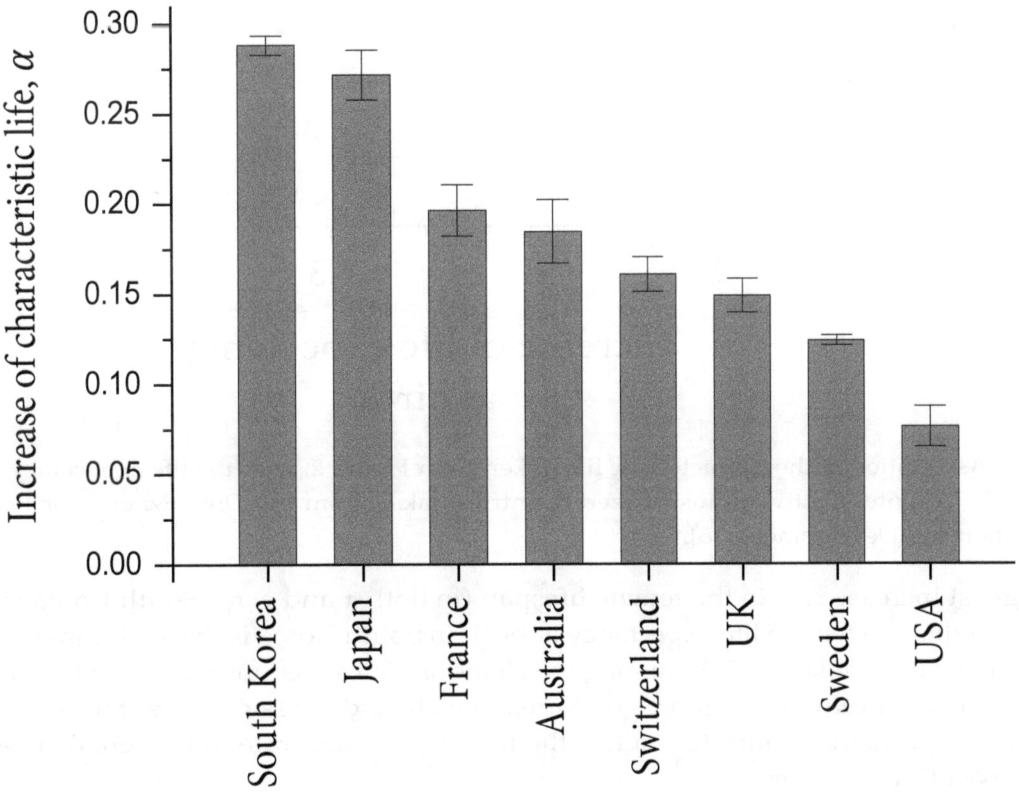


**Figure 2.** Comparison in the increase rate of the characteristic life per decade among representative industrialized countries. The data were taken for South Korea (1987–2016) from the Korean Statistical Information Service (http://kosis.kr/eng) and for other countries (1980–2010) from the Human Mortality Database (http://www.mortality.org).

To demonstrate the association of the characteristic life ($\alpha$), taken from Figure 2, with the life expectancy at birth ($\varepsilon$), the annual increase rates of $\alpha$ and $\varepsilon$ are compared in Figure 3. The $\varepsilon$ values for 1980–2015 were taken from the Organization for Economic Cooperation and Development [16] and the increase rates of the ε values were achieved by linear fits (the error bars taken from the standard errors: some of the error bars are smaller than the symbol sizes). The increase rates of the ε values per decade were evaluated as ~4.15 years for South Korea, ~2.33 years for Japan, ~2.15 years for France, ~1.96 years for Australia, ~1.78 years for Switzerland, ~1.93 years for UK, ~1.43 years for Sweden, and ~1.06 years for USA. The annual increase rate of the ε values (marked by $m$) is proportionally correlated with the annual increase rate of the $\alpha$ values (marked by $n$) as $n \approx 1.173\ m - 0.046$ (adj. $R^2 \sim 0.85243$) except for South Korea. This analysis result suggests that the annual increase rate of the ε values for South Korea looks an extraordinary case among the representative high-income countries.

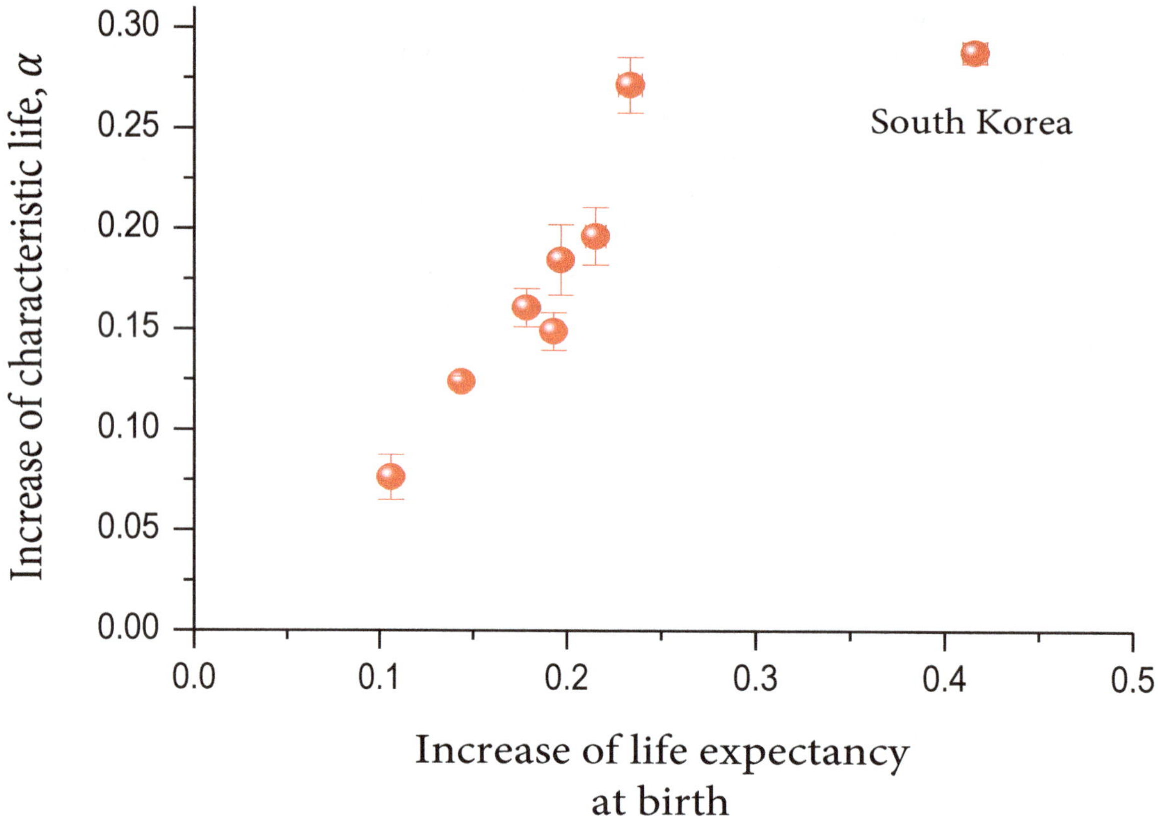


**Figure 3.** Association of the characteristic life, taken from Figure 2, with the life expectancy at birth per decade in representative industrialized countries, taken from the Organization for Economic Cooperation and Development [16].

The highest increase rate in the female lifespan (in both $\alpha$ and ε) for South Korea in Figure 3 is consistent with that the female life expectancy at birth in South Korea is the sixth ranked in 2010 and expected to be the first ranked in 2030 among the 35 industrialized countries [4]. So far, little attention has been given to South Korea in research on human health and longevity except for a few reports [4]. This analysis supports that South Korea has the highest increase rate in the female lifespan in the world in the past three decades.

### *3.3. Maximum Lifespan Analysis*

The term *lifespan* describes how long an individual can live and the (observed) maximum lifespan is the age reached by the longest-lived member of a species, while the life expectancy is a population-based estimate of expected duration of life for individuals at any age, based on a statistical life table [3]. Our methodology enables us to estimate the characteristic life ($\alpha$) and the (mathematical) maximum lifespan ($\omega$) as good measures of the human lifespan. The estimates of $\alpha$ and $\omega$ for Korean female (data from the Korean Statistical Information Service, http://kosis.kr/eng) are summarized in Figure 4. The estimates of $\omega$ are obtained by the mathematical constraint of $\frac{ds(x)}{dx} \to 0$ [5,14]. The fitting of $\beta(x)$ with the quadratic formula enables us to determine the estimates of $\omega$ at the specific age of $\gamma(x) = -x\ln(x/\alpha)\frac{d\beta(x)}{dx}$ which corresponds to the intercept point $\beta(x) = \gamma(x)$ [5]. This estimation is practically available if and only if the phase transition exists in old-age $\beta(x)$ curves. Indeed, the estimates of $\omega$ are significant over the calendar year of 2002, as shown in Figure 4.

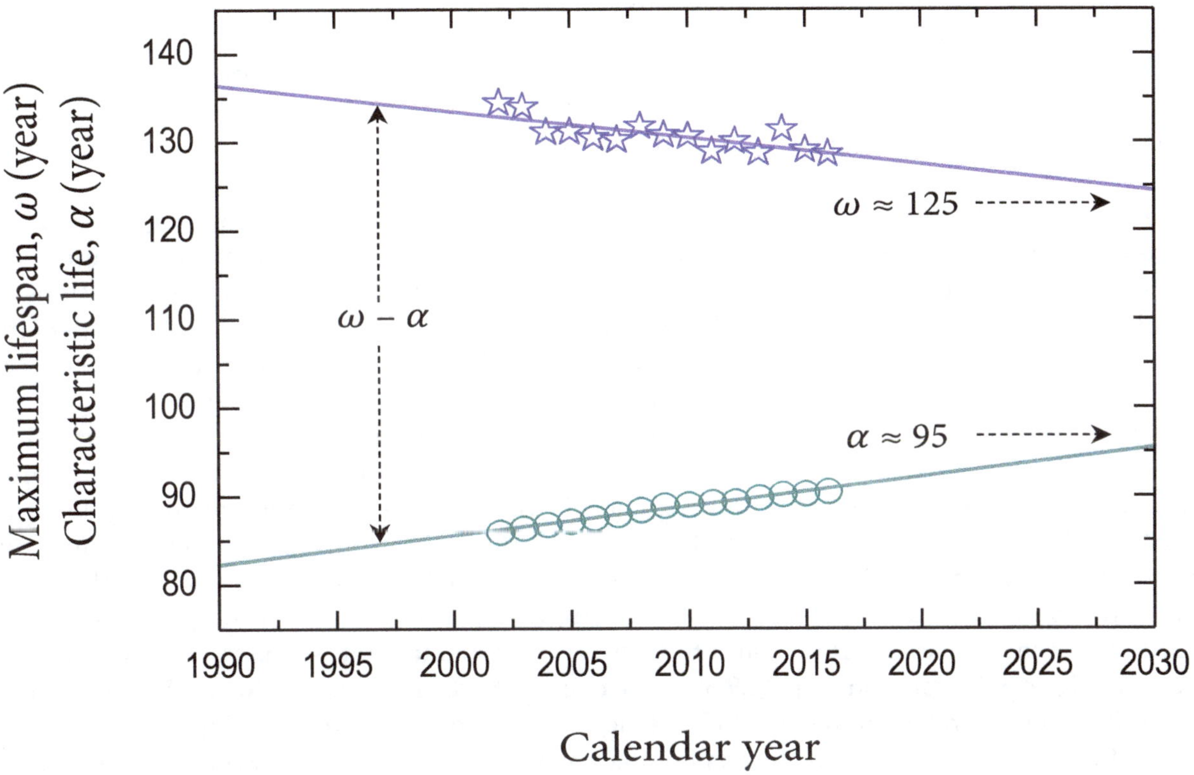


**Figure 4.** Estimation of the maximum lifespan and the characteristic life for Korean female (data from the Korean Statistical Information Service, http://kosis.kr/eng). The maximum lifespan gradually decreases at a constant rate of ~2.99 years per decade and the characteristic life gradually increases at a constant rate of ~3.30 years per decade.

Looking at the recent trends in $\omega$ and $\alpha$ for the South Korean female in Figure 4, the estimates of $\omega$ gradually decrease at a constant rate of ~2.99 years per decade and the estimates of $\alpha$ gradually increase at a constant rate of ~3.30 years per decade. Assuming continuity in the increments, the estimates of $\omega$ and $\alpha$ are predicted to reach ~125 years and ~95 years respectively around 2030. The change rates for South Korean female are much higher than those of ~1.6 years per decade in the $\omega$ values and ~1.2 years per decade in the $\alpha$ values for Swedish female [5]. The estimates of $\omega$ and $\alpha$ eventually become closer together over time: this tendency for South Korean female is consistent with Swedish female [5]. This result indicates that the survival curves have been increasingly concentrated at old ages, demonstrating the population aging [17,18]. As $\alpha$ becomes closer to $\omega$ (Figure 4), the survival curves tend to become strongly concentrated at very old ages, corresponding to the retangularization of survival curves [13,19]. This result would be relevant to the compression of morbidity, which is responsible for the accumulation of the very old populations in the population configuration [5].

### 3.4. Discussion

Now, it is noteworthy that the stretched exponential survival analysis enables the quantitative and comparative study of female lifespan between South Korea and other countries, particularly quantifying the survival rate, the characteristic life, and the maximum lifespan. All evidence suggests that South Korea has a remarkable rapid increase in female lifespan during the three recent decades (from 1987 to 2016), as demonstrated from the characteristic life analysis in Figures 2 and 3. An interesting question is why South Korea exhibits the highest increase rate in female lifespan. Economic development in South Korea is supposed to be beneficial to health care improvement, presumably provoking many potential social or cultural changes that are favorable for healthy daily habits and welfare. Obviously, health is the result of a combination of individual, social, and environmental factors [20]. In general, the recent increase in the numbers of older people in developed countries is a consequence of advances in hygiene and biomedicine as well as an artefact of human civilization [21]. In particular, South Korea has experienced rapid economic development and a substantial increase in life expectancy in an extremely short period, between 1970 and 2010, mainly due to the rapid processes of industrialization and urbanization [22,23].

Specifically, South Korea is expected to become the first country where the life expectancy at birth will exceed 90 years for women [24]. The recent industrialization and the subsequent improvements in living standards, nutrition, and health care have often been cited as major contributions to the remarkable improvements in health for South Korea [25]. The rapid increases in life expectancy in South Korea could be mostly achieved by reductions in infant mortality and in decreases related to infections and blood pressure [25]. More recent gains in South Korea have been largely due to postponement of death from chronic diseases [25]. These gains were mainly due to broad-based inclusive improvements in economic status and social capital (including education), which improved childhood and adolescent nutrition [26], expanded access to primary and secondary health care, and facilitated rapid scale-up of new medical technologies [25]. South Korea has also maintained lower body-mass index and blood pressure than other industrialized countries [27,28], and lower smoking in women. Additionally, South Korea might have lower health inequalities (for cancer and cardiovascular disease mortality, and for self-reported health status) than some of their western counterparts, especially for women [24,29,30]. The death rates from all causes in South Korea decreased significantly in both genders in the last three decades except for a period following the economic crisis in the late 1990s [31]. Looking at the trends in infectious disease mortality for South Korea, 1983—2015, infant mortality caused by infectious diseases has substantially decreased, while death rates from infectious disease for elderly populations with lower education levels and subgroups susceptible to respiratory infections and sepsis has not decreased overall [32]. The potential reasons for South Korea may be plausible but not for other countries.

Finally, the lifespan trends for Korean female may give a clue for the question regarding if there is a biological or social limit to human lifespan [3,33–36]. The heterogeneity in population and the dynamics of heterogeneous populations would become important in interpreting human lifespan [37,38]. The question about whether the upper limit to the maximum lifespan is fixed or flexible has been topics of continuous debate [34,39–45]. The decrease of the $\omega$ estimate in Figure 4 means that more people can reach the biological lifespan limit as expected to be 125 years [12]. The mathematical evaluation for female survival curves would be useful in achieving reliability and reproducibility in aging research [6–8] as well as in demonstrating the effectiveness of anti-aging therapies to slow the aging process [46]. Finding the appropriate mathematical model is quite important to accurately evaluate the human survival curves that exhibit a variety of heterogeneity and complexity. The practical implication of this study is that the potential reasons of South Korea may be useful to improve human lifespan, suggesting a further application of the stretched exponential survival analysis to identify personal, social, and environmental factors on human lifespan.

## 4. Conclusions

A steady increase in female lifespan is obvious in recent decades for most industrialized countries. This study shows the quantitative and comparative evidence for a remarkable rapid increase of female lifespan in South Korea during three recent decades, from 1987 to 2016, by applying the stretched exponential survival analysis. Based on the estimation of the increase rate of female lifespan for South Korea, the comparative analysis with Japan, France, Australia, Switzerland, UK, Sweden, and USA implies that South Korea would have the highest increase rate of female lifespan during recent three decades. This result suggests that Korean female datasets would be a representative population dataset for further study on what contributions would be essential to human longevity. Further application would be feasible for a better estimation of human aging statistics, which will be useful for future population prediction and policy making.

## References


1. Wilmoth, J.R.; Deegan, L.J.; Lundström, H.; Horiuchi, S. Increase of maximum life-span in Sweden, 1861–1999. *Science* **2000**, *289*, 2366–2368. [CrossRef] [PubMed]
2. Oeppen, J.; Vaupel, J.W. Broken limits to life expectancy. *Science* **2006**, *296*, 1029–1031. [CrossRef] [PubMed]
3. Olshansky, S.J. Ageing: Measuring our narrow strip of life. *Nature* **2016**, *538*, 175–176. [CrossRef] [PubMed]
4. Kontis, V.; Bennett, J.E.; Mathers, C.D.; Li, G.; Foreman, K.; Ezzati, M. Future life expectancy in 35 industrialised countries: Projections with a Bayesian model ensemble. *Lancet* **2017**, *389*, 1323–1335. [CrossRef]
5. Weon, B.M. A solution to debates over the behavior of mortality at old ages. *Biogerontology* **2015**, *16*, 375–381. [CrossRef] [PubMed]
6. Petrascheck, M.; Miller, D.L. Computational analysis of lifespan experiment reproducibility. *Front. Genet.* **2017**, *8*, 92. [CrossRef] [PubMed]
7. Ruby, J.G.; Smith, M.; Buffenstein, R. Naked mole rat mortality rates defy Gompertzian laws by not increasing with age. *eLife* **2018**, *7*, e31157. [CrossRef] [PubMed]
8. Beltrán-Sánchez, H.; Finch, C. Life expectancy: Age is just a number. *eLife* **2018**, *7*, e34427. [CrossRef] [PubMed]
9. Weibull, W.A. A statistical distribution function of wide applicability. *J. Appl. Mech.* **1951**, *18*, 293–297.
10. Kohlrausch, R. Theorie des elektrischen rückstandes in der leidener flasche. *Pogg. Ann. Phys. Chem.* **1854**, *91*, 179–214. [CrossRef]
11. Williams, G.; Watts, D.C. Non-symmetrical dielectric relaxation behavior arising from a simple empirical decay function. *Trans. Faraday Soc.* **1970**, *66*, 80–85. [CrossRef]
12. Weon, B.M.; Je, J.H. Theoretical estimation of maximum human lifespan. *Biogerontology* **2009**, *10*, 65–71. [CrossRef] [PubMed]
13. Weon, B.M.; Je, J.H. Plasticity and rectangularity in survival curves. *Sci. Rep.* **2011**, *1*, 104. [CrossRef] [PubMed]
14. Weon, B.M.; Je, J.H. Trends in scale and shape of survival curves. *Sci. Rep.* **2012**, *2*, 504. [CrossRef] [PubMed]
15. Wrycza, T.; Baudisch, A. The pace of aging: Intrinsic time scales in demography. *Demogr. Res.* **2014**, *30*, 1571–1590. [CrossRef]
16. OECD. *Health at a Glance 2017: OECD Indicators*; OECD Publishing: Paris, France, 2017. [CrossRef]
17. Anderson, G.F.; Hussey, P.S. Population aging: A comparison among industrialized countries. *Health Aff.* **2000**, *19*, 191–203. [CrossRef] [PubMed]
18. Robine, J.M.; Michel, J.P. Looking forward to a general theory on population aging. *J. Gerontol. A Biol. Sci. Med. Sci.* **2004**, *59*, 590–597. [CrossRef]
19. Fries, J.F. Aging, natural death, and the compression of morbidity. *N. Engl. J. Med.* **1980**, *303*, 130–135. [CrossRef]
20. Shkrabtak, N.; Frolova, N.; Kiseleva, T.; Sergeeva, I.; Pomozova, V. Impact of environmental conditions on the health of the Far Eastern region population. *Appl. Sci.* **2019**, *9*, 1354. [CrossRef]

21. Hayflick, L. The future of ageing. *Nature* **2000**, *408*, 267–269. [CrossRef]
22. Kim, I.K.; Liang, J.; Rhee, K.O.; Kim, C.S. Population aging in Korea: Changes since the 1960s. *J. Cross Cult. Gerontol.* **1996**, *11*, 369–388. [CrossRef] [PubMed]
23. Bahk, J.; Lynch, J.W.; Khang, Y.H. Forty years of economic growth and plummeting mortality: The mortality experience of the poorly educated in South Korea. *J. Epidemiol. Community Health* **2017**, *71*, 282–288. [CrossRef] [PubMed]
24. Khang, Y.H.; Bahk, J.; Yi, N.; Yun, S.C. Age- and cause-specific contributions to income difference in life expectancy at birth: Findings from nationally representative data on one million South Koreans. *Eur. J. Public Health* **2016**, *26*, 242–248. [CrossRef] [PubMed]
25. Yang, S.; Khang, Y.H.; Harper, S.; Davey Smith, G.; Leon, D.A.; Lynch, J. Understanding the rapid increase in life expectancy in South Korea. *Am. J. Public Health* **2010**, *100*, 896–903. [CrossRef] [PubMed]
26. NCD-RisC. A century of trends in adult human height. *eLife* **2016**, *5*, e13410. [CrossRef] [PubMed]
27. NCD-RisC. Trends in adult body-mass index in 200 countries from 1975 to 2014: A pooled analysis of 1698 population-based measurement studies with 19.2 million participants. *Lancet* **2016**, *387*, 1377–1396. [CrossRef]
28. NCD-RisC. Worldwide trends in blood pressure from 1975 to 2015: A pooled analysis of 1479 population-based measurement studies with 19.1 million participants. *Lancet* **2017**, *389*, 37–55. [CrossRef]
29. Di Cesare, M.; Khang, Y.H.; Asaria, P.; Blakely, T.; Cowan, M.J.; Farzadfar, F.; Guerrero, R.; Ikeda, N.; Kyobutungi, C.; Msyamboza, K.P.; et al. Inequalities in non-communicable diseases and effective responses. *Lancet* **2013**, *381*, 585–597. [CrossRef]
30. OECD. *Health at a Glance 2015: OECD Indicators*; OECD Publishing: Paris, France, 2015. [CrossRef]
31. Lim, D.; Ha, M.; Song, I. Trends in the leading causes of death in Korea, 1983–2012. *J. Korean Med. Sci.* **2014**, *29*, 1597–1603. [CrossRef]
32. Choe, Y.J.; Choe, S.A.; Cho, S.I. Trends in infectious disease mortality, South Korea, 1983–2015. *Emerg. Infect. Dis.* **2018**, *24*, 320–327. [CrossRef]
33. Carnes, B.A.; Witten, T.M. How long must humans live? *J. Gerontol. A Biol. Sci. Med. Sci.* **2014**, *69*, 965–970. [CrossRef]
34. Dong, X.; Milholland, B.; Vijg, J. Evidence for a limit to human lifespan. *Nature* **2016**, *538*, 257–259. [CrossRef] [PubMed]
35. Newman, S.; Easteal, S. The dynamic upper limit of human lifespan [version 1; referees: 1 approved, 1 approved with reservations]. *F1000Research* **2017**, *6*, 569. [CrossRef] [PubMed]
36. Marck, A.; Antero, J.; Berthelot, G.; Saulière, G.; Jancovici, J.M.; Masson-Delmotte, V.; Boeuf, G.; Spedding, M.; Le Bourg, E.; Toussaint, J.F. Are we reaching the limits of homo sapiens? *Front. Physiol.* **2017**, *8*, 812. [CrossRef] [PubMed]
37. Carnes, B.A.; Olshansky, S.J. Heterogeneity and its biodemographic implications for longevity and mortality. *Exp. Gerontol.* **2001**, *36*, 419–430. [CrossRef]
38. Vaupel, J.W. Biodemography of human ageing. *Nature* **2010**, *464*, 536–542. [CrossRef]
39. Ben-Haim, M.S.; Kanfi, Y.; Mitchel, S.J.; Maoz, N.; Vaughan, K.; Amariglio, N.; Lerrer, B.; de Cabo, R.; Rechavi, G.; Cohen, H.Y. Breaking the ceiling of human maximal lifespan. *J. Gerontol. A Biol. Sci. Med. Sci.* **2018**, *73*, 1465–1471. [CrossRef]
40. Brown, N.J.L.; Albers, C.J.; Ritchie, S.J. Contesting the evidence for limited human lifespan. *Nature* **2017**, *546*, E6–E7. [CrossRef]
41. De Beer, J.; Bardoutsos, A.; Janssen, F. Maximum human lifespan may increase to 125 years. *Nature* **2017**, *546*, E16–E17. [CrossRef]
42. Hughes, B.G.; Hekimi, S. Many possible maximum lifespan trajectories. *Nature* **2017**, *546*, E8–E9. [CrossRef]
43. Lenart, A.; Vaupel, J.W. Questionable evidence for a limit to human lifespan. *Nature* **2017**, *546*, E13–E14. [CrossRef] [PubMed]
44. Rozing, M.P.; Kirkwood, T.B.L.; Westendorp, R.G.J. Is there evidence for a limit to human lifespan? *Nature* **2017**, *546*, E11–E12. [CrossRef] [PubMed]
45. Rootzen, H.; Zholud, D. Human life is unlimited–but short. *Extremes* **2017**, *20*, 713–728. [CrossRef]
46. De Magalhães, J.P.; Stevens, M.; Thornton, D. The business of anti-aging science. *Trends Biotechnol.* **2017**, *35*, 1062–1073. [CrossRef] [PubMed]

# 10

# Realizing an Integrated Multistage Support Vector Machine Model for Augmented Recognition of Unipolar Depression

**Kathiravan Srinivasan [1], Nivedhitha Mahendran [1], Durai Raj Vincent [1], Chuan-Yu Chang [2,*] and Shabbir Syed-Abdul [3,4,*]**

1 School of Information Technology and Engineering, Vellore Institute of Technology (VIT), Vellore 632 014, India; kathiravan.srinivasan@vit.ac.in (K.S.); nivedhitha.m2019@vitstudent.ac.in (N.M.); pmvincent@vit.ac.in (D.R.V.)
2 Department of Computer Science and Information Engineering, National Yunlin University of Science and Technology, Yunlin 64002, Taiwan
3 International Center for Health Information Technology (ICHIT), Taipei Medical University, Taipei 110, Taiwan
4 Graduate Institute of Biomedical Informatics, Taipei Medical University, Taipei 110, Taiwan
* Correspondence: chuanyu@yuntech.edu.tw (C.-Y.C.); drshabbir@tmu.edu.tw (S.S.-A.)

**Abstract:** Unipolar depression (UD), also referred to as clinical depression, appears to be a widespread mental disorder around the world. Further, this is a vital state related to a person's health that influences his/her daily routine. Besides, this state also influences the person's frame of mind, behavior, and several body functionalities like sleep, appetite, and also it can cause a scenario where a person could harm himself/herself or others. In several cases, it becomes an arduous task to detect UD, since, it is a state of comorbidity. For that reason, this research proposes a more convenient approach for the physicians to detect the state of clinical depression at an initial phase using an integrated multistage support vector machine model. Initially, the dataset is preprocessed using multiple imputation by chained equations (MICE) technique. Then, for selecting the appropriate features, the support vector machine-based recursive feature elimination (SVM RFE) is deployed. Subsequently, the integrated multistage support vector machine classifier is built by employing the bagging random sampling technique. Finally, the experimental outcomes indicate that the proposed integrated multistage support vector machine model surpasses methods such as logistic regression, multilayer perceptron, random forest, and bagging SVM (majority voting), in terms of overall performance.

**Keywords:** multistage support vector machine model; multiple imputation by chained equations; SVM-based recursive feature elimination; unipolar depression

## 1. Introduction

In recent years, depression seems to be a very prevalent disorder around the globe, having a presence among approximately 264 million individuals. Psychiatrists usually claim that this disorder is unique, and it is unlike mood swings or ephemeral emotions and their reactions. Usually, when such a depressive condition is prevalent for a long duration among individuals, it might be a somber state of health. Additionally, the causes and effects of such cases are severe, and it critically rescinds the day to day functioning of individuals. In the worst scenario, it might stimulate suicidal tendencies in an individual.

In the millennial (born 1981–1996) era, depression is found to be on the rise; the reason is not apparent. Research shows that depression is greater among the younger Millennials, which results in many risk factors such as substance abuse and behavioral failures [1]. It is found that the depression symptoms have gone to 15 percent from 9 percent between 2005 and 2015, which is very shocking [1]. The three main parts of the brain that are affected by depression are the hypothalamus, the prefrontal cortex, and the amygdala. Some of the common reasons for being depressed are hormonal imbalance, stress, or genetic [2]. The symptoms of depression involve prolonged feelings of regret, sadness and hopelessness, irregular appetite, weight gain or weight loss, and many others. These days, more than the physical health issues, mental health issues are increasing exponentially [3]. It seems like almost everyone is affected by stress, anxiety, and depression [4].

More than physical health, mental health is essential, as it would directly affect physical health too. It will be easier if we have proper techniques to identify mental health as well [5]. There are few significant issues in diagnosing and treating the individual affected with unipolar depression such as, it is not easy for a depressed individual to seek expert help due to motivation and cost, and in some cases, the individual fails to take the mental health seriously [6].

In order to treat the depressed individuals better, we have proposed a machine learning classification algorithm, integrated multistage support vector machine model. It is an ensemble-based classification algorithm, where the support vector machine (SVM) classifiers are integrated with the help of the SVR-based weighted voting method to produce the outcome. Machine learning techniques are the best in identifying the patterns in the dataset and predict the outcome. We gathered data with the help of a questionnaire and preprocessed it to handle the missing values. The preprocessed data is then processed with a feature selection technique to select the relevant features.

The key contributions of this work include the following:

- The multiple imputation by chained equations (MICE) method is deployed for preprocessing and cleaning the gathered dataset
- The feature selection process is accomplished by employing the support vector machine-based recursive feature elimination (SVM RFE).
- The UD classification is performed using the proposed integrated multistage support vector machine classifier, which is built by employing the bagging random sampling approach.

The significant motivation of this research is to devise a random sampling-based integrated multistage SVM model for classifying the unipolar depression dataset, and we also attempt to enhance the overall performance of the proposed model. The rest of this research work is organized as follows. Section 2 elucidates the methodology formulation process and provides a detailed outlook into the individual modules of the proposed integrated multistage SVM model. Section 3 focuses on the experimental results. Section 4 provides information regarding the conclusion and future work.

## 2. Materials and Methods

### *2.1. Utilized Dataset*

The dataset we used in this study was collected from various individuals with an average age of 30. We framed a questionnaire based on the "Hamilton Depression Rating Scale" [7] and prepared a self-rating report. The dataset collected had 3040 samples with 22 features, including the target variable. The features are the demographic attributes and symptom scores. For processing, we split the dataset into training and testing sets (75-25 rule). The model was trained with the training set then tested with the test set and evaluated with specific performance metrics. Essential features are portrayed in Table 1.

**Table 1.** The portrayal of essential features.

| Features | Description |
|---|---|
| Age | Average Age 30. |
| Gender | Male/Female. |
| Sleep Quotient | Time taken to fall asleep. |
| Early Wake-Up | The irregular waking uptime. |
| Sleeping excessively | Irregular sleep hours. |
| Gloomy | Prolonged feelings of sadness, sometimes in the day or all the time. |
| Exasperation | Prolonged feelings of irritation, sometimes in the day or all the time. |
| Apprehensive or Nervous | Prolonged feelings of anxiousness or tension, sometimes in the day or all the time. |
| Response of the Individual to Preferred Happenings | Reactions, mood-wise to the events happening in life. |
| Relation between an Individual's Mood and Time | Moods at different time of the day. |
| Mood Quality | If the individual is sad, is it because of something happened or sad for no reason. |
| Reduced Desire for food | Not eating enough food. |
| Augmented Desire for food | Eating more than enough food. |
| Weight Reduction | Losing more weight in two weeks without any reason. |
| Weight Increase | Gaining weight at a specific time. |
| Ability to make Decisions/Attentiveness | Failure in making decisions and losing focus. |
| Future Perspective | Positive and Negative thoughts about the future. |
| Suicidal Contemplations | Attempting to harm oneself. |
| Happiness Quotient | Feeling good or extremely annoyed with pleasure and enjoyment in life. |
| Fidgety | Constant pacing and difficulty in concentrating. |
| Physical Indications | Sweating, increased heartbeat, blurred vision, shivering, chest pain or none at all. |
| Paranoid Signs | Constant panic attacks or none at all. |
| Result | Depressed or Not Depressed. |

### 2.2. *Data Cleaning and Preprocessing*

The data cleaning and preprocessing were performed by utilizing the multivariate imputation by chained equations (MICE) [8]. MICE is a flexible, advanced method in handling the missing values [9]. This technique handles the missing values by imputing multiple values [10]. The primary assumption in MICE is that the imputation variables were from the observed values, not from the unobserved values [11]. The process of chained equations involves various steps as follows,

Step 1: For every missing value in the dataset, the mean imputation technique was performed. These mean imputations were considered as placeholders.

Step 2: The mean imputation placeholder for any one of the variables say "var" was set back to null.

Step 3: In Step 2, the values that were observed for the "var" variable, which was made null, were regressed with other variables present in the imputation model and might or might not have all the variables from the dataset. In simpler terms, in this regression model, "var" was considered to be the dependent variable, and the other variables were considered to be independent.

Step 4: The variable "var", which was made as null, was now replaced with the actual imputations or predictions from the regression model. In the later stages, when "var" was used as an independent variable for other variables in the regression model, the observed values, as well as the imputed values, were used.

Step 5: For every missing value in the dataset, steps 2–4 were repeated to impute values. This process was continued to one iteration or one cycle. At the end of the first cycle, all the missing values would have been handled and imputed with the predictions from the regression model that can be seen in the observed data.

Step 6: Steps 2–4 were repeated for several cycles; the iterations depend on one's requirement. The imputation values would be updated at the end of each cycle. The final imputation values were retained at the end, which formed an imputed dataset. The most common number of cycles used was ten.

### 2.3. *Selection of Features*

In the dataset we collected the Hamilton Depression Rating Scale based self-rating report, there were about 22 features, including the target variable with 3040 samples. In the dataset, we found that there were features that interacted with each other. The features that were dependent on each other directly affected the accuracy of the model. In order to reduce the interaction between the features and remove the irrelevant or redundant variables, we implemented a wrapper based feature selection algorithm, support vector machine-based recursive feature elimination (SVM RFE).

Using this approach, nine features were selected. Alternatively, it has to be witnessed that choosing extra features will not assure higher accuracy levels in classification scenarios. Table 2 demonstrates the selected features and their indices for UD classification.

**Table 2.** Selected features and their indices for unipolar depression (UD) classification.

| Selected Features | Index |
|---|---|
| Gloomy | 1 |
| Exasperation | 2 |
| Apprehensive or Nervous | 3 |
| Response of the Individual to Preferred Happenings | 4 |
| Relation between an Individual's Mood and Time | 5 |
| Suicidal Contemplations | 6 |
| Happiness Quotient | 7 |
| Physical Indications | 8 |
| Paranoid Signs | 9 |

### 2.4. *Machine Learning Approaches Considered*

#### 2.4.1. Logistic Regression Approach

Logistic regression (LR) is a statistical approach, borrowed by machine learning in predictive analysis. This approach is mainly used when the dependent or the target variable is categorical. In logistic regression, the dependent variable must be dichotomous (i.e., Binary, Yes or No) [12]. The main assumptions made in logistic regression are that there are no outliers in the data, and that there is no multicollinearity between the predictor variables. Logistic regression is an extension of linear regression when the target variable seems to be categorical [13]. In this work, the penalized logistic regression uses a Glmnet in RStudio for predicting the unipolar depression. Table 3 presents the parameter settings for the logistic regression approach. Logistic regression is calculated through the probability of event occurrence with the help of the following the logistic function.

$$logit(p) = log\left(\frac{p(z=1)}{1-(p=1)}\right) = \alpha_0 + \alpha_1 y_{j2} + \cdots \alpha_x y_{jn} \tag{1}$$

where, $p$ is the probability of event occurrence, for $j = 1, \ldots, n$.

**Table 3.** Logistic regression approach—parameter settings.

| Parameters | Settings |
|---|---|
| fdev | 0.00001 |
| devmax | 0.999 |
| eps | 0.000001 |
| big | $9.9 \times 10^{35}$ |
| mnlam | 5 |
| pmin | 0.00001 |
| exmx | 250 |
| prec | 0.0000000001 |
| mxit | 100 |
| factory | FALSE |

### 2.4.2. Multilayer Perceptron Approach

Usually, when there is an increase in the complexity of the problem, the complexity of the theoretical understanding of the problem also upsurges. In that case, traditional statistical approaches are sought after. Currently, the studies show that neural networks, multilayered perceptron (MLP) in particular, seem to be replacing traditional statistical approaches. Multilayered perceptron does not make any prior assumptions about the data distribution, unlike the statistical models, and it can model even a highly non-linear function to accuracy by training it with new unseen data [14]. Multilayered perceptron is a model with interconnected nodes or neurons, which are connected by connection links with weights and the output signals [14]. We implemented the MLP in RStudio by deploying the RSNNS package. Table 4 shows the parameter settings for the multilayer perceptron approach. The input and the output signals are connected with the help of these neurons and connection links. The net input is calculated by,

$$PA = \sum_{k=1}^{n} Wt_k I_k + b \tag{2}$$

where,

$PA$—preactivation function or Net input;
$Wt_k$—the weight associated with the connection link;
$I_k$—inputs $(I_1, I_2, \ldots, I_n)$;
$B$—bias.

Based on the error rate at every iteration, the weights of the neurons can be adjusted. The perceptron weight adjustment is calculated by,

$$\Delta Wt = L \times P \times I \tag{3}$$

where

$\Delta Wt$—change in weights of the neurons;
$L$—learning rate;
$P$—predicted or desired output.

**Table 4.** Multilayer perceptron approach—parameter settings.

| Parameters | Settings |
|---|---|
| Max. output unit error | 0.2 |
| Learning function | Rprop Backprop |
| Modification | None |
| Print covariance and error | No |
| Cache the unit activations | No |
| Prune new hidden unit | No |
| Min. covariance change | 0.040 |
| Candidate patience | 25 |
| Max. no. of covariance updates | 200 |
| Activation function | LogSym |
| Error change | 0.010 |
| Output patience | 50 |
| Max. no. of epochs | 200 |

### 2.4.3. Random Forest Approach

In this work, we utilized the tuneRanger package in RStudio for the quick deployment of the random forests. Table 5 presents the hyperparameter settings of the random forest (RF) approach in this work. Random forest is an ensemble approach; it uses a recursive partitioning method to produce numerous trees, which are then aggregated to get the results [15–17]. Every tree in the random forest was constructed independently with the help of bootstraps of the training data. In random forest, each tree was constructed using two-thirds of the training data and the remaining one-third was used for testing the tree. The error rate of the forest depends on the strength of the individual trees and the correlation between each tree. The main advantage of using random forest is that there is no need to use any cross-validation methods, as the random forest approach itself has a built-in method called the out-of-bag errors to determine the test set errors in an unbiased manner. When compared with decision tree, random forest seems to have better accuracy and was less dependent on the training set and more tolerant to noise.

**Table 5.** Random forest approach—hyperparameter settings.

| Hyperparameter | Settings |
|---|---|
| mtry | 3 |
| sample size | 3040 |
| replacement | TRUE |
| node size | 1 |
| number of trees | 1000 |
| splitting rule | random |

#### 2.4.4. SVM Classifier

Support vector machine (SVM) is a machine learning algorithm that can be modeled for both regression and classification problems but it is majorly used for classification of a binary class problem [18,19]. In this work, we utilized the e1071package in RStudio for the deployment of the SVM classifier. Table 6 illustrates the hyperparameter settings for the SVM classifier in this work.

**Table 6.** Support vector machine (SVM) classifier—hyperparameter settings.

| Hyperparameter | Settings |
|---|---|
| Kernel | RBF |
| Problem type | Classification |
| $\log_2 C$ | −5, 15, 2 |
| $\log_2 \gamma$ | 3, −15, −2 |

When a labeled training data is given as an input, the model gives an optimal hyperplane as an output, which categorizes the samples. It is easy to maintain a linear hyperplane between two classes. However, when there is no precise classification between the vector points, manual separation is not possible [20]. For such situations, SVM has a strategy called the kernel. Kernel techniques convert a non-separable space to a separable space, which is called kernels used in non-linear separation models. Some of the commonly used kernel techniques are Gaussian kernel, Polynomial kernel, and many more [21,22].

### *2.5. Integrated MultiStage Support Vector Machine Classification Model*

The proposed integrated multistage support vector machine classification model comprises of two segments: the first one being the design of the SVM classifier, and the second is the UD feature selecting and ranking.

#### 2.5.1. Design of Integrated Multistage Support Vector Machine Classifier

In the proposed model, we were combining the individual SVM classifiers into a stronger and accurate model to improve the robustness and the generality of the SVM classifier. The deployment of this integration model depends on two factors: (i) the efficient way to build the member classifiers, aligning with the integration technique, and (ii) how to make all the member classifiers fuse to end up with a robust classifier. Therefore, to form a group of member classifiers, a random sampling method based on bagging is applied repeatedly [23]. For every individual SVM classification member classifier, around 75% from the original data sample is selected randomly for the training set, and the rest of the samples are used as a test or validation set to evaluate the performance of the model. A grid search utilizing the factor ranges $C = \{1, 2, 3, 4, 5, \ldots, 30\}$ and $\gamma = \{0.1, 0.2, 03, 0.4, 0.5, \ldots, 5\}$ is accomplished, for determining the optimimum values of C and $\gamma$. Later, without considering the optimal number of members in an integrated classifier, in this study, we implemented 10 different SVM classifiers with data from 10 random samplings and validated using the 10-fold cross-validation. This technique uses SVM RFE as the base learner. Thus, we constructed an SVM classifier with ten members in this study. In the SVM RFE, the features will be selected by the member classes based on their rankings in the support vector ratio-based ranking criteria. As the member classifiers are built with different random samples, they tend to have behaviors different from each other, and also, they will have different classification outcomes for the same data. As the final step, to integrate all the decisions by the individual classifiers to form ensemble SVM classifiers, the SVR-based weighted voting technique is implemented. The overall design of the proposed method is shown in Figure 1. Once the integrated classifier is built, it can be used for any classification tasks, as shown in Figure 1. In Figure 1, we can see that, once the member classifier was trained, the rest of the samples, which was 25% from the training set, was used as a temporary validation set for evaluating the performance of the model. In order to maintain the diversity of the classifiers and the simplicity of the integrated model, we used m = 10 member classifiers in this study.

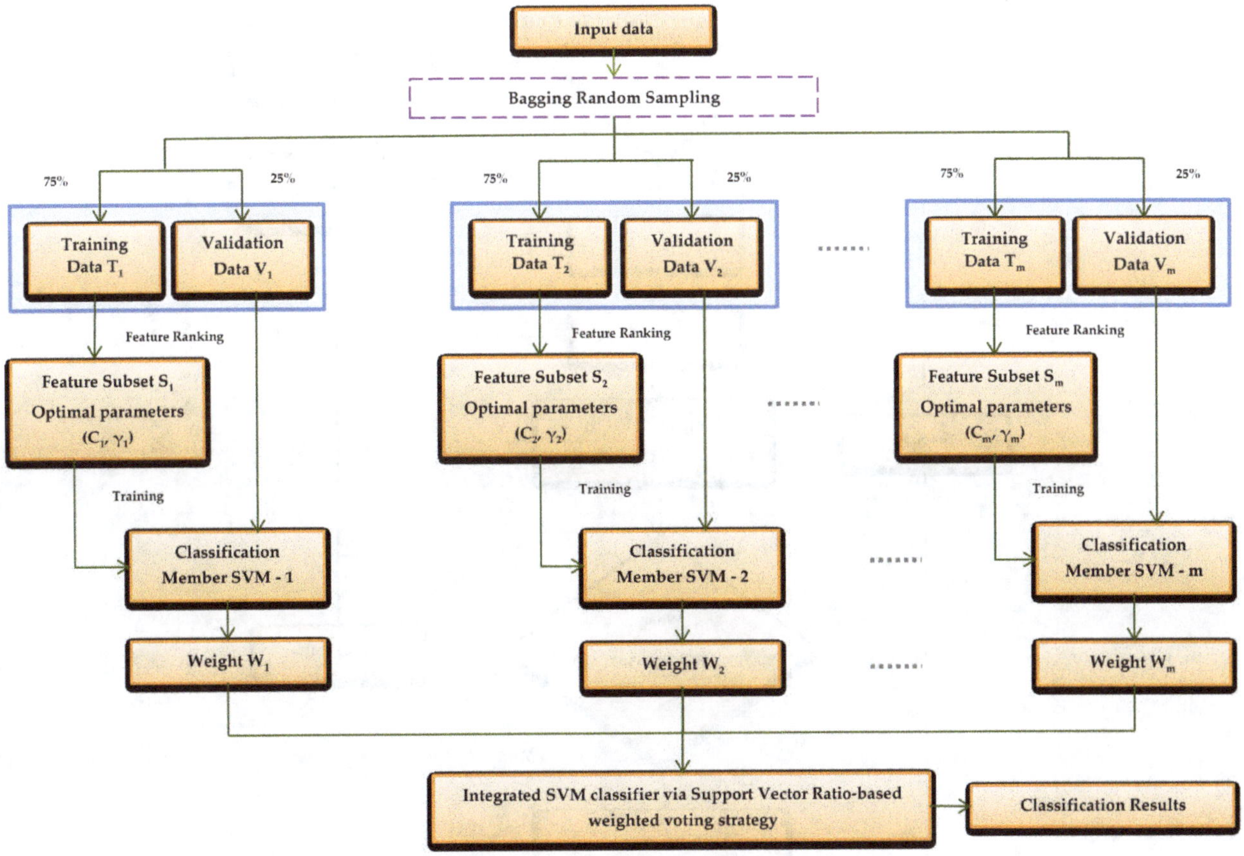


**Figure 1.** Proposed support vector ratio-based integrated multistage support vector machine classification model—architectural framework.

### 2.5.2. Ranking and Selection of Features

The essential step in implementing the integrated multistage SVM classification model is selecting the feature subset, which eventually enhances the performance of the member classifiers. Figure 2 represents the flow diagram of the support vector ratio-based support vector machine recursive feature ranking—the irrelevant variables and the variables that interact with each other usually slow down the overall performance of the model concerning computation and storage, during training or prediction. Sometimes, the irrelevant features can make drastic effects on the learning phase of the model. To improve the performance of the SVM classifier, we implemented an effective feature ranking and feature selection method to remove the irrelevant features from the 22 available features in the dataset, which can be seen in Table 1. The commonly used feature selection algorithms come under two categories, the filter methods and wrapper methods [24]. As simple as the filter methods look, they are not considered most of the time because they do not take into account the interaction between the features, which reduces the optimality of the feature subset, though they are computationally effective. On the other hand, wrapper methods evaluate the features jointly and iteratively, which results in effective capturing of interaction between the features [25].

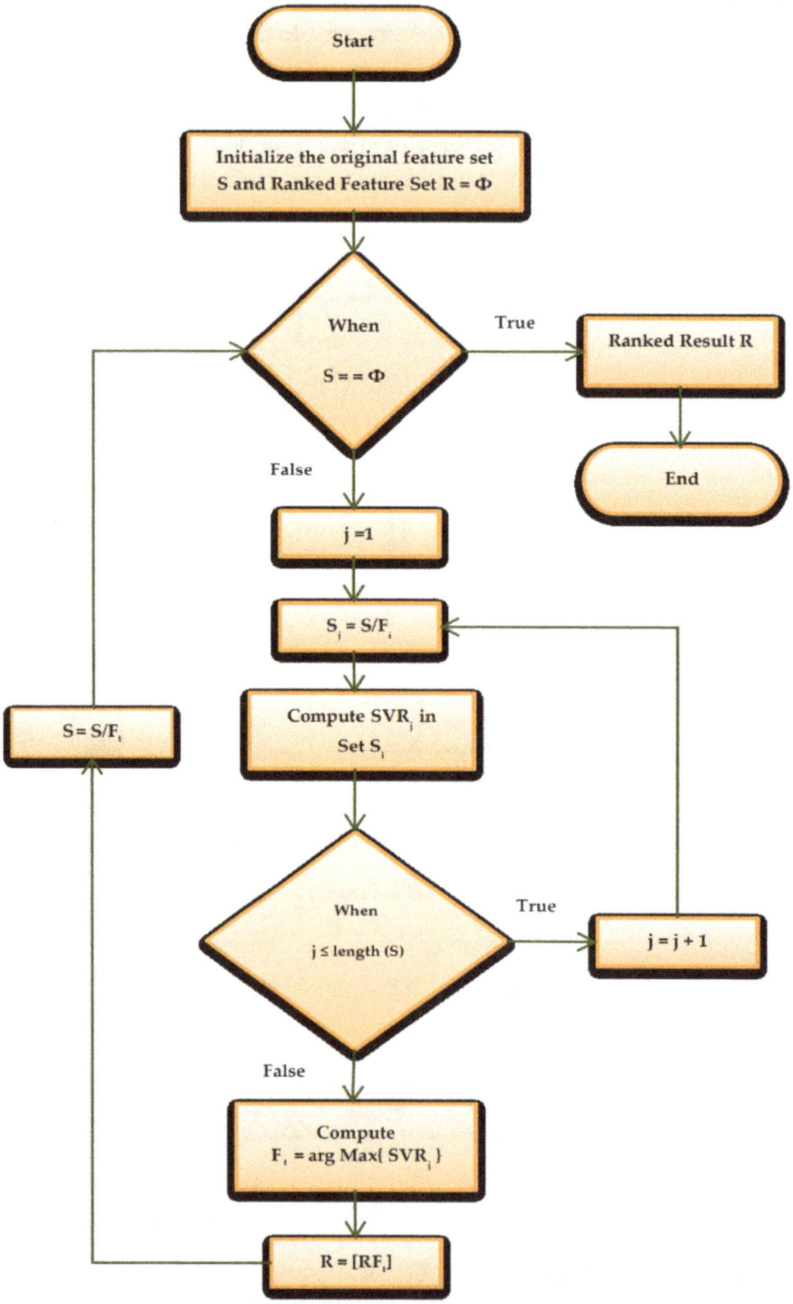


**Figure 2.** Support vector ratio-based support vector machine recursive feature ranking—flow diagram.

Due to the above-mentioned advantage, we used a wrapper method for feature selection in constructing the ensemble-based SVM classifier. Among all the existing wrapper-based feature selection methods, SVM RFE is considered as the most effective [26]. In this study, we implemented RFE as a part of the RBF SVM classification with the help of the support vector rate (SVR) metric for ranking all the 22 features shown in Table 1. The SVR is given by,

$$Support\ Vector\ Ratio = \frac{\text{The number of support vectors}}{\text{the number of total training samples}} \times 100\% \qquad (4)$$

The features are the support vectors in SVM; it is known that some of the support vectors help in minimizing the computational load of SVM and also improve its efficiency during the training. The ranking process is illustrated in Figure 2. The algorithm for the ranking process is as follows,

Step 1: Initialize the feature set, define S with all the 22 features from the dataset.

Step 2: Assume the ranked feature set as R.

Step 3: Eliminate one feature from the set and train the SVM model with 21 features. The classifier is initialized with empirical parameters, in order to calculate the SVR, which allows us to find out the contribution of the removed feature.

Step 4: Repeat step 3 for all the 22 features in the dataset. The feature with higher SVR after removal is placed in the ranked set R. It implies that the feature is not a support vector and is far away from the hyperplane.

## 3. Results and Discussion

The collected dataset had 3040 samples with 22 features, including the outcome variable. We preprocessed the dataset for removing the missing values using the MICE technique. Once the missing values were handled, we applied a wrapper-based feature selection technique, SVM RFE, to eliminate the less relevant and low performing features from the set. The algorithm removed the features in iteration and ranked them based on the SVR score. From the total 22 features, the algorithm selected nine features as the most important ones. These nine features did not depend on each other and also there was no interaction among them. The dataset was then divided into training and testing sets, where the model was trained with a training set and evaluated with the testing set. The composition was 75-25 for the training and testing dataset, respectively, with 10-fold cross-validation. In the numerical implementation, we implemented the proposed method with 10-member SVM classifiers and then integrated them with the help of the SVR-based weighted voting technique, as explained in the previous section.

To evaluate the proposed model, we have used the confusion matrix [27]. The confusion matrix was used to validate the performance of the model, which was tested with test data and whose true values were known. The technical terms involved in the confusion matrix are the true positive TP (model prediction—positive, actual outcome—positive), true negative TN (model prediction—negative, actual outcome—negative), false positive FP (model prediction—positive, actual outcome—negative), and false negative FN (model predicted—negative, actual outcome—positive). From the confusion matrix, different performance metrics can be calculated, such as accuracy, specificity, precision, sensitivity, and FMeasure [27]. The respective formulas for the metrics can be seen in Table 7. The results are tabulated in Table 8; the proposed model was compared with other methods such as logistic regression (LR), multilayer perceptron (MLP), random forest (RF), and bagging SVM (majority voting). Figure 3 represents the confusion matrix for LR, MLP, RF, and bagging SVM (majority voting), the proposed model, respectively. A comparison of evaluation metrics of the proposed model with other approaches is illustrated in Figure 4. It can be witnessed that the proposed model surpasses all other compared approaches in terms of performance and superior accuracy. The receiver operating characteristic (ROC) curve for the LR, MLP, RF, bagging SVM (majority voting), and the proposed model is depicted in Figure 5, Figure 6, Figure 7, Figure 8, and Figure 9, respectively. Stability comparison between the integrated SVM classifier and the member classifiers is shown in Figure 10.

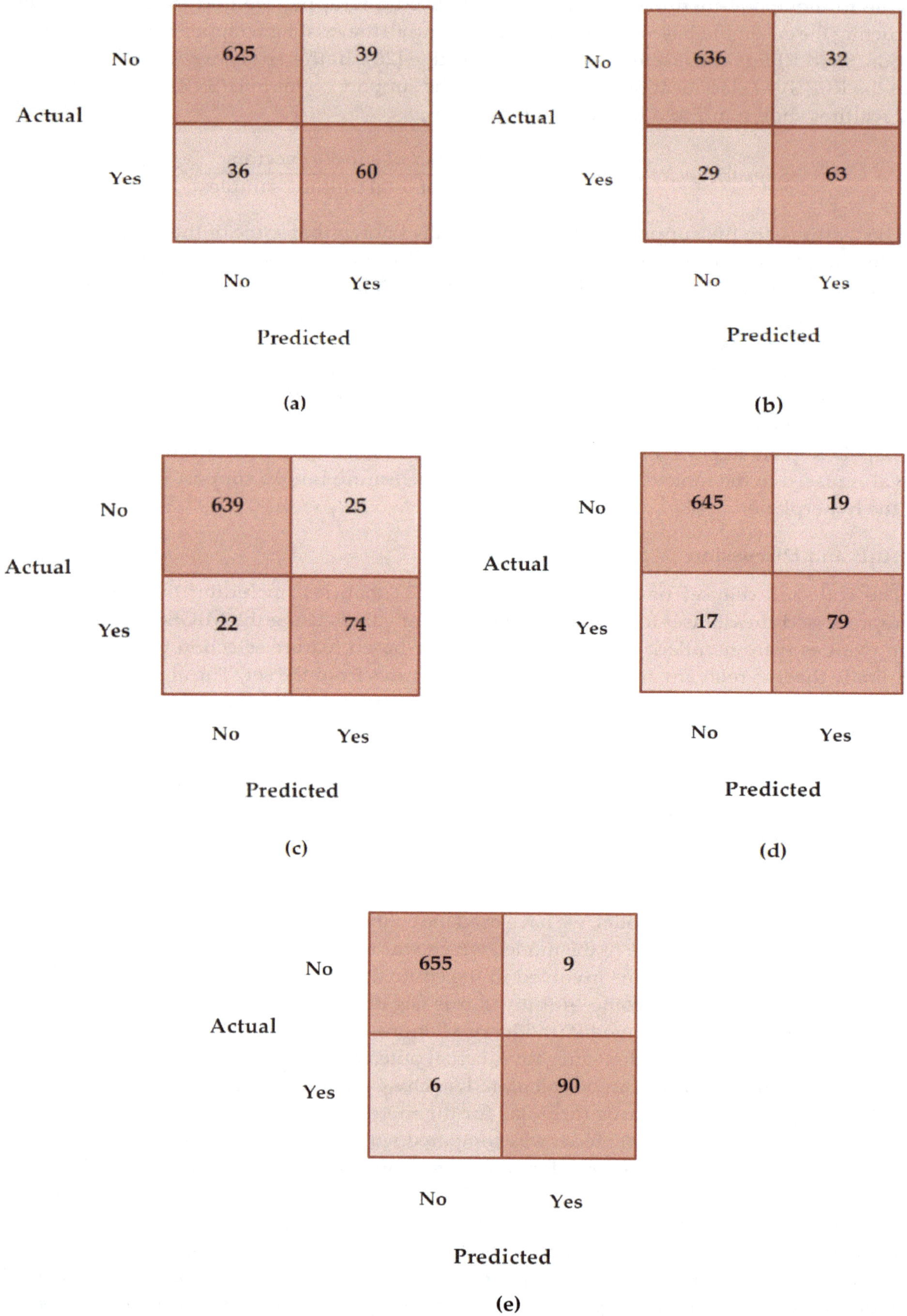


**Figure 3.** Confusion matrix: (**a**) Logistic regression (LR), (**b**) multilayer perceptron (MLP), (**c**) Random Forest (RF), (**d**) bagging SVM (majority voting), and the (**e**) proposed model.

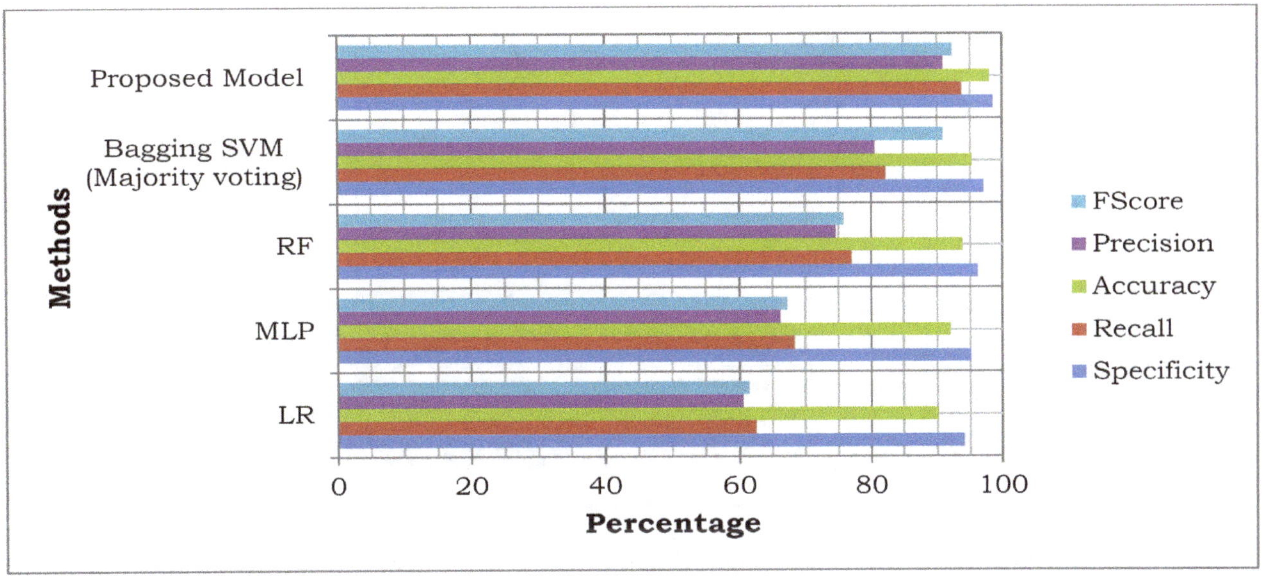


**Figure 4.** Comparison of evaluation metrics of the proposed model with other approaches.

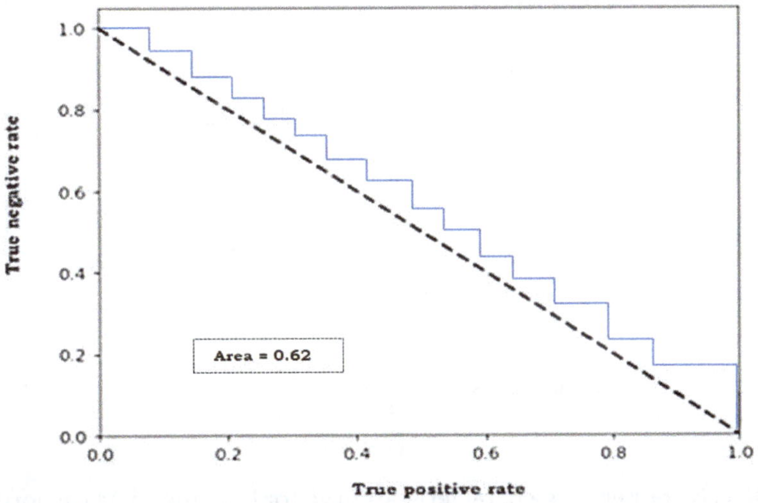


**Figure 5.** Receiver operating characteristic (ROC) curve for logistic regression.

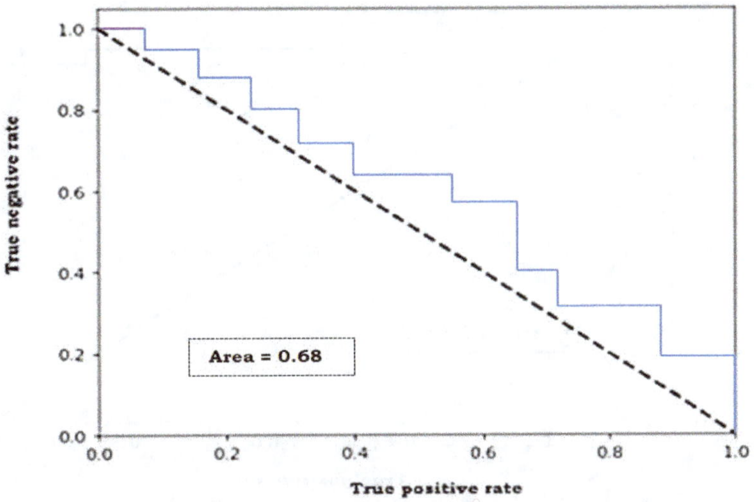


**Figure 6.** Receiver operating characteristic curve for multilayer perceptron.

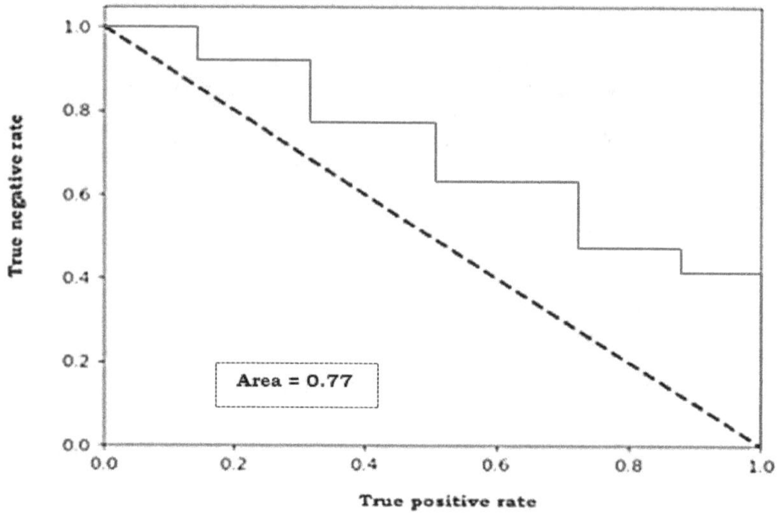


**Figure 7.** Receiver operating characteristic curve for random forest.

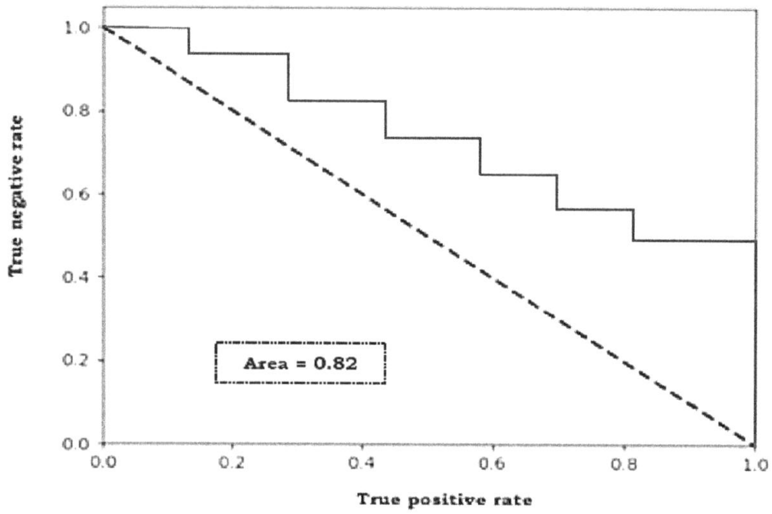


**Figure 8.** Receiver operating characteristic curve for bagging SVM (majority voting).

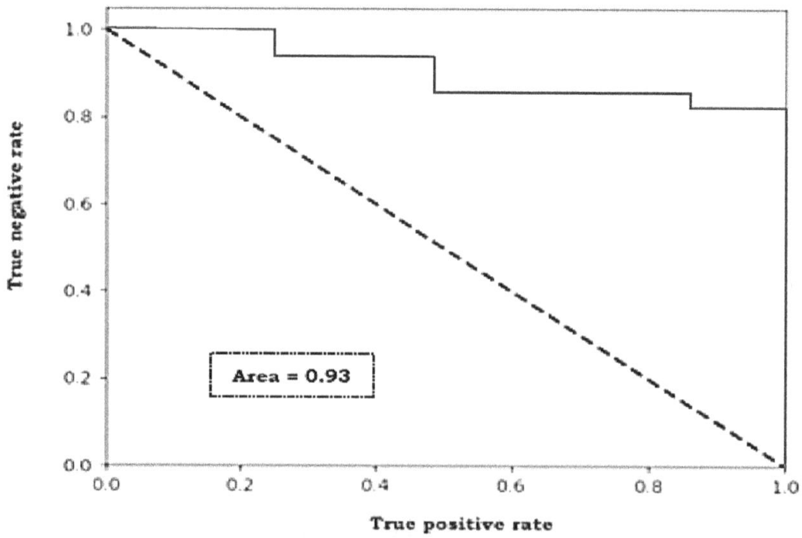


**Figure 9.** Receiver operating characteristic curve for the proposed model.

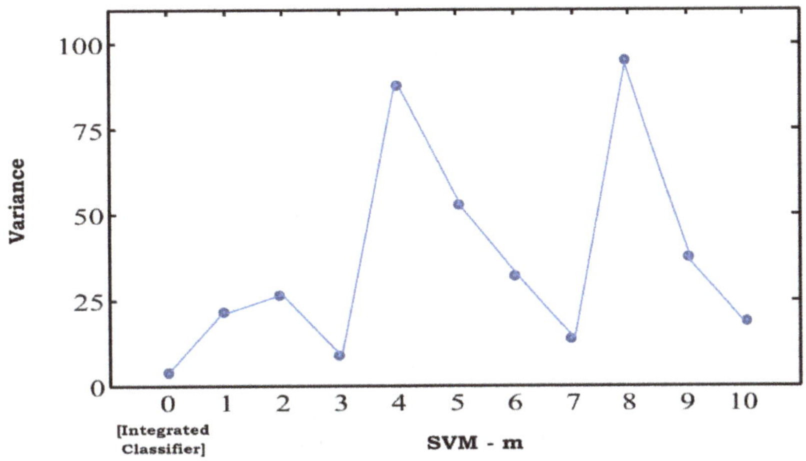


**Figure 10.** Stability comparison between the integrated SVM classifier and the member classifiers.

**Table 7.** Confusion matrix related metrics.

| Confusion Matrix | Formula |
|---|---|
| Specificity | TN/TN + FP |
| Recall | TP/TP + FN |
| Accuracy | TN + TP/TP + FP + TN + FN |
| Precision | TP/TP + FP |
| FScore | 2 × (Precision × Recall)/(Recall + Precision) |

**Table 8.** Comparison of evaluation metrics of the proposed model with other approaches.

| Evaluation Metric | LR (%) | MLP (%) | RF (%) | Bagging SVM (Majority Voting) | Proposed Model (%) |
|---|---|---|---|---|---|
| Specificity | 94.12 | 95.20 | 96.23 | 97.13 | 98.64 |
| Recall | 62.5 | 68.47 | 77.08 | 82.29 | 93.75 |
| Accuracy | 90.13 | 91.97 | 93.81 | 95.26 | 98.02 |
| Precision | 60.6 | 66.31 | 74.74 | 80.61 | 90.91 |
| FScore | 61.53 | 67.37 | 75.89 | 81.44 | 92.31 |

## 4. Conclusions

In this study, we proposed an effective ensemble-based classification model, integrated multistage support vector machine classification model for enhancing the predicting accuracy of UD. As the first step, we cleaned the data with MICE for handling the missing values. Then we implemented SVM RFE, a wrapper-based feature selection technique in order to reduce the feature dimension and select the necessary features, which are not dependent on each other, which eventually improves the accuracy of the model. The initial number of features in the original dataset was 22 on which the feature selection technique was applied. We used a 75-25 composition for training and testing datasets. The results proved that the proposed methodology had improved the prediction accuracy of UD when compared with other classification models. It could be observed that the proposed model was better than all other compared approaches in terms of performance and also offered greater accuracy.

**Author Contributions:** Conceptualization, K.S., N.M. and D.R.V.; Methodology, K.S. and N.M.; Software, K.S.; Validation, C.-Y.C. and S.S.-A.; Formal Analysis, K.S.; Investigation, K.S.; Resources, C.-Y.C. and S.S.-A.; Data Curation, N.M. and D.R.V.; Writing—Original Draft Preparation, K.S.; Writing—Review & Editing, K.S., N.M., C.-Y.C., and S.S.-A; Visualization, K.S.; Supervision, C.-Y.C.; Project Administration, C.-Y.C. and S.S.-A.; Funding Acquisition, C.-Y.C. and S.S.-A. All authors have read and agreed to the published version of the manuscript.

## References


1. Patalay, P.; Gage, S.H. Changes in millennial adolescent mental health and health-related behaviours over 10 years: A population cohort comparison study. *Int. J. Epidemiol.* **2019**, *48*, 1650–1664. [CrossRef] [PubMed]
2. McElroy, E.; Fearon, P.; Belsky, J.; Fonagy, P.; Patalay, P. Networks of Depression and Anxiety Symptoms Across Development. *J. Am. Acad. Child Adolesc. Psychiatry* **2018**, *57*, 964–973. [CrossRef] [PubMed]
3. Fried, E.I.; Nesse, R.M.; Zivin, K.; Guille, C.; Sen, S. Depression is more than the sum score of its parts: Individual DSM symptoms have different risk factors. *Psychol. Med.* **2013**, *44*, 2067–2076. [CrossRef]
4. Fried, E.I.; Nesse, R.M. Depression is not a consistent syndrome: An investigation of unique symptom patterns in the STAR*D study. *J. Affect. Disord.* **2014**, *172*, 96–102. [CrossRef]
5. Klakk, H.; Kristensen, P.L.; Andersen, L.B.; Froberg, K.; Møller, N.C.; Grøntved, A. Symptoms of depression in young adulthood is associated with unfavorable clinical- and behavioral cardiovascular disease risk factors. *Prev. Med. Rep.* **2018**, *11*, 209–215. [CrossRef] [PubMed]
6. Papakostas, G.I.; Petersen, T.; Mahal, Y.; Mischoulon, D.; Nierenberg, A.A.; Fava, M. Quality of life assessments in major depressive disorder: A review of the literature. *Gen. Hosp. Psychiatry* **2004**, *26*, 13–17. [CrossRef] [PubMed]
7. Hamilton, M. A Rating Scale For Depression. *J. Neurol. Neurosurg. Psychiatry* **1960**, *23*, 56–62. [CrossRef] [PubMed]
8. Azur, M.; Stuart, E.; Frangakis, C.; Leaf, P.J. Multiple imputation by chained equations: What is it and how does it work? *Int. J. Methods Psychiatr. Res.* **2011**, *20*, 40–49. [CrossRef]
9. Raghunathan, T.W.; Lepkowksi, J.M.; Van Hoewyk, J.; Solenbeger, P. A multivariate technique for multiply imputing missing values using a sequence of regression models. *Surv. Methodol.* **2001**, *27*, 85–95.
10. Van Buuren, S. Multiple imputation of discrete and continuous data by fully conditional specification. *Stat. Methods Med. Res.* **2007**, *16*, 219–242. [CrossRef]
11. Schafer, J.L.; Graham, J.W. Missing data: Our view of the state of the art. *Psychol. Methods* **2002**, *7*, 147–177. [CrossRef] [PubMed]
12. Peduzzi, P.; Concato, J.; Kemper, E.; Holford, T.R.; Feinstein, A.R. A simulation study of the number of events per variable in logistic regression analysis. *J. Clin. Epidemiol.* **1996**, *49*, 1373–1379. [CrossRef]
13. Press, S.J.; Wilson, S. Choosing between logistic regression and discriminant analysis. *J. Am. Stat. Assoc.* **1978**, *73*, 699–705. [CrossRef]
14. Gardner, M.; Dorling, S. Artificial neural networks (the multilayer perceptron)—A review of applications in the atmospheric sciences. *Atmos. Environ.* **1998**, *32*, 2627–2636. [CrossRef]
15. Breiman, L. Random Forests. *Mach. Learn.* **2011**, *45*, 5–32. [CrossRef]
16. Kandaswamy, K.K.; Chou, K.-C.; Martinetz, T.; Möller, S.; Suganthan, P.N.; Sridharan, S.; Pugalenthi, G. AFP-Pred: A random forest approach for predicting antifreeze proteins from sequence-derived properties. *J. Theor. Boil.* **2011**, *270*, 56–62. [CrossRef]
17. Zhou, Q.; Zhou, H.; Zhou, Q.; Yang, F.; Luo, L. Structure damage detection based on random forest recursive feature elimination. *Mech. Syst. Signal Process.* **2014**, *46*, 82–90. [CrossRef]
18. Hamed, T.; Dara, R.; Kremer, S.C. An Accurate, Fast Embedded Feature Selection for SVMs. In Proceedings of the 2014 13th International Conference on Machine Learning and Applications, Detroit, MI, USA, 3–5 December 2014; pp. 135–140.
19. Cortes, C.; Vapnik, V. Support-Vector Networks. *Mach. Learn.* **1995**, *20*, 273–297. [CrossRef]
20. Jarrett, K.; Kavukcuoglu, K.; Ranzato, M.A.; LeCun, Y. What is the best multi-stage architecture for object recognition? In Proceedings of the 2009 IEEE 12th International Conference on Computer Vision, Kyoto, Japan, September 27–October 4 2009; pp. 2146–2153.
21. Chang, C.-Y.; Srinivasan, K.; Chen, M.-C.; Chen, S.-J. SVM-Enabled Intelligent Genetic Algorithmic Model for Realizing Efficient Universal Feature Selection in Breast Cyst Image Acquired via Ultrasound Sensing Systems. *Sensors* **2020**, *20*, 432. [CrossRef]
22. Guyon, I.; Weston, J.; Barnhill, S.; Vapnik, V. Gene Selection for Cancer Classification using Support Vector Machines. *Mach. Learn.* **2002**, *46*, 389–422. [CrossRef]
23. Breiman, L. Bagging Predictors. *Mach. Learn.* **1996**, *24*, 123–140. [CrossRef]

24. Tuia, D.; Pacifici, F.; Kanevski, M.; Emery, W.J. Classification of Very High Spatial Resolution Imagery Using Mathematical Morphology and Support Vector Machines. *IEEE Trans. Geosci. Remote. Sens.* **2009**, *47*, 3866–3879. [CrossRef]
25. Ataş, M.; Yardimci, Y.; Temizel, A. A new approach to aflatoxin detection in chili pepper by machine vision. *Comput. Electron. Agric.* **2012**, *87*, 129–141. [CrossRef]
26. Wang, R.; Li, R.; Lei, Y.; Zhu, Q. Tuning to optimize SVM approach for assisting ovarian cancer diagnosis with photoacoustic imaging. *Bio-Med. Mater. Eng.* **2015**, *26*, S975–S981. [CrossRef] [PubMed]
27. Sokolova, M.; Lapalme, G. A systematic analysis of performance measures for classification tasks. *Inf. Process. Manag.* **2009**, *45*, 427–437. [CrossRef]

# 11

# Classification Maps in Studies on the Retirement Threshold

**Agnieszka Bielińska [1], Dorota Bielińska-Wąż [2,*] and Piotr Wąż [3]**

1 Department of Quality of Life Research, Medical University of Gdańsk, 80-210 Gdańsk, Poland
2 Department of Radiological Informatics and Statistics, Medical University of Gdańsk, 80-210 Gdańsk, Poland
3 Department of Nuclear Medicine, Medical University of Gdańsk, 80-210 Gdańsk, Poland
* Correspondence: djwaz@gumed.edu.pl

**Abstract:** The aim of this work is to present new classification maps in health informatics and to show that they are useful in data analysis. A statistical method, correspondence analysis, has been applied for obtaining these maps. This approach has been applied to studies on expectations and worries related to the retirement threshold. For this purpose two questionnaires formulated by ourselves have been constructed. Groups of individuals and their answers to particular questions are represented by points in the classification maps. The distribution of these points reflects psychological attitudes of the considered population. In particular, we compared structures of the maps searching for factors such as gender, marital status, kind of work, economic situation, and intellectual activity related to the attendance the University of the Third Age, which are essential at the retirement threshold. Generally, in Polish society, retirement is evaluated as a positive experience and the majority of retirees do not want to return to their professional work. This result is independent of the kind of work and of the gender.

**Keywords:** medical informatics; statistical computing; data analysis; retirement threshold

---

## 1. Introduction

Classification studies are a valuable source of information in various areas of science. The problem of classification is related to the problem of similarity of objects. Objects arranged in simple, one-dimensional sets may be classified in a unique way according to one, properly chosen, aspect of similarity. The problem becomes more complicated if we consider multidimensional sets, i.e., objects characterized by several different aspects. The degree of similarity depends on the selected aspects, on the number of aspects considered and on the mathematical measure establishing the relations between different properties.

One of class of objects considered by us is biological sequences. Both graphical and numerical classification of these objects is possible using methods based on *Graphical Representations* [1,2]. Within these methods, one can create a large number of different types of numerical characteristics (descriptors) of the plots representing the sequences. One kind of descriptors we propose are the distribution moments related to different statistical distributions describing the DNA sequences. We have shown that using these descriptors a pair of the sequences that differ by only one base can be distinguished. The coordinates of the descriptors representing these sequences are different in the classification maps [1]. The distribution moments we have also introduced as new descriptors of another class of objects—the molecular spectra [3,4]. The applications of the theory of molecular similarity are broad. Except for the studies of the properties of the systems explicitly considered in our works, the new descriptors may have broad range of interdisciplinary applications. For example, they may be applied in computational pharmacology and toxicology [5]. Our new descriptors have also found their application in the classification of the solutions in the chaotic systems [6], or in the classification of the stellar spectra [7,8]. Another kind of descriptor we propose are values used in the classical dynamics such as coordinates of center of mass or the moments of inertia. Examples of the classification studies using these descriptors may be found in the theory of molecular similarity [9] or in bioinformatics [10].

A class of objects considered in this work are groups of individuals. The studies are focused on the *retirement threshold*. A graphical representation of the results known as the *Correspondence Analysis* (CA) proves to be very useful in this kind of study [11]. Recently, CA was applied for studies on a variety of problems, for example, on high school dropouts [12], and also in archeology [13], in food science [14], etc. In the CA the information about the whole system is stored on maps in which objects under consideration are represented by points located in a specific way. The classification of the objects is here performed by studying distances between the points and, in particular, by identifying clusters of the points. Objects corresponding to the points which form a cluster are similar in some way.

Progress of medicine and lower fertility rate caused significant changes in the structure of modern societies. The number of seniors in developed countries is growing dynamically. In Poland in 2010 the percentage of people aged 65 and over was 19%. According to Eurostat forecasts, in 2030 the ratio of elderly people to the population aged 15–64 will be 36%, and in 2050—56% [15].

Due to acceleration of aging process, it seems reasonable to study the quality of life of older people. An important role in shaping the quality of life of seniors plays the retirement threshold, which is described in literature as symbolic moment—starting a new chapter in life. It involves many negative changes such as loss of professional status, deterioration of the economic situation, as well as reduction in the number of social interactions. On the other hand, pensioners have much free time for family life and hobby. Therefore, despite losing one of the most important roles in life, one can set new goals and develop non-professional passions. The change of social role from employee to retiree is a natural process, but such a big change in life may lead to negative psychological effects [16–19]. Changes in different aspects of life due to the retirement threshold have been studied in many countries. For example, changes in the sleep duration were studied in the United States [20] and Finland [21]; changes in the physical activity were studied in Canada [22], Belgium [23], and Finland [24–26]; and changes in the body mass index were studied in the United States [27] and Finland [28]. A variety of changes in the quality of life in different domains have been observed, for example, in the subjective wellbeing [29], in the use of time, activity patterns, in health and wellbeing [30], in the health-related quality of life [31], in the enjoyment of everyday activities [32], and in mobility [33]. The observed changes at the retirement threshold are not unique. Different factors, e.g., sex, social background, and education level, may determine whether they are positive or negative. Education is one of the most important factors determining worry-free retirement [34]. Recently, the Universities of the Third Age (U3A) became popular in many countries, and their positive influence has been broadly discussed [35–39]. The International Association of Universities of the Third Age (AU3A) is a global international organization. The AU3A network includes institutions from Asia, both Americas, Europe, and Australia. The attendance of U3A grows exponentially in the global scale. In China alone the number of universities for senior citizens has grown from 19,000 in 2002 to 70,000 in 2017. The corresponding numbers of students of U3A in China is even more impressive: from 1.8 million to 8 million.

In the present work, we study the influence of factors, such as gender, kind of work, marital status, intellectual activity related to the attendance the University of the Third Age, economic situation, on the expectations and on the worries related to the retirement threshold from the Polish perspective. Some pilot studies on the changes of the quality of life related to the retirement threshold using the World Health Organization Quality of Life-BREF (WHOQOL-BREF) questionnaire, and this graphical representation of the results we have already published [40–45]. The WHOQOL-BREF questionnaire is a standard tool in the quality of life research and many versions of this questionnaire have been created in different countries,for example, the Polish version [46], the Bangla version [47], the Spanish version [48], or the Finnish version [49]. This questionnaire is composed of 26 questions. Two questions are related to *Overall Quality of Life and General Health*. The remaining 24 questions concern four domains: *Physical Health*, *Psychological*, *Social Relationships*, and *Environment*. Using this questionnaire, we have shown that CA classification maps are a convenient tool for the studies on the role of different factors in changing the quality of life after the retirement threshold, such as gender [42] and marital status [43] in four domains, job position in *Physical Health* and *Psychological* domains [44], or in *Social Relationships* and *Environment* domains [45]. In most of cases, these factors play an important role. The considered factors are particularly important in the *Psychological* and in the *Social Relationships* domains. The influence of different factors, such as age, education, marital status, and job position on the *Overall Quality of Life and General Health* has also been studied by us using this graphical approach and WHOQOL-BREF questionnaire [40,41].

## 2. Materials and Methods

In the present work, the points forming clusters in CA maps correspond to subgroups of all individuals and to their answers to the questions. We used two our own questionnaires: *Questionnaire for an Employed or a Self-Employed Person* and *Questionnaire for a Retiree* (see Appendix A).

The studies have been performed in the period from February 2017 to May 2017 in Bydgoszcz, the eighth largest city in Poland (~350,000 inhabitants). We considered 449 individuals (older than 50): 160 employees (100 females and 60 males) and 289 retirees (186 females and 103 males).

We split the group of the retirees to two subgroups: students of U3A denoted in the figures as *retirees2* and non-students of U3A denoted as *retirees1* (Appendix A, question No. 9R). We also split all the subgroups (*employees, retirees1, retirees2*) according to the marital status. We consider two subgroups: *married* and *others* (Appendix A, question No. 7ER). In subgroup *others* are those individuals who are single, separated, divorced, or widowed.

Groups of individuals and their answers to particular questions (e.g., answer No. 1: *A1*) are represented by points in the classification maps. In this way, we can classify different subgroups, i.e., we can find subgroups of these individuals who answer in a similar way to some specific questions considered in the questionnaires.

The clusters of points are defined by the angles between vectors and the lengths of these vectors. The initial points of all vectors are located at the central point (CP) of the map, i.e., at the crossing point of the dotted lines marked in the maps. The terminal points of the vectors are denoted in the figures by empty squares (groups of individuals) and by full circles (answers). The squares and the circles belong to one cluster if the angles between the vectors (CP-square and CP-circle) are small. The longer are the vectors, the stronger is the positive association. Angles close to 90 degrees indicate no relationship. It the angles are close to 180 degrees, then they indicate a negative association. The longer are the vectors, the stronger is the negative association.

The final results have been generated using the *R* statistics language [50].

## 3. Results and Discussion

Figures 1–4 show the results (maps) obtained using CA.

Figure 1 shows maps related to the answers to questions about emptiness after the retirement (Appendix A, questions No. 21E and 18R). The structure of the maps for *males* and for *females* (top panels) are different. For *females* (top right panel), the angles between the vectors CP-*employees* and CP-*A4*, between CP-*retirees2* and CP-*A2* are small. Consequently, we can extract two clusters:

- *employees—A4*,
- *retirees2—A2*.

The lengths of all of the vectors CP-*employees*, CP-*A4*, CP-*retirees2*, and CP-*A2* are large. Then, the two associations are strong.

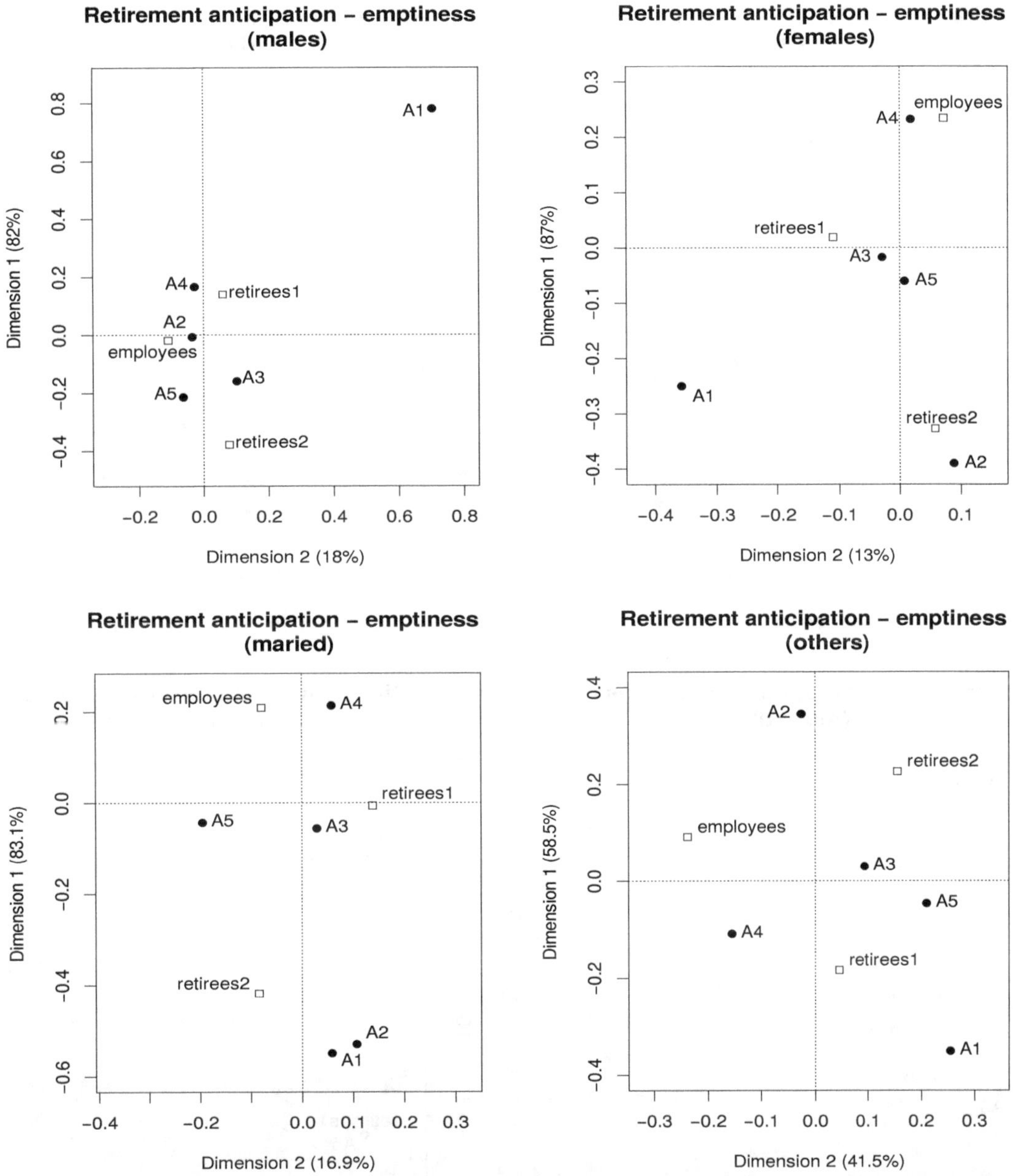


**Figure 1.** Classification maps (questions No. 21E and 18R).

For *males* (top left panel), the angles are nearly 180 degrees between vectors CP-*retirees2* and CP-*A4*, between CP-*retirees1* and CP-*A5*. Therefore, in this case, we have negative associations:

- *retirees2—A4*,
- *retirees1—A5*.

If the spread between the number of answers to different questions is large then the least common answers usually correspond to the negative associations. The least common answer about emptiness after retirement given by *retirees2* is A4 "I was not afraid". The least common answer about emptiness after retirement given by *retirees1* is A5 "I was not afraid at all". Depending on the lengths of the corresponding vectors, the strengths of the association may vary. In this case, the negative association for *males* is weak since the lengths of these vectors are smaller than for *females*. The point representing *employees (males)* is located close to the central point, so there are no strong associations of this group with any of the answers, while the most frequent answer for the *employees (females)* is A4 "I am not afraid" (cluster *employees—A4*).

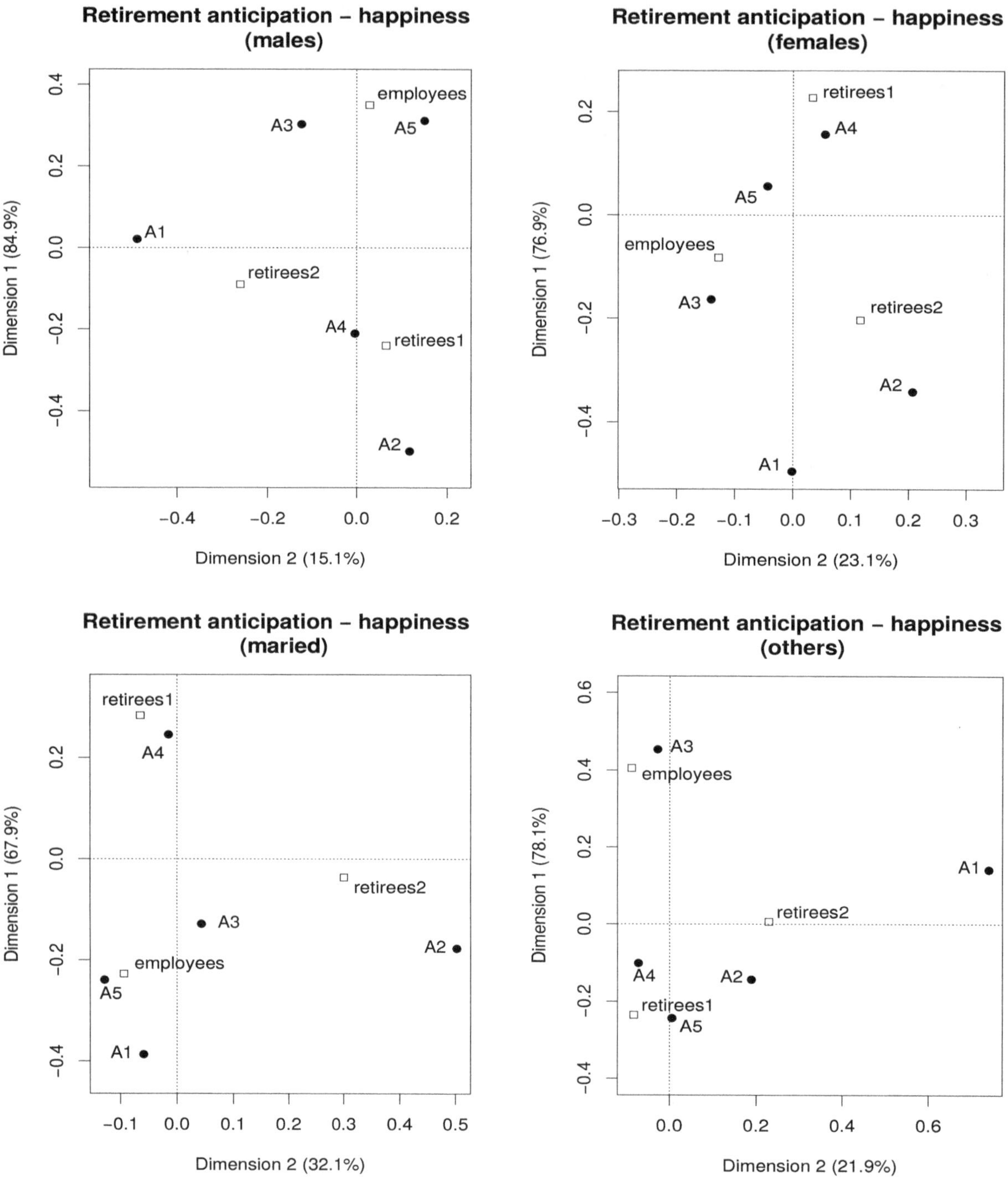


**Figure 2.** Classification maps (questions No. 15E and 15R).

Transition to retirement is a key moment when an individual must redefine his or her social roles, which is not always successful. Women more often define their social role as a family member: housewife and mother. After the end of their professional activity they find themselves in the role of grandmothers, participating in the family life of their children [51]. According to opinion polls in Polish society men are less involved in family life and performing household duties so after they terminate professional life they would stay without any activities and many of them may feel emptiness [52].

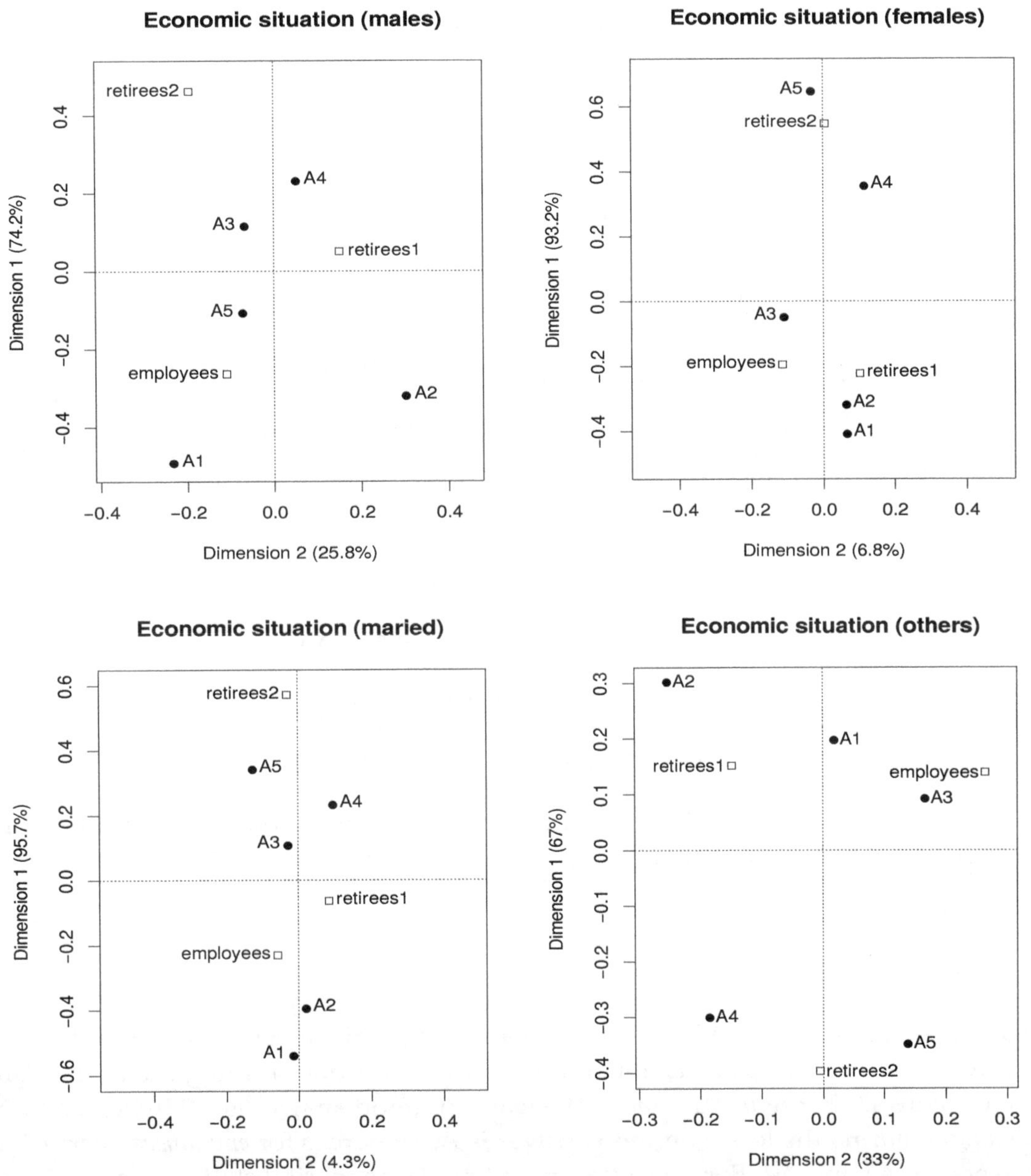


**Figure 3.** Classification maps (questions No. 19E and 20R).

If we consider the marital status, we observe negative associations for *married* (Figure 1, bottom left panel):

- *employees—A1,*
- *employees—A2,*
- *retirees2—A4,*
- *retirees1—A5.*

The angles between the vectors CP-*employees* and CP-*A1*, between CP-*employees* and CP-*A2*, between CP-*retirees2* and CP-*A4*, and between CP-*retirees1* and CP-*A5* are close to 180 degrees. The least common answers for *employees (married)* about emptiness after the retirement are A1 "Yes, I am very much afraid" and A2 "Yes, I am slightly afraid". The least common answer to this question of *retirees2 (married)* is A4 "I was not afraid". The least common answer to this question of *retirees1 (married)* is A5 "I was not afraid at all". As the lengths of CP-*A5* and CP-*retirees1* are smaller comparing to other vectors, the association for *retirees1* is the weakest.

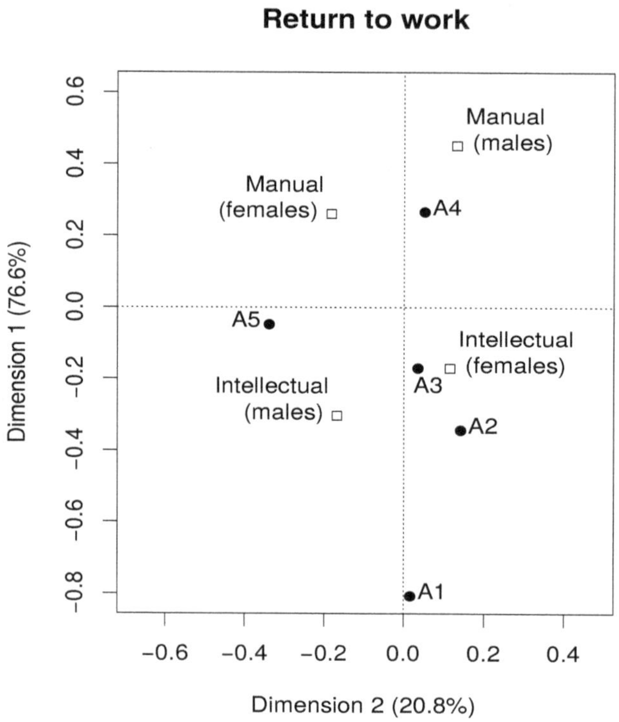


**Figure 4.** Classification map (question No. 25R).

For *others* (Figure 1, bottom right panel), the structure of the map is different than for *married*. We observe different negative associations:

- *employees—A5,*
- *retirees2—A4,*
- *retirees1—A2.*

Analogously, as for *married*, the least common answer to this question of *retirees2 (others)* is A4 "I was not afraid". The marital status is not an important factor determining the kind of answer to this question for *retirees2*. For *retirees1 (others)* the least common answer is A2, whereas for married is A5. For *employees (others)* the least common answer is A5, whereas for *employees (married)* the least common answers are A1 and A2. For *employees* and *retirees1*, the marital status changes the results of the classification.

Similar studies can be performed for other aspects, for example, satisfaction with retirement (Appendix A, questions No. 15E and 15R). The results are shown in Figure 2: *males* (Figure 2, top left panel), *females* (Figure 2, top right panel), *married* (Figure 2, bottom left panel), and *others* (Figure 2, bottom right panel). The answer A1 corresponds to "Very unhappy", whereas A5 corresponds to "Very happy". We observe different clusters for *males* and *females*, so gender is an important factor influencing the kind of answer to this question. In particular, for *males* we observe the following clusters:

- *retirees1—A2,*
- *employees—A5.*

For *females* the clusters are:

- *retirees1—A4,*
- *retirees2—A2.*

The most frequent answer of *females* attending the U3A (*retirees2*) is the same as *retirees1 (males)*, i.e., A2. There are also several negative associations for *males*:

- *employees—A4,*
- *retirees1—A3.*

The least common answer for *retirees1 (males)* is A3. For *females* the negative associations are:

- *retirees2—A5,*
- *retirees1—A1.*

The least common answer for *retirees1 (females)* is A1. A5 is located close to the central point so the association for *retirees2 (females)* is weak.

If we consider the marital status, for this question, we also observe different clusters for *married* and for *others*. The marital status is an important factor influencing the results of the classification in this case. In particular, for *married* we observe the clusters (Figure 2, bottom left panel):

- *employees—A5,*
- *retirees1—A4,*

and for *others* (Figure 2, bottom right panel)

- *employees—A3,*
- *retirees1—A5,*
- *retirees2—A1.*

The associations *retirees1—A5* and *retirees2—A1* are weak for *others*. The most frequent answer for *employees (married)* is A5 "Very happy", while for *employees (others)* the least common answer is A5 (negative association).

Figure 3 is concerned about the question on the adequate amount of money after retirement (Appendix A, questions No. 19E and 20R). Analogously to Figures 1 and 2, the top panels refer to *males* and to *females* and the bottom ones to *married* and to *others*. A1 corresponds to the answer "Not at all", and A5 to "Quite enough". For *males* (top left panel) the clusters are the following:

- *employees—A5,*
- *retirees2—A3,*

and for *females* (Figure 3, top right panel)

- *retirees1—A1,*
- *retirees1—A2,*
- *retirees2—A5.*

The negative associations for *males* are:

- *employees—A4,*
- *retirees2—A2,*

and for *females*

- *employees—A4,*
- *retirees2—A1,*
- *retirees1—A5.*

Employees and retirees estimate in a different way the economic situation during the retirement. Some differences are also between *males* and *females*. Considering the marital status, the clusters are also different. In particular, the group *employees (married)* clusters with A1, whereas *employees (others)* clusters with A3.

The summary is contained in the question about the return to the professional work (Appendix A, question No. 25R). The results are shown in Figure 4. The groups are split according to the kind of work—*Manual labor* and *Intellectual labor* (Appendix A, question No. 4ER)—and according to the gender. Finally, four subgroups are considered and denoted in the figure as *Manual (females)*, *Manual (males)*, *Intellectual (females)*, and *Intellectual (males)*. The answer A1 is "Yes, full-time", and the answer A5 is "Absolutely not". We observe the cluster

- *Manual (males)—A4.*

The negative associations are as follows:

- *Manual (females)—A2,*
- *Manual (males)—A1,*
- *Intellectual (males)—A4.*

The most frequent answer of *Manual (males)* is A4 "No". The associations of *Intellectual (females)* with A3 and A2 are weak. None of the groups clusters with A1 "Yes, full-time". Our analysis shows that in Poland in 2017, reaching the retirement threshold is rather a positive experience.

In line with social expectations, the retirement age was reduced to 60 for females and 65 for males in October 2017.

## 4. Conclusions

Summarizing, we described a non-standard approach to deriving information about objects met in the medical sciences based on an analysis of classification maps. We demonstrate that the graphical representation of the considered data (of the answers to some questions in the case of groups of individuals) is useful in health informatics, i.e., a lot of information is stored on one map. Searching for the so-called *clusters of points*, we can classify the objects. In this way, one can discover new properties of the considered objects. In the case of groups of individuals, we search for factors such as gender, marital status, kind of work, intellectual activity related to the attendance the University of the Third Age, economic situation, and determining the psychological attitudes of the considered population. For the creation of the classification maps, a statistical method, *Correspondence Analysis*, is used. New applications of the method are proposed: studies on expectations and worries related to the *retirement threshold*. Using standard methods, some considerable part of information may be lost. In particular, the commonly used Pearson's coefficients measure the strength of the linear correlation between the variables. If the correlation is strong but nonlinear, for example, quadratic or exponential, then the standard methods, contrary to the CA, may show that there is no correlation or that the correlation is weak. Similar classification maps we are also going to apply in other medical informatics areas in forthcoming papers related to the studies on the quality of life and to bioinformatics.

**Author Contributions:** Conceptualization, A.B., D.B.-W., and P.W.; methodology, A.B., D.B.-W., and P.W.; software, P.W., formal analysis, D.B.-W.; data curation, A.B.; writing—original draft preparation, D.B.-W. and A.B.; visualization, P.W. All authors have read and agreed to the published version of the manuscript.

**Funding:** This research received no external funding.

**Conflicts of Interest:** The authors declare no conflicts of interest.

## Appendix A

*Appendix A.1. Questionnaire for an Employed or a Self-Employed Person*

I. Personal information

1ER. Gender:

| A1. Male | A2. Female |
|---|---|

2ER. Age (years):

3ER. Education:

| A1. Elementary school | A2. Vocational education | A3. High school | A4. University education | A5. Doctor's degree |
|---|---|---|---|---|

4ER. Kind of work:

| A1. Manual labor | A2. Intellectual labor |
|---|---|

5ER. Business position:

| A1. Staff | A2. Supervisor/manager | A3. Director/president | A4. Business owner |
|---|---|---|---|

6ER. In how many years do you plan to retire?

7ER. Marital status

| A1. Single | A2. Married | A3. Separated | A4. Divorced | A5. Widowed |
|---|---|---|---|---|

8ER. Are you chronically ill?

| A1. Yes | A2. No |
|---|---|

If yes, which disease you suffer from?

II. Questions about your current satisfaction level

9E. Are you satisfied with your job?

| A1. Very dissatisfied | A2. Dissatisfied | A3. Neither satisfied nor dissatisfied | A4. Satisfied | A5. Very satisfied |
|---|---|---|---|---|

10E. Does your job make your life meaningful?

| A1. Not at all | A2. Slightly | A3. Moderately | A4. Very much | A5. Essentially |
|---|---|---|---|---|

11E. How do you rate the interpersonal relations in your work?

| A1. Very bad | A2. Bad | A3. Neither bad nor good | A4. Good | A5. Very good |
|---|---|---|---|---|

12E. Are you satisfied with your salary?

| A1. Very dissatisfied | A2. Dissatisfied | A3. Neither satisfied nor dissatisfied | A4. Satisfied | A5. Very satisfied |
|---|---|---|---|---|

13E. Do you feel that you have enough energy to perform your work?

| A1. Not at all | A2. Slightly enough | A3. Moderately enough | A4. Nearly enough | A5. Quite enough |
|---|---|---|---|---|

14E. Are you satisfied with your social life?

| A1. Very dissatisfied | A2. Dissatisfied | A3. Neither satisfied nor dissatisfied | A4. Satisfied | A5. Very satisfied |
|---|---|---|---|---|

III. Retirement-related questions

15E. Are you happy that in several years/months you will retire?

| A1. Very unhappy | A2. Unhappy | A3. Neither happy nor unhappy | A4. Happy | A5. Very happy |
|---|---|---|---|---|

16E. Do you think that after the retirement you will have enough energy to implement your aims?

| A1. Not at all | A2. Slightly enough | A3. Moderately enough | A4. Nearly enough | A5. Quite enough |
|---|---|---|---|---|

17E. Are you afraid that after the retirement you may not be self-sufficient?

| A1. Yes, I am very much afraid | A2. Yes, I am slightly afraid | A3. I do not think of it | A4. I am not afraid | A5. I am not afraid at all |
|---|---|---|---|---|

18E. Are you afraid that after the retirement you will feel lonely?

| A1. Yes, I am very much afraid | A2. Yes, I am slightly afraid | A3. I do not know yet | A4. I am not afraid | A5. I am not afraid at all |
|---|---|---|---|---|

19E. Do you expect to have enough retirement income to support yourself?

| A1. Not at all | A2. Slightly enough | A3. Moderately enough | A4. Nearly enough | A5. Quite enough |
|---|---|---|---|---|

20E. Do you think that you will be satisfied having a lot of free time during retirement?

| A1. Very dissatisfied | A2. Dissatisfied | A3. Neither satisfied nor dissatisfied | A4. Satisfied | A5. Very satisfied |
|---|---|---|---|---|

21E. Are you afraid of emptiness after the retirement, because you will not be so active as before?

| A1. Yes, I am very much afraid | A2. Yes, I am slightly afraid | A3. I do not think of it | A4. I am not afraid | A5. I am not afraid at all |
|---|---|---|---|---|

22E. Are you afraid that during the next several years your health is going to deteriorate?

| A1. Yes, I am very much afraid | A2. Yes, I am slightly afraid | A3. I do not think of it | A4. I am not afraid | A5. I am not afraid at all |
|---|---|---|---|---|

*Appendix A.2. Questionnaire for a Retiree*

I. Personal information

1ER, 2ER, . . . 8ER (see Appendix A.1)
9R. Do you attend classes at the University of the Third Age?

| A1. Yes | A2. No |
|---|---|

II. Professional work-related questions

10R. Were you satisfied with your job?

| A1. Very dissatisfied | A2. Dissatisfied | A3. Neither satisfied nor dissatisfied | A4. Satisfied | A5. Very satisfied |
|---|---|---|---|---|

11R. Did your job make your life meaningful?

| A1. Not at all | A2. Slightly | A3. Moderately | A4. Very much | A5. Essentially |
|---|---|---|---|---|

12R. How did you rate the interpersonal relations in your work?

| A1. Very bad | A2. Bad | A3. Neither bad nor good | A4. Good | A5. Very good |
|---|---|---|---|---|

13R. Were you satisfied with your salary?

| A1. Very dissatisfied | A2. Dissatisfied | A3. Neither satisfied nor dissatisfied | A4. Satisfied | A5. Very satisfied |
|---|---|---|---|---|

III. Just before retirement-questions

14R. Did you have enough energy to perform your work?

| A1. Not at all | A2. Slightly enough | A3. Moderately enough | A4. Nearly enough | A5. Quite enough |
|---|---|---|---|---|

15R. Were you happy that in several years/months you would retire?

| A1. Very unhappy | A2. Unhappy | A3. Neither happy nor unhappy | A4. Happy | A5. Very happy |
|---|---|---|---|---|

16R. Were you afraid that you would have not enough retirement income to support yourself?

| A1. Yes, I was very much afraid | A2. Yes, I was slightly afraid | A3. I did not think of it | A4. I was not afraid | A5. I was not afraid at all |
|---|---|---|---|---|

17R. Were you satisfied that after the retirement you would have a lot of free time?

| A1. Very dissatisfied | A2. Dissatisfied | A3. Neither satisfied nor dissatisfied | A4. Satisfied | A5. Very satisfied |
|---|---|---|---|---|

18R. Were you afraid of emptiness after the retirement, because you would not be so active as before?

| A1. Yes, I was very much afraid | A2. Yes, I was slightly afraid | A3. I did not think of it | A4. I was not afraid | A5. I was not afraid at all |
|---|---|---|---|---|

IV. Questions about your current satisfaction level

19R. Do you think that after the retirement your health deteriorated?

| A1. Yes, it did very much | A2. Yes, it did a little | A3. It is the same | A4. It is not worse | A5. On the contrary, I feel better |
|---|---|---|---|---|

20R. Do you have enough retirement income to support yourself?

| A1. Not at all | A2.Slightly enough | A3. Moderately enough | A4. Nearly enough | A5. Quite enough |
|---|---|---|---|---|

21R. Are you afraid that due to your bad health you will not manage with your housework?

| A1. Yes, I am very much afraid | A2. Yes, I am slightly afraid | A3. I do not think of it | A4. I am not afraid | A5. I am not afraid at all |
|---|---|---|---|---|

22R. Do you feel lonely?

| A1. Yes, very much | A2. Yes, a little | A3. Neither yes nor no | A4. No | A5. Absolutely not |
|---|---|---|---|---|

23R. Are you satisfied with your social life?

| A1. Very dissatisfied | A2. Dissatisfied | A3. Neither satisfied nor dissatisfied | A4. Satisfied | A5. Very satisfied |
|---|---|---|---|---|

24R. Are you satisfied with relations with your children and grandchildren (emotional relations, frequency of visits)?

| A1. Very dissatisfied | A2. Dissatisfied | A3. Neither satisfied nor dissatisfied | A4. Satisfied | A5. Very satisfied |
|---|---|---|---|---|

25R. Would you like to return to your professional work?

| A1. Yes, full-time | A2. Yes, part-time | A3. I do not think of it | A4. No | A5. Absolutely not |
|---|---|---|---|---|

## References

1. Bielińska-Wąż, D. Graphical and numerical representations of DNA sequences: Statistical aspects of similarity. *J. Math. Chem.* **2011**, *49*, 2345–2407. [CrossRef]
2. Randić, M.; Novič, M.; Plavšić, D. Milestones in graphical bioinformatics. *Int. J. Quant. Chem.* **2013**, *113*, 2413–2446. [CrossRef]
3. Bielińska-Wąż, D.; Wąż, P.; Basak, S.C. Similarity studies using statistical and genetical methods. *J. Math. Chem.* **2007**, *42*, 1003–1013. [CrossRef]
4. Bielińska-Wąż, D.; Wąż, P. Correlations in Spectral Statistics. *J. Math. Chem.* **2008**, *43*, 1287–1300. [CrossRef]
5. Bielińska-Wąż, D.; Wąż, P.; Jagiełło, K.; Puzyn, T. Spectral Density Distribution Moments as Novel Descriptors for QSAR/QSPR. *Struct. Chem.* **2014**, *25*, 29–35. [CrossRef]
6. Wąż, P.; Bielińska-Wąż, D. Asymmetry Coefficients as Indicators of Chaos. *Acta Phys. Pol. A* **2009**, *116*, 987–991. [CrossRef]
7. Wąż, P.; Bielińska-Wąż, D.; Pleskacz, A.; Strobel, A. Identification of Stellar Spectra Using Methods of Statistical Spectroscopy. *Acta Phys. Polon. B* **2008**, *39*, 1993–2001.
8. Wąż, P.; Bielińska-Wąż, D.; Strobel, A.; Pleskacz, A. Statistical indicators of astrophysical parameters. *Acta Astronom.* **2010**, *60*, 283–293.
9. Wąż, P.; Bielińska-Wąż, D. Moments of Inertia of Spectra and Distribution Moments as Molecular Descriptors. *MATCH Commun. Math. Comput. Chem.* **2013**, *70*, 851–865.
10. Wąż, P.; Bielińska-Wąż, D.; Nandy, A. Descriptors of 2D-dynamic graphs as a classification tool of DNA sequences. *J. Math. Chem.* **2014**, *52*, 132–140. [CrossRef]
11. Beh, E.J.; Lombardo, R. *Correspondence Analysis: Theory, Practice and New Strategies*; John Wiley & Sons: Oxford, UK, 2014.
12. Ziemer, K.S.; Pires, B.; Lancaster, V.; Keller, S.; Orr, M.; Shipp, S. A New Lens on High School Dropout: Use of Correspondence Analysis and the Statewide Longitudinal Data System. *Am. Stat.* **2018**, *72*, 191–198. [CrossRef]
13. Beh, E.J.; Lombardo, R.; Alberti, G. Correspondence analysis and the Freeman-Tukey statistic: A study of archaeological data. *Comput. Stat. Data Anal.* **2018**, *128*, 73–86. [CrossRef]
14. Frost, S.C.; Blackman, J.W.; Ebeler, S.E.; Heymann, H. Analysis of temporal dominance of sensation data using correspondence analysis on Merlot wine with differing maceration and cap management regimes. *Food Qual. Prefer.* **2018**, *64*, 245–252. [CrossRef]
15. Parnowski, T. Medyczne i psychologiczne problemy wieku podeszłego. *Probl. Rodz.* **1996**, *5*, 41–50. (In Polish)
16. Skarborn, M.; Nicki, R. Worry in pre- and post-retirement persons. *Int. J. Aging Hum. Dev.* **2000**, *50* 61–71. [CrossRef]
17. Hershey, D.A.; Henkens, K.; van Dalen, H.P. What drives retirement income worries in Europe? A multilevel analysis. *Eur. J. Ageing* **2010**, *7*, 301–311. [CrossRef]
18. Gutierrez, H.C.; Hershey, D.A. Impact of Retirement Worry on Information Processing. *J. Neurosci. Psychol. Econ.* **2013**, *6*, 264–277. [CrossRef]
19. Kail, B. The Mental and Physical Health Consequences of Changes in Private Insurance Before and After Early Retirement. *J. Gerontol. B Psychol. Sci. Soc. Sci.* **2016**, *71*, 358–368. [CrossRef]
20. Hagen, E.W.; Barnet, J.H.; Hale, L.; Peppard, P.E. Changes in Sleep Duration and Sleep Timing Associated with Retirement Transitions. *Sleep* **2016**, *39*, 665–673. [CrossRef]
21. Myllyntausta, S.; Salo, P.; Kronholm, E.; Aalto, V.; Kivimaki, M.; Vahtera, J.; Stenholm, S. Changes in Sleep Duration During Transition to Statutory Retirement: A Longitudinal Cohort Study. *Sleep* **2017**, *40*. [CrossRef]
22. Regan, K.; Intzandt, B.; Swatridge, K.; Myers, A.; Roy, E.; Middleton, L.E. Changes in Physical Activity and Function with Transition to Retirement Living: A Pilot Study. *Can. J. Aging* **2016**, *35*, 526–532. [CrossRef] [PubMed]
23. Van Dyck, D.; Cardon, G.; De Bourdeaudhuij, I. Longitudinal changes in physical activity and sedentary time in adults around retirement age: What is the moderating role of retirement status, gender and educational level? *BMC Public Health* **2016**, *16*, 1125. [CrossRef] [PubMed]
24. Manty, M.; Kouvonen, A.; Lallukka, T.; Lahti, J.; Lahelma, E.; Rahkonen, O. Pre-retirement physical working conditions and changes in physical health functioning during retirement transition process. *Scand. J. Work Environ. Health* **2016**, *42* 405–412. [CrossRef] [PubMed]

25. Stenholm, S.; Pulakka, A.; Kawachi, I.; Oksanen, T.; Halonen, J.I.; Aalto, V.; Kivimaki, M.; Vahtera, J. Changes in physical activity during transition to retirement: A cohort study. *Int. J. Behav. Nutr. Phys. Act.* **2016**, *13*, 51. [CrossRef]
26. Holstila, A.; Manty, M.; Rahkonen, O.; Lahelma, E.; Lahti, J. Statutory retirement and changes in self-reported leisure-time physical activity: A follow-up study with three time-points. *BMC Public Health* **2017**, *17*, 528. [CrossRef]
27. Gueorguieva, R.; Sindelar, J.L.; Wu, R.; Gallo, W.T. Differential changes in body mass index after retirement by occupation: Hierarchical models. *Int. J. Public Health* **2011**, *56* 111–116. [CrossRef]
28. Stenholm, S.; Solovieva, S.; Viikari-Juntura, E.; Aalto, V.; Kivimaki, M.; Vahtera, J. Change in body mass index during transition to statutory retirement: An occupational cohort study. *Int. J. Behav. Nutr. Phys. Act.* **2007**, *14*, 85. [CrossRef]
29. Barrett, G.F.; Kecmanovic, M. Changes in subjective well-being with retirement: Assessing savings adequacy. *Appl. Econ.* **2013**, *45*, 4883–4893. [CrossRef]
30. Maher, C.A.; Burton, N.W.; van Uffelen, J.G.Z.; Brown, W.J.; Sprod, J.A.; Olds, T.S. Changes in use of time, activity patterns, and health and wellbeing across retirement: Design and methods of the life after work study. *BMC Public Health* **2013**, *13* 952. [CrossRef]
31. Vercambre, M.N.; Okereke, O.I.; Kawachi, I.; Grodstein, F.; Kang, J.H. Self-Reported Change in Quality of Life with Retirement and Later Cognitive Decline: Prospective Data from the Nurses' Health Study. *J. Alzheimers Dis.* **2016**, *52*, 887–897. [CrossRef]
32. Olds, T.S.; Sprod, J.; Ferrar, K.; Burton, N.; Brown, W.; van Uffelen, J.; Maher, C. Everybody's working for the weekend: Changes in enjoyment of everyday activities across the retirement threshold. *Age Ageing* **2016**, *45*, 850–855. [CrossRef]
33. Berg, J. Mobility changes during the first years of retirement. *Qual. Ageing Older Adults* **2016**, *17* 131–140. [CrossRef]
34. Cho, H.; Suh, W.; Lee, J.; Jang, Y.; Kim, M. A worry-free retirement in Korea: Effectiveness of retirement coaching education. *Educ. Gerontol.* **2016**, *42*, 785–794. [CrossRef]
35. Jun, S.K.; Evans, K. The learning cultures of Third Age participants: Institutional management and participants' experience in U3A in the UK and SU in Korea. *KEDI J. Educ. Policy* **2007**, *4*, 53–72.
36. Hebestreit, L. The role of the University of the Third Age in meeting needs of adult learners in Victoria, Australia. *Aust. J. Adult Learn.* **2008**, *48*, 547–565.
37. Sonati, J.G.; Modeneze, D.M.; Vilarta, R.; Maciel É.S.; Boccaletto, E.M.A.; da Silva, C.C. Body composition and quality of life (QoL) of the elderly offered by the "University Third Age" (UTA) in Brazil. *Arch. Gerontol. Geriatr.* **2011**, *52*, e31–e35. [CrossRef]
38. Mackowicz, J.; Wnek-Gozdek, J. "It's never too late to learn"—How does the Polish U3A change the quality of life for seniors? *Educ. Gerontol.* **2016**, *42*, 186–197. [CrossRef]
39. Nascimento, M.D.; Giannouli E. Active aging through the University of the Third Age: The Brazilian model. *Educ. Gerontol.* **2019**, *45*, 11–21. [CrossRef]
40. Bielińska, A.; Majkowicz, M.; Wąż, P.; Bielińska-Wąż, D. Overall Quality of Life and General Health—Changes Related to the Retirement Threshold. In Proceedings of the eTELEMED 2018, The Tenth International Conference on eHealth, Telemedicine, and Social Medicine, Rome, Italy, 25–29 March 2018; XPS IARIA Press: Copenhagen, Denmark, 2018; pp. 1–5.
41. Bielińska, A.; Majkowicz, M.; Bielińska-Wąż, D.; Wąż, P. Influence of the Education Level on Health of Elderly People. In Proceedings of the eTELEMED 2018, The Tenth International Conference on eHealth, Telemedicine, and Social Medicine, Rome, Italy, 25–29 March 2018; XPS IARIA Press: Copenhagen, Denmark, 2018; pp. 6–11.
42. Bielińska, A.; Majkowicz, M.; Bielińska-Wąż, D.; Wąż, P. Classification Studies in Various Areas of Science. In *Numerical Methods and Applications*; NMA 2018, Lecture Notes in Computer Science; Nikolov, G., Kolkovska, N., Georgiev, K.; Eds.; Springer: Cham, Switzerland, 2019; Volume 11189, pp. 326–333.
43. Bielińska, A.; Majkowicz, M.; Wąż, P.; Bielińska-Wąż D. Mathematical Modeling: Interdisciplinary Similarity Studies. In *Numerical Methods and Applications*; NMA 2018, Lecture Notes in Computer Science; Nikolov, G., Kolkovska, N., Georgiev, K.; Eds.; Springer: Cham, Switzerland, 2019; Volume 11189, pp. 334–341.
44. Bielińska, A.; Majkowicz, M.; Bielińska-Wąż, D.; Wąż, P. A New Method in Bioinformatics—Interdisciplinary Similarity Studies. *AIP Conf. Proc.* **2019**, *2116*, 450013.

45. Bielińska, A.; Majkowicz, M.; Wąż, P.; Bielińska-Wąż, D. A New Computational Method: Interdisciplinary Classification Analysis. *AIP Conf. Proc.* **2019**, *2116*, 450014.
46. Jaracz, K.; Kalfoss, M.; Bączyk, G. Quality of life in Polish respondents: Psychometric properties of the Polish WHOQOL—Bref. *Scand. J. Caring Sci.* **2006**, *20*, 251–260. [CrossRef] [PubMed]
47. Tsutsumi, A.; Izutsu, T.; Kato, S.; Islam, A.; Yamada, H.S.; Kato, H.; Wakai, S. Reliability and validity of the Bangla version of WHOQOL-BREF in an adult population in Dhaka, Bangladesh. *Psychiatry Clin. Neurosci.* **2006**, *60*, 493–498. [CrossRef] [PubMed]
48. Benitez-Borrego, S.; Guardia-Olmos, J.; Urzua-Morales, A. Factorial structural analysis of the Spanish version of WHOQOL-BREF: An exploratory structural equation model study. *Qual. Life Res.* **2014**, *23*, 2205–2212. [CrossRef] [PubMed]
49. Siljander, E.; Luoma, M.L.; Merilainen-Porras, S. Validity and reliability of Finnish version of WHOQOL-Bref on adult population in Finland. *IJHD* **2015**, *2*, 52–68. [CrossRef]
50. R Core Team. *R: A Language and Environment for Statistical Computing*; R Foundation for Statistical Computing: Vienna, Austria, 2018.
51. Kim, J.E.; Moen, P. Is Retirement Good or Bad for Subjective Well-Being? *Curr. Dir. Psychol. Sci.* **2001**, *10*, 83–86. [CrossRef]
52. Bożewicz, M. Kobiety i Mężczyźni w Domu. *CBOS, Komunikat z Badań* **2018**, *127*. Available online: https://www.cbos.pl/SPISKOM.POL/2018/K_127_18.PDF (accessed on 1 December 2019). (In Polish)

# 12

# Leukemia Image Segmentation Using a Hybrid Histogram-Based Soft Covering Rough K-Means Clustering Algorithm

**Hannah Inbarani H.** [1], **Ahmad Taher Azar** [2,3,*] **and Jothi G** [4]

1 Department of Computer Science, Periyar University, Tamil Nadu, Salem 636 011, India; hhinba@gmail.com
2 Robotics and Internet-of-Things Lab (RIOTU), Prince Sultan University, Riyadh 11586, Saudi Arabia
3 Faculty of Computers and Artificial Intelligence, Benha University, Benha 13511, Egypt
4 Department of Computer Science and Engineering, Sona College of Technology (Autonomous), Salem 636005, India; jothiys@gmail.com
* Correspondence: aazar@psu.edu.sa or ahmad.azar@fci.bu.edu.eg

**Abstract:** Segmenting an image of a nucleus is one of the most essential tasks in a leukemia diagnostic system. Accurate and rapid segmentation methods help the physicians identify the diseases and provide better treatment at the appropriate time. Recently, hybrid clustering algorithms have started being widely used for image segmentation in medical image processing. In this article, a novel hybrid histogram-based soft covering rough k-means clustering (HSCRKM) algorithm for leukemia nucleus image segmentation is discussed. This algorithm combines the strengths of a soft covering rough set and rough k-means clustering. The histogram method was utilized to identify the number of clusters to avoid random initialization. Different types of features such as gray level co-occurrence matrix (GLCM), color, and shape-based features were extracted from the segmented image of the nucleus. Machine learning prediction algorithms were applied to classify the cancerous and non-cancerous cells. The proposed strategy is compared with an existing clustering algorithm, and the efficiency is evaluated based on the prediction metrics. The experimental results show that the HSCRKM method efficiently segments the nucleus, and it is also inferred that logistic regression and neural network perform better than other prediction algorithms.

**Keywords:** leukemia nucleus image; segmentation; soft covering rough set; clustering; machine learning algorithm; soft computing

---

## 1. Introduction

Due to the growth of advanced medical imaging modalities, it is very difficult to analyze the medical images manually. For this reason, an advanced and efficient computer-aided system is needed to diagnose the diseases. This will help the hematologist to begin the treatment at the right time and increase the patient's survival rate. Leukemia is a cancer of blood-forming tissues that affects the bone marrow. Leukemia is caused by the proliferation of abnormal white blood cells in the body. Leukemia is mostly affected by people living in developed countries and children aged 14 or under. As per the National Cancer Institute (NCI) statistics, in the United States, it is expected that there will be 62,130 persons as new cases for cancer treatment and 245,000 cases that are fatal or very serious [1]. In India, leukemia stands at ninth position among diseases (tumors) among children [2,3]. Leukemia is identified into two broad categories such as acute and chronic. Acute forms of leukemia occur when the number of immature blood cells increases, and it is the most common type of leukemia in children. Segmenting an image of a nucleus is one of the major challenging tasks in leukemia diagnosis. Recently, soft computing plays an important role in many research areas such as medical image processing, pattern recognition, big data analytics, Internet of Things (IoT) analysis, bioinformatics, and so on.

The rough set theory [4] was proposed by Pawlak in 1982. This concept is an extension of set theory for the study of intelligent systems characterized by insufficient and incomplete information. This classical rough set theory is based on equivalence relations, but it can also be extended to covering based rough sets [5–7]. In 1999, Molodtsov [8] proposed the concept of a soft set, which can be seen as a new mathematical approach to vagueness. The absence of any restrictions on the approximate description in soft set theory makes this theory very versatile and easily applicable in practice. Maji et al. [9] improved Molodtsov's idea by introducing several operations in soft set theory. In [10], the researcher investigated a soft covering-based rough set as a new kind of soft rough set. This method is a combination of a covering soft set and rough set. In [11], a covering-based rough k-means clustering approach is applied to segment the leukemia nucleus. The advantage of covering-based subsets is that they generate upper and lower approximations by using the covering feature, which brings about more roughness. Since different clusters give rise to different results, determination of the number of clusters is a difficult task in clustering-based segmentation. To overcome this limitation, the hybrid histogram-based soft covering rough k-means clustering algorithm (HSCRKM) is introduced to segment the image of the leukemia nucleus. In this algorithm, the peak values of the histogram of an image are identified and the number of clusters is initialized. This will avoid the random initialization of a number of clusters. Here, soft covering approximation space is also included. The term 'covering soft set' is more accurate than 'soft rough set.' It also combines the strengths of covering soft set theory and the rough k-means clustering algorithm to effectively segment the image of the nucleus. Soft covering rough approximation is utilized to find the lower and upper approximation values. The performance of the HSCRKM algorithm is evaluated using existing algorithms such as k-means clustering, fuzzy c-means clustering, and particle swarm optimization (PSO)-based clustering. Different types of features such as GLCM-0, GLCM-45, GLCM-90, GLCM-135, and shape color-based features are extracted from the segmented leukemia nucleus image. Nowadays, a lot of machine learning algorithms are applied to predict the degree of sickness. The state-of-art machine learning prediction algorithms such as neural networks (NN) [12], logistic regression (LR) [13], support vector machine (SVM) [14], naive Bayes (NB) [15], k-nearest neighborhood (KNN) [13], decision tree (DT) [13], and random forest (RF) [16] are applied to classify the cancerous and non-cancerous leukemia cells. The empirical results show that logistic regression and neural network efficiently predict the blast and non-blast cells when compared with other prediction algorithms.

The main objective of this research work is to develop a diagnostic approach for the identification of acute lymphoblastic leukemia blast cells using image processing and computational intelligence techniques. In experimental analysis, relevant image processing and computational intelligence techniques are applied in order to select the most suitable approach for the delineation of acute lymphoblastic leukemia cells. The following objectives have been formulated in order to predict leukemia: to apply computational intelligence-based algorithms for the segmentation of acute lymphoblastic leukemia blast cells in images and to apply machine learning algorithms to evaluate the performance of the proposed method.

The contribution of this study is summarized as follows. To find the number of clusters using the peak value of a histogram image and compute the lower and upper approximation values based on the soft covering approximation space, three clustering methods—k-means, FCM, and PSO-based clustering—are preferred for segmentation comparison. Through these methods, different kinds of features are extracted, and the efficiency of the proposed algorithm is assessed using machine learning prediction algorithms. The HSCRKM achieves the successful results i.e., above 80% when compared with the existing clustering algorithms. Therefore, it can be concluded that the HSCRKM clustering algorithm works effectively with the other clustering algorithms.

In the clustering algorithm, defining the number of clusters is a very difficult task. To overcome this limitation, the proposed algorithm identifies the peak values of the histogram of an image and initializes the number of clusters. This is one of the advantages of our proposed method, which avoids the random initialization of a number of clusters. The next advantage of the HSCRKM algorithm is that it combines the strengths of covering soft set theory and the rough k-means clustering algorithm to effectively segment the image of the nucleus. Based on a literature review, the term 'covering soft set' is more accurate than 'soft rough set', since it gives a better result than the soft rough set for several applications. In covering rough sets, the lower and upper approximation values are computed based on the soft covering approximation space.

Morphologically, a lymphoblast consists of a massive nucleus of irregular shape and size. In blood sample images, it is difficult to identify the cytoplasm, because it appears rarely and even if it does, it looks intensely colored. The nucleus and cytoplasm of lymphoblast cells reflect the morphological and functional changes. Feature extraction plays a main role in the assessment of leukemia in blood samples. After segmenting the nucleus using the proposed HSCRKM algorithm, salient features are extracted. It reduces the amount of data space and the working time of an image. In this research, different kinds of features are extracted such as gray level co-occurrence matrix (GLCM), color, and shape-based features. These were measured from every channel of the segmented nucleus image. The efficiency of the proposed algorithm is assessed using machine learning prediction algorithms. The performance of the segmentation algorithms was analyzed in the light of different machine learning (ML) prediction methods. With respect to HSCRKM clustering algorithms, most of the ML methods (except naive Bayes) achieved greater than 80% prediction accuracy compared with the existing clustering algorithms, viz., k-means clustering, fuzzy c-means clustering, and rough k-means clustering. It is inferred that the proposed clustering algorithms are more effective in segmenting the nucleus image. Due to the effective segmentation process, the extracted features have increased the prediction accuracy. To evaluate the experimental results, we have empirically set the best accuracy to be greater than 80%. The outline of the proposed system is shown in Figure 1.

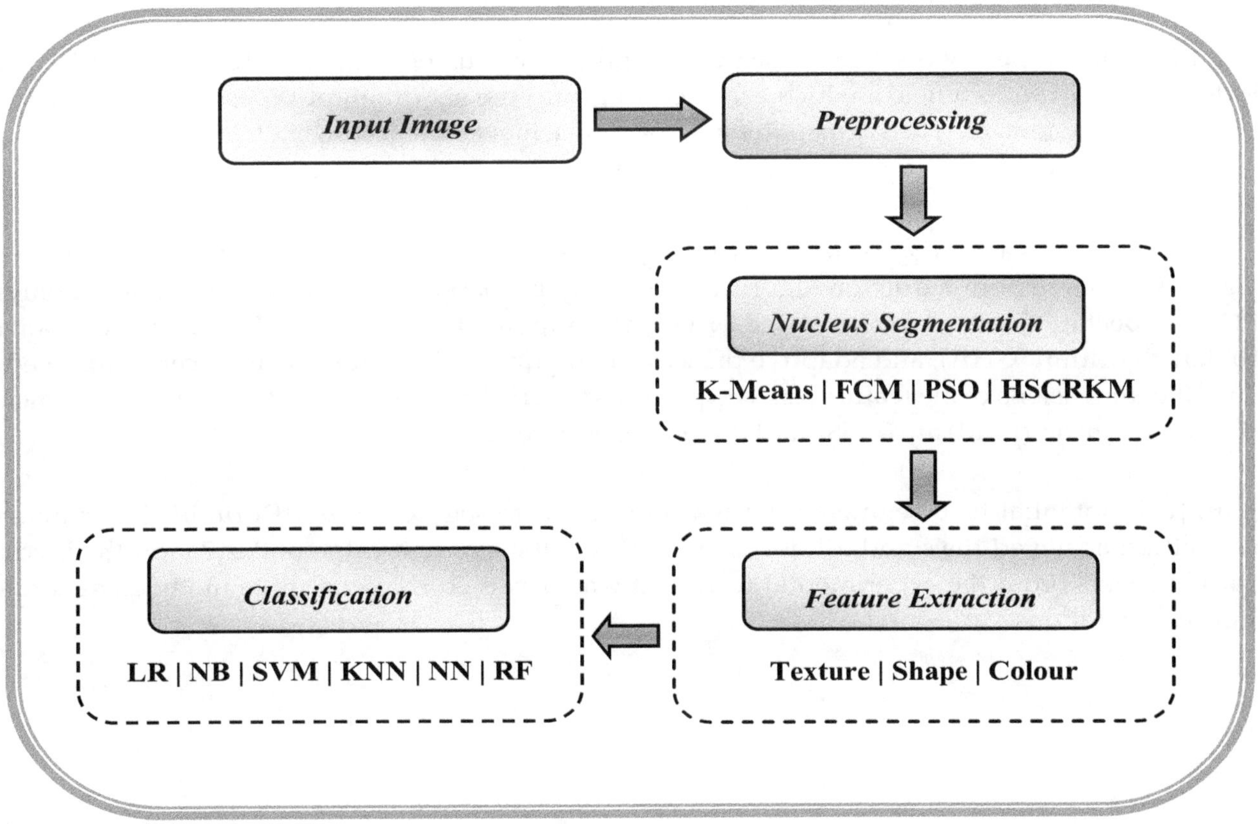


**Figure 1.** Outline of the proposed image segmentation process.

The rest of the research report is organized as follows. Section 2 reviews the related literature on clustering-based segmentation algorithms. Section 3 describes the methods of the proposed algorithm and its results. The empirical results are discussed in Section 4. Section 5 states the conclusion and indicates the future direction of this research.

## 2. Related Literature

In recent years, a lot of clustering algorithms have been developed for segmenting medical images.

Petal [17] applied k-means clustering for segmentation and the Zack algorithm for clustered white blood cells (WBCs). The features—namely, the mean, standard deviation, area, elongation, perimeter, color etc.—are extracted, and support vector machine (SVM) was used to classify the cells. The proposed algorithm effectively segmented the WBCs, which produced 93.57% accuracy. For this experiment, 27 images from the Acute Lymphoblastic Leukemia Image Database (ALL-IDB) were utilized.

Two bare-bones particle swarm optimization (BBPSO) algorithms with and without subswarms were introduced by Srisukkham et al. in 2017 [18] to diagnosis the leukemia cells. A stimulating discriminant measure (SDM)-based clustering algorithm that combined with the genetic algorithm (GA) was employed to segment the nucleus, cytoplasm, and background regions. The relevant features were extracted; then, various feature selection methods such as particle swarm optimization (PSO), cuckoo search (CS), and dragonfly algorithm (DA) were applied to select the optimal features and reduce the dimensions. An average geometric mean was computed with different sizes of training and test samples to evaluate the performance of the proposed methods. The BBPSO and binary BBPSO algorithms produced 91% to 96% of the geometric mean value.

Su [19] developed two stages of segmentation process using k-means clustering and HMRF (hidden Markov random field), which are used to group the six different types of AML cells from the bone marrow images. The segmentation algorithm achieved an accuracy of 96% to 98% (average) when compared with other existing segmentation methods.

In [20], k-means and fuzzy c-means clustering algorithms were applied to segment the brain tumor images. Various feature reduction algorithms, namely probabilistic principal component analysis (PPCA), expectation maximization-based principal component analysis (EM-PCA), the generalized Hebbian algorithm (GHA), and adaptive principal component extraction (APEX) were employed to reduce the dimensions of the feature set. The produced coefficient of variance (CV) values for k-means and Fuzzy C-mean (FCM) are 0.4582 and 0.1224, respectively.

In [21], potential field segmentation was employed to segment the MRI brain tumor images. This method achieved the standard deviation of 0.283, the average value of 0.517, and the median values of 0.644. From the experimental results, it was observed that ensemble methods generated better segmentations.

Küçükkülahlı [22] and Namburu [23] identified the number of cluster values in the clustering algorithm using the peak value of the histogram of an image. In [22], the automatic segmentation method using the histogram-based k-means clustering algorithm was developed. In [23], the soft fuzzy rough c-means clustering algorithm (SFRCM) was used to segment the MRI brain tumor images. The proposed SRFCM algorithm achieved a better Jaccard coefficient value of 0.97 for without noise and 0.79 for with 9% Gaussian noise when compared with the existing clustering algorithms namely, k-means, rough k-means (RKM), rough fuzzy c-means (RFCM), and generalized rough c-means (GFCM).

Ali [24] introduced a new clustering algorithm based on neutrosophic orthogonal matrices (CANOM) to segment the dental X-ray images. The experimental results show that the CANOM simplified silhouette width criterion (SSWC) index is 0.941 and the FCM is 0.02. CANOM is also better than Otsu and eSFCM with the values being 0.657 and 0.647, respectively. The value of CANOM is 47 times larger than that of FCM and 1.43 times larger than those of Otsu and eSFCM.

In [25], the unsupervised fuzzy c-means (FCM) clustering technique was employed for prostate cancer MRI images. The derived average dice similarity, Jaccard index, sensitivity, specificity, mean absolute difference, and Hausdorff distance is 88.68, 81.26, 90.71, 88.09, 88.09, 3.5, and 4.1 respectively.

In [26], the proposed multi-Otsu thresholding-based segmentation method can successfully segmented the CT image stacks. In addition, it sows the distribution characteristics of different components in three dimensions.

In [27], the enhanced adaptive fuzzy k-means (AFKM) algorithm was used to detect the three regions such as white matter (WM), gray matter (GM), and cerebrospinal fluid spaces (CSF) in the brain images. AFKM performed better than FCM, which produced a minimum mean square error (MSE) value of 2.2441.

In [28], the clustering method intuitionistic fuzzy c-means (IFCM) was applied for medical image segmentation. It is observed from the experimental results that the proposed method outperformed other algorithms that achieved the average quantitative index 0.95. The chronic wound region was detected using fuzzy spectral clustering in [29]. The proposed method produced 91.5% segmentation accuracy, an 86.7% Dice index, a Jaccard score of 79.0%, 87.3% sensitivity, and 95.7% specificity.

In [30], the convolutional neural networks (CNN) approach is applied to identify the subtypes of leukemia. It is observed from the experimental results that the CNN model achieves 88.25% and 81.74% accuracy for leukemia and healthy cells, respectively. From the literature review, it is inferred that the clustering-based algorithms were applied to segment the tumor region. A brief review of the literature on various clustering methods in image segmentation and their performances appears in Table 1.

**Table 1.** Overview of the literature on clustering algorithms.

| Author | Used Methods | Objective | Type of Diseases | Imaging Modalities/Dataset Used | No. of IMAGES | Performance Metrics and Accuracy % |
|---|---|---|---|---|---|---|
| Patel et al., 2015 [17] | K-mean clustering Zack algorithm, Support vector machines (SVM) | The K-means clustering algorithm was used to detect the white blood cells and the Zack algorithm was applied to categorize the cells. | Leukemia | Microscopic image (ALL-IDB) | 27 | Classification accuracy 93.57% |
| Srisukkham et al., 2017 [18] | Spatial Data Mining (SDM)-based clustering, Genetic Algorithm (GA), particle swarm optimization (PSO), Bare Bones PSO (BBPSO) | This optimization method was utilized to diagnose leukemia. | Acute lymphoblastic leukemia (ALL) | Microscopic image (ALL-IDB) | 180 | Geometric mean 91 to 96% |
| Su et al., 2017 [19] | K-means, Hidden Markov random field | This algorithm segmented the nucleus from the background, extracted the features, and then classified the blast cells. | Acute myeloid leukemia | Microscopic image (AML Patient) | 61 | Segmentation accuracy 96 to 98% (average) |
| Kaya et al., 2017 [20] | K-means, fuzzy c-means | Comparative analysis of various types of PCA algorithms on MRIs for two cluster methods. | Brain tumor | MRI (Hospital) | - | Average reconstruction error rates, Euclidean distance error rate, CV of K-Means = 0.4582 FCM = 0.1224 |
| Cabria et al., 2017 [21] | Potential field clustering | The algorithm is based on an analogy with the concept of potential field in physics and views the intensity of a pixel in an MRI as a "mass" that creates a potential field. | Brain tumor | MRI (BRATS) | 30 | SD = 0.283, Average = 0.517, Median = 0.644. |
| Küçükkülahlı et al., 2016 [22] | Histogram-based k-means clustering | This method to find the optimum cluster number based on the histogram of an image. | MATLAB media | Image Dataset | 10-15 | Derived metrics |
| Ali et al., 2017 [23] | Fuzzy clustering based on neutrosophic orthogonal matrix | This algorithm transforms image data into a neutrosophic set and computes the inner products of the cutting matrix of input. Then, pixels are segmented using the orthogonal principle to form clusters. | Dental | X-Ray (Hospital) | 22 | DB index Silhouette index = 0.941 |

**Table 1.** *Cont.*

| Author | Used Methods | Objective | Type of Diseases | Imaging Modalities/Dataset Used | No. of IMAGES | Performance Metrics and Accuracy % |
|---|---|---|---|---|---|---|
| Rundo et al., 2018 [24] | Fuzzy c-means (FCM) | This approach automatically segments the prostate and image computes the gland volume. | Prostate cancer | MRI (Hospital) | 7 (Patients) | Dice Similarity = 88.68, Jaccard index = 81.26, Sensitivity = 90.71, Specificity = 88.09, Mean Absolute Difference = 3.5, Hausdorff distance = 4.1 |
| Zhang et al., 2017 [25] | Multi-Otsu thresholding algorithm | This segmentation method can successfully segment CT image stacks. In addition, it sows the distribution characteristics of different components in three dimensions. | Backscattered electron images | X-ray CT (Hospital) | 1571 (Slice) | Derived metrics |
| Namburu et al., 2017 [26] | classical k-means (KM), rough k-means (RKM), rough fuzzy c-means (RFCM), and generalized rough c-means (GFCM). | In this method, soft fuzzy rough approximations are applied to obtain the rough regions of an image and compute the similarity of the clusters using soft set similarity coefficient. | Brain tumor | MRI (BRATS) | 20 | Jaccard's coefficient = 0.97 Accuracy |
| Ganesh et al., 2017 [27] | Enhanced adaptive fuzzy k-means algorithm | This approach is used to classify the three important regions in brain: namely, white matter, gray matter, and cerebrospinal fluid spaces. | Brain tumor | MRI (Brain Image) | 3 | MSE 2.2441 |
| Kaur 2017 [28] | Intuitionistic fuzzy sets-based credibilistic fuzzy c-means clustering | In this method, the hesitation factor and fuzzy entropy were utilized to improve the noise sensitivity of fuzzy c-means. | Brain tumor | MRI (brainweb) | 3 | Quantitative index 0.95 |
| Dhane et al., 2017 [29] | Fuzzy spectral clustering gray-based fuzzy similarity measure | This approach is adopted to compute the ulcer boundary demarcation and estimation. | Chronic wound | Digital Camera | 70 | Sensitivity = 87.3% Specificity = 95.7% Accuracy = 91.5% Dice index = 86.7% Jaccard score = 79.0% |
| Ahmed et al., 2019 [30] | Convolutional neural network (CNN) | This approach is identify the subtypes of leukemia. | Leukemia | Microscopic image (ALL-IDB) ASH Image Bank | 903 | Accuracy = 88.25% (Leukemia) Accuracy = 81.74% (Healthy cell) |

## 3. Methods

### 3.1. Basics of Soft Covering Based Rough Set

This section describes the basic properties of soft covering-based rough approximation [11].

**Definition 1.** *Let $C_G = (F, A)$ be a covering soft set over $U$ if $F(a) \neq \varnothing$, $\forall a \in A$. The pair $S = (U, C_G)$ is known as soft covering approximation space. For a set $X \subseteq U$, the soft covering lower and upper approximations are, respectively, defined as*

$$\underline{S}_*(X) = \cup_{a \in A}\{F(a) : F(a) \subseteq X\} \tag{1}$$

$$\overline{S}^*(X) = \cup\{Md_S(x) : x \in X\}. \tag{2}$$

*In addition,*

$$S_{pos}\,(X) = \underline{S}_*(X) \tag{3}$$

$$S_{neg}(X) = U - \overline{S}^*(X) \tag{4}$$

$$S_{bon}\,(X) = \overline{S}^*(X) - \underline{S}_*(X) \tag{5}$$

*are called the soft covering positive, negative, and boundary regions of X, respectively [11].*

**Definition 2.** *Let $S = (U, C_G)$ be a soft covering approximation space. If $\overline{S}^*(X) = \underline{S}_*(X)$, then subset $X \subseteq U$ is called soft covering. X is said to be a soft covering based rough set if $\overline{S}^*(X) \neq \underline{S}_*(X)$.*

The soft covering based rough set can be applied to image segmentation with the following considerations.

- The set of pixels in the input image is denoted as $U$ $U = X = \{xi/xi$ is the value of the ith pixel in the image$\}$.
- Let $C_G = (F,\ A)$ be the covering soft set to be constructed containing the pixels belonging to clusters.
- The set of parameter $A$ is considered as the number of clusters $Cl_G$ $\{i = 1, 2, 3, \ldots, k\}$ to which the pixels fit.
- For example, let a set of pixels in an image be denoted as $U = \{x_1, x_2, x_3, x_4,\}$ and the parameter set $A$ be denoted as number of clusters $\{Cl_{G1}, Cl_{G2}, Cl_{G3}\}$ to which the pixels belong. The distance between each pixel and the centroids are calculated. Based on the minimum distance, the pixels are grouped to the clusters. Assume that the input pixels are grouped in one cluster or more than one clusters as follows.
$$F(Cl_{G1}) = \{x_2, x_3, x_4\}$$
$$F(Cl_{G2}) = \{x_1, x_4,\}$$
$$F(Cl_{G3}) = \{x_1, x_3\}$$

Let $(F,\ A)$ be represented as $(F,\ A) = \{F\ (Cl_G) \mid Cl_G \in A\}$. The soft covering based rough set representation of the above example is given by

$$(F, A) = \left\{ \begin{array}{c} Cl_{G1} = \{x_2, x_3, x_4\} \\ Cl_{G2} = \{x_1, x_4,\} \\ Cl_{G3} = \{x_1, x_3\} \end{array} \right\}.$$

A tabular presentation of soft sets appears in Table 2. If $x_i \in F(Cl_{Gi})$, then the value is one; else, it is zero.

**Table 2.** Soft covering-based rough set representation of an image.

| U | $Cl_{G1}$ | $Cl_{G2}$ | $Cl_{G3}$ |
|---|---|---|---|
| $x_1$ | 0 | 1 | 1 |
| $x_2$ | 1 | 0 | 0 |
| $x_3$ | 1 | 0 | 1 |
| $x_4$ | 1 | 1 | 0 |

### 3.2. *The Proposed Histogram-Based Soft Covering Rough K-Means Clustering*

The proposed histogram-based soft covering rough k-means clustering is summarized in Algorithm 1. The combination of the covering soft set and rough set gives rise to a new kind of soft rough sets. Based on the covering soft sets, soft covering rough approximation was proposed by Yüksel et al. in 2014 [11,31], which is more accurate than the soft rough set. Here, we establish a rough k-means clustering using soft covering-based rough approximation to segment the image of the leukemia nucleus. Let $\underline{S}_*(X)$, $\overline{S}^*(X)$ be denoted as soft covering lower and upper approximation, and for $\underline{S}_*(X) \in \overline{S}^*(X)$ *i.e.*, in soft covering-based rough k-means clustering, the lower approximation is a subset of the upper approximation. The pixel data $X_n = (x_1, x_2, \ldots \ldots .x_n)$ of the lower approximation surely belong to the cluster; in this way, they can not have a place with some other cluster. The pixel data $X_n = (x_1, x_2, \ldots \ldots .x_n)$ in an upper approximation may belong to the cluster. Since their participation is dubious, they should be an individual set from an upper approximation of at least another cluster. The distance between the pixel data $X_n$ and the mean $sm_k$ is defined as [32]

$$d(X_n, sm_k) = ||X_n - sm_k||. \tag{6}$$

The cluster center $sm_k$ i.e., the mean, is computed using the following equation:

$$sm_k = \begin{cases} w_{low} \sum\limits_{X_n \in \underline{S}_*} \frac{X_n}{|\underline{S}_{*k}|} + w_{upp} \sum\limits_{X_n \in \overline{S}^*} \frac{X_n}{|\overline{S}^*_k|} \, for \; \underline{S}_* \neq \phi \\ \sum\limits_{X_n \in \overline{S}^*} \frac{X_n}{|\overline{S}^*_k|} \; otherwise, \end{cases} \tag{7}$$

where $|\underline{S}_{*k}|$ indicates the numbers of pixels in the lower approximation of the cluster $k$ and $|\overline{S}^*_k|$ is the number of pixels in the upper approximation of the cluster $k$. The weight parameters $w_{low}$ and $w_{upp}$ stress the significance of the lower and upper approximation of the cluster.

Explanation: In this algorithm, identify the peak value of a histogram image and use it to define the number of clusters $k$. Initially, assign each pixel $X_n = (x_1, x_2, \ldots \ldots .x_n)$ to exactly one lower approximation. Here, soft covering-based rough approximation is applied instead of rough approximation. Determine the new means $sm_k$ using Equation (7). Assign each pixel data to its closest mean using Equation (6). Compute the distance between each pixel $X_n$ with centroid $sm_k$ i.e., $d(X_n, sm_k)$. For each pixel, compute the relative distance (RD). If it is greater than the threshold, then the pixel is put into the upper approximation of the cluster $k$; otherwise, put it into the lower approximation of the cluster $h$. This algorithm is continued until all the data objects close to the cluster remain unchanged. Finally, the clustered image is labeled by the cluster index, and the segmented image of the nucleus is extracted.

**Algorithm 1: Based Soft Covering Rough K − Means Clustering Algorithm**

**Input**: $Img\ (X_n),\ k,\ w_{low},\ w_{upp},\ \delta$
**Output**: Segmented Nucleus Image $(Seg_{neu})$
**Initialization**:

$$X_n = (x_1, x_2, \ldots \ldots .x_n)\ //\ n = \text{no. of pixels in an image}$$

K = hist($Img(X_n)$) *No. of Clusters found using the peak value of a histogram image*
$w_{low}$ = *Lower Approximation Weight*
$w_{upp}$ = *Upper Approximation Weight*
$\delta$ = *Threshold Value*
*Randomly assign each pixel into exactly one lower approximation.*
**Procedure**:
**Step1**: *Randomly assign each pixel's data to the soft covering approximations*
**Step2**: *Compute cluster centers* $sm_k$ *using Equation* (7)
**Step3**: *Assign the pixels to the approximations.*
*The pixel data* $X_n$ *determine its closest mean* $sm_h$.

$$sd_{n,h}^{min} = d(X_n, sm_h) = \min_{k=1,2,\ldots K} d(X_n, sm_k)$$

*Assign* $X_n$ *to the upper approximation of the cluster* $h$: $X_n \in \overline{S}^*_h$.
**Step4**: *The relative distance is defined as*

$$RD = d(X_n, sm_k) - d(X_n, sm_h)$$

$ST = \{t : RD \leq \delta \cup h \neq k\}$.
*If* $ST \neq \phi$ *then* $X_n \epsilon \overline{S}^*_t\ \forall t \in T$.
*Else,* $X_n \epsilon \underline{S}_{*h}$.
**Step5**: *Check the convergence of the algorithm; if not, make it converge, and then continue with Step* 1.
**Step6**: *Lable the image by cluster index and extract the leukemia nucleus* $(Seg_{neu})$.

### 3.3. *Performance Assessment for Segmentation Algorithms*

After preprocessing, a novel HSCRKM algorithm is applied for leukemia nucleus image segmentation. The peak values of histogram are identified, and these values will automatically be assigned the number of clusters (K). In each iteration, the k value will change. The range of weight of the lower and boundary region in rough k-means algorithms is ($0.0 <= w_{low}, w_{bon} <= 1.0$). The relative threshold in the HSCRKM algorithm is defined as $\delta <= 1.0$. The parameters' values are assigned as $w_{low} = 0.7$, $w_{bon} = 0.3$, and $\delta = 0.5$. These values give possible stable results in rough k-means [30]. Figure 2 illustrates the segmentation results produced by the proposed HSCRKM algorithm.

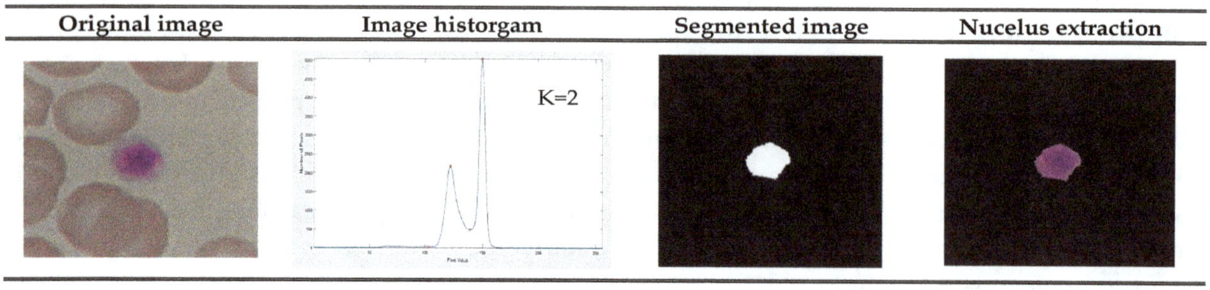


**Figure 2.** *Cont.*

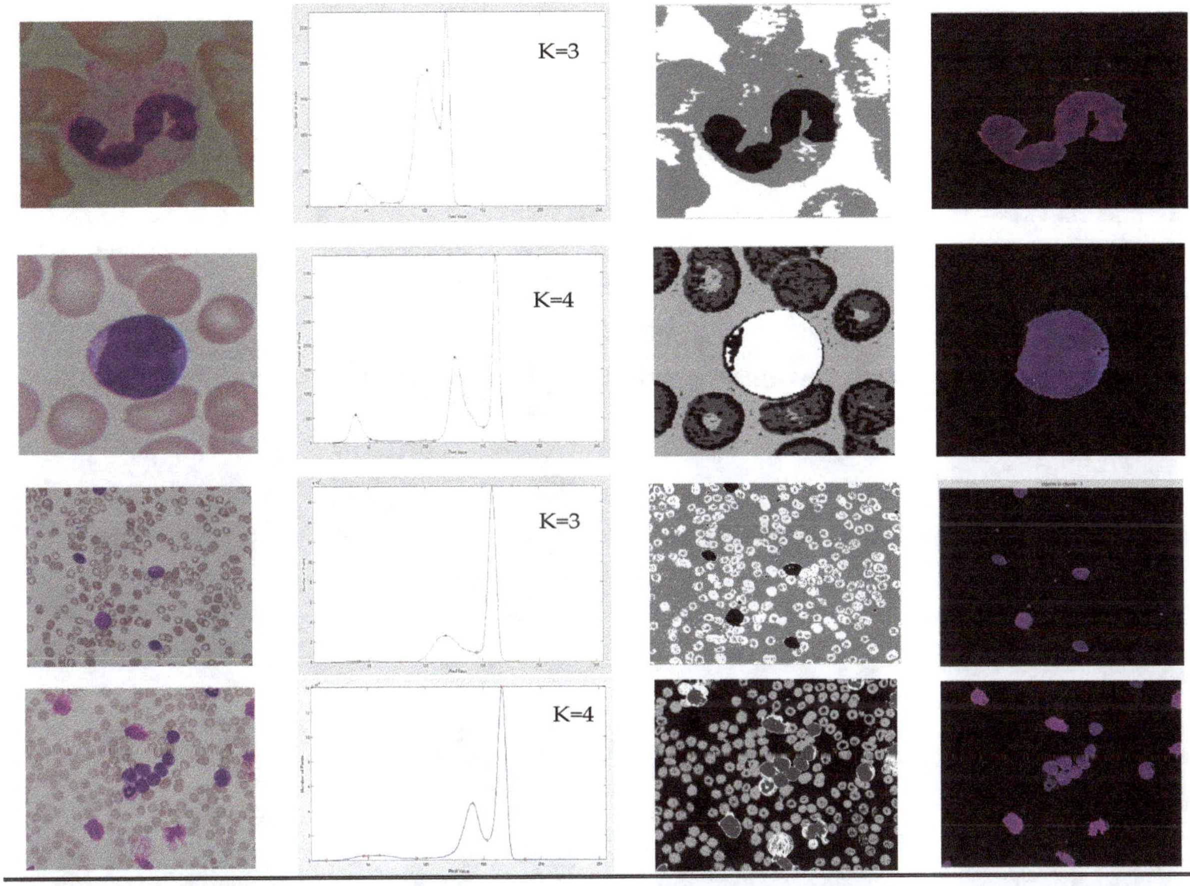


**Figure 2.** Segmentation results produced by the proposed histogram-based soft covering rough k-means clustering (HSCRKM) algorithm.

In Figure 2, the first column displays the original image, the second column shows the histogram of an image that helps find the number of clusters (K), the third column displays the clustered image, and the last column displays the extracted nucleus. It is observed that if the k value is at its minimum, we get a better segmentation result. This helps reduce the processing time. The parameters utilized in the clustering algorithms are presented in Figure 3.

| | |
|---|---|
| K-Means Clustering | •K=3, Max Iteration = 500 |
| FCM Clustering | •K=3, υ=0.000001, m=2 |
| PSO-based Clustering | •K= 3 |
| HSCRKM Clustering | •$K$ = $Peak\ value\ of\ Histogram\ image$,<br>• $w_{low}$= 0.7, $w_{bon}$= 0.3, and $\delta$ = 0.5 |

**Figure 3.** Parameters utilized in clustering algorithms.

Figure 4 shows the sample output of leukemia image segmentation using existing clustering algorithms such as k-means clustering, FCM clustering, and PSO-based clustering algorithms. Here, the number of clusters k is assigned as three using the elbow method.

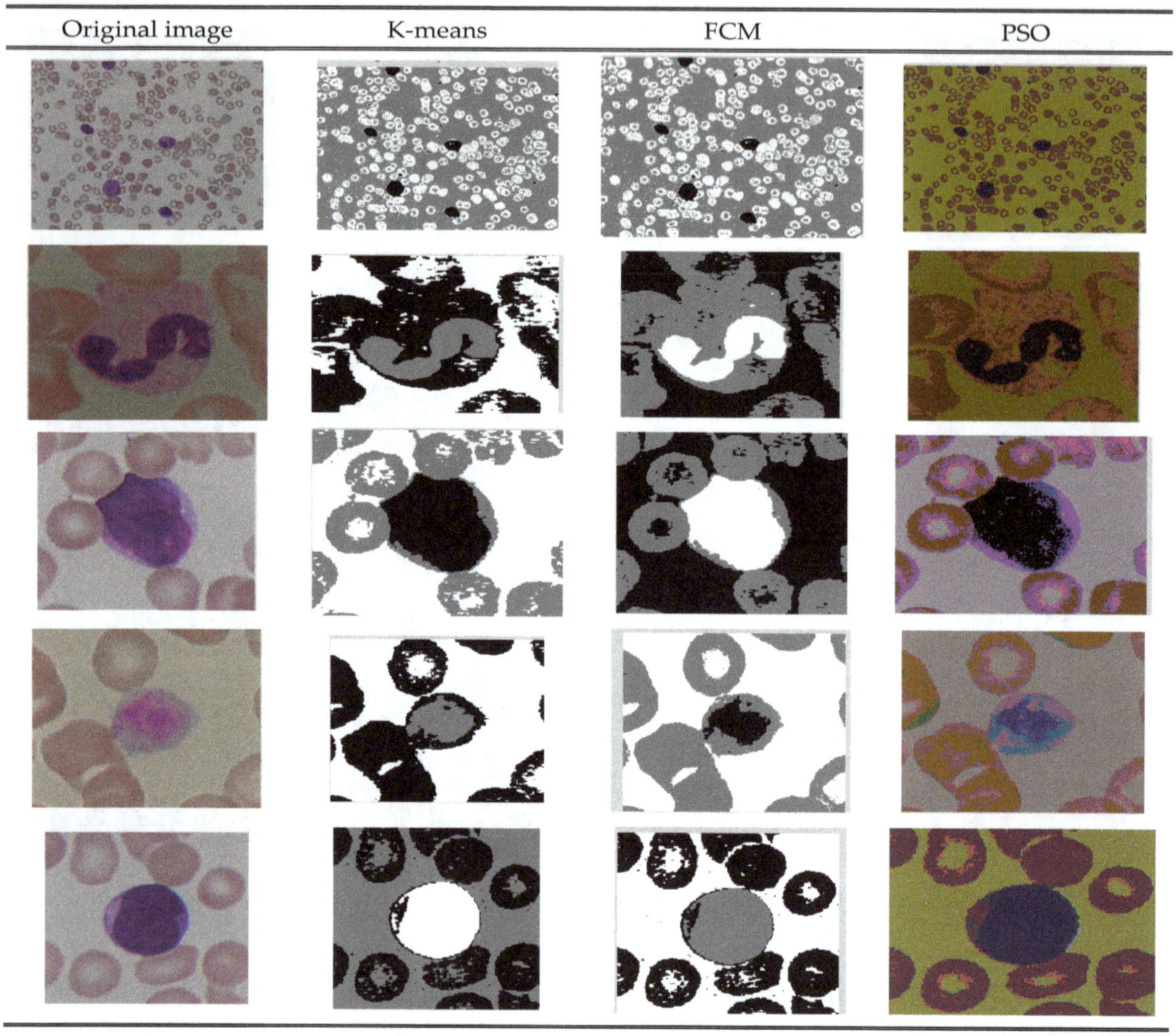


**Figure 4.** Segmentation results by k-means, FCM, and particle swarm optimization (PSO) algorithms.

## 4. Results and Discussion

### *4.1. Dataset*

The Acute Lymphoblastic Leukemia Image Database (ALL-IDB) datasets were used for this experiment. These data were downloaded from the website www.dti.unimi.it/fscotti/all/ [33–36]. There were 368 images—175 benign and 193 malignant—taken for this experimental analysis. Digital microscopes are not suitable, since they are usually designed to work in the RGB color space. In the preprocessing step, all the RGB input images are converted into a LAB color space.

### *4.2. Feature Extraction*

The segmented image data were too large, and it was very difficult to process them. Feature extraction is a technique to extract the relevant informative data of a segmented image. This will reduce the processing speed, time, and dimensionality of an image. In this research, 21 shape and color-based features—namely, the area, perimeter, roundness, elongation, form_factor, length_to_diameter_ratio, compactness, discrete_fourier_transform, mean_of_harra_coefficient, h_coefficient, v_coefficient, variance_of_harra_coefficient, h_coefficient, v_coefficient, mean_colour_intensity for red, green, and blue, hue, saturation, value component, and class attribute—were extracted [37]. Twenty-three texture-based features—namely, angular_second_moment, entropy, dissimilarity, contrast, inverse_difference, correlation, homogeneity, autocorrelation, cluster_shade, cluster_prominence, maximum_probability, sum_of_squares, sum_average, sum_variance, sum_entropy, difference_variance, difference_entropy, information_measures_correlation1, information_measures_correlation2, maximal_correlation_ coefficient, inverse_difference_normalized, inverse_difference_moment_normalized, and class attribute were extracted. These features are derived from the gray level co-occurrence matrix (GLCM) in directions 0°, 45°, 90°, and 135° [38,39]. From the literature review, we found that these features are widely used for leukemia image analysis.

### 4.3. Performance Assessments of Segmentation Algorithms

The empirical results are interpreted in two ways. First, we analyze the efficiency of various clustering-based segmentation algorithms through state-of-the-art machine learning algorithms. Secondly, we compare the machine learning methods using some evaluation measures such as receiver operating characteristic (ROC) curve analysis and kappa statistics. The extracted feature set was fed into the machine learning (ML) prediction algorithms to classify the segments indicating the tumor and non-tumor leukemia in the image. In this experiment, there were seven ML algorithms—namely, logistic regression (LR), naive Bayes (NB), support vector machine (SVM), k-nearest neighborhood (KNN), neural network (NN), random forest (RF), and decision tree (DT)—were used to evaluate the performance of the clustering algorithms.

The performance of the machine learning prediction algorithm was analyzed using various evaluation metrics such as accuracy (A), precision (P), recall (R), F1 measure, area under the ROC Curve (AUC), mean absolute error (MAE), and coefficient of determination ($R^2$) [40,41]. It is noted that the prediction value of $R^2$ lies between 0 and 1 for no-fit and perfect fit, respectively.

The classification results of k-means clustering, FCM clustering, PSO-based clustering, and the proposed HSCRKM clustering algorithms are presented in Tables 3–6, respectively. The performance of the segmentation algorithms was analyzed through different machine learning prediction methods. The experimental results show that the proposed method HSCRKM clustering algorithm performs better than the existing algorithms. On a closer look at the overall performance of the proposed method, it is believed that logistic regression and neural network perform well when compared to other prediction algorithms and also produce the highest classification accuracy i.e., 93%. It is also observed that the naive Bayes method produces the lowest classification accuracy rate i.e., 58%.

Table 3 presents the performance analysis of k-means clustering. The LR, NN, and RF algorithms produce the highest classification accuracy of 79%. The NB algorithm gives the minimum accuracy of 65%. KNN and DT produce 72% accuracy and SVM produces 74% accuracy. The overall performance of k-means clustering was 69%, which is computed by the average accuracy of all the datasets with all the ML algorithms.

Table 5 presents the performance analysis of FCM clustering. The LR, DT, and RF algorithms achieve the maximum accuracy value of 88%. Obviously, it gives the lowest mean absolute error (MAE) value. Similar to k-means clustering, the NB algorithm gives the lowest accuracy value of 81% when compared to other algorithms. The SVM and NN give the accuracy of 83% and 84%, respectively. The overall accuracy of FCM clustering is 77%.

**Table 3.** Performance analysis of k-means clustering. A: accuracy, AUC: area under the receiver operating characteristic curve, DT: decision tree, KNN: k-nearest neighborhood, LR: logistic regression, MAE: mean absolute error, NB: naive Bayes, NN: neural network, P: precision, R: recall, RF: random forest.

| ML Algorithms | Dataset | P | R | F1 | AUC | MAE | $R^2$ | A |
|---|---|---|---|---|---|---|---|---|
| LR | GLCM-0 | 81.00 | 77.00 | 78.00 | 0.821 | 0.134 | 0.195 | 76.74 |
| | GLCM045 | 79.00 | 79.00 | 78.00 | 0.660 | 0.087 | 0.076 | **79.07** |
| | GLCM-90 | 60.00 | 66.00 | 68.00 | 0.706 | 0.112 | 0.097 | 65.17 |
| | GLCM-135 | 70.00 | 66.00 | 67.00 | 0.805 | 0.128 | 0.159 | 67.44 |
| | SC | 76.00 | 74.00 | 75.00 | 0.805 | 0.115 | 0.152 | 74.42 |
| NB | GLCM-0 | 61.00 | 60.00 | 61.00 | 0.738 | 0.082 | 0.193 | 60.47 |
| | GLCM045 | 62.00 | 61.00 | 58.00 | 0.880 | 0.093 | 0.068 | 60.60 |
| | GLCM-90 | 54.00 | 51.00 | 50.00 | 0.799 | 0.128 | 0.162 | 51.16 |
| | GLCM-135 | 60.00 | 56.00 | 57.00 | 0.710 | 0.088 | 0.132 | 55.81 |
| | SC | 68.00 | 65.00 | 65.00 | 0.618 | 0.110 | 0.047 | **65.11** |
| SVM | GLCM-0 | 77.00 | 74.00 | 71.00 | 0.805 | 0.073 | 0.106 | **74.41** |
| | GLCM045 | 80.00 | 72.00 | 72.00 | 0.871 | 0.113 | 0.323 | 72.09 |
| | GLCM-90 | 82.00 | 70.00 | 73.00 | 0.792 | 0.032 | 0.143 | 69.77 |
| | GLCM-135 | 65.00 | 65.00 | 65.00 | 0.750 | 0.130 | 0.372 | 65.11 |
| | SC | 73.00 | 70.00 | 67.00 | 0.692 | 0.113 | 0.090 | 69.78 |
| KNN | GLCM-0 | 71.00 | 72.00 | 72.00 | 0.928 | 0.119 | 0.083 | **72.09** |
| | GLCM045 | 71.00 | 67.00 | 39.00 | 0.819 | 0.062 | 0.169 | 67.44 |
| | GLCM-90 | 69.00 | 67.00 | 67.00 | 0.817 | 0.138 | 0.162 | 67.44 |
| | GLCM-135 | 63.00 | 63.00 | 63.00 | 0.787 | 0.135 | 0.162 | 62.79 |
| | SC | 67.00 | 67.00 | 67.00 | 0.839 | 0.112 | 0.135 | 67.44 |
| NN | GLCM-0 | 79.00 | 79.00 | 76.00 | 0.821 | 0.077 | 0.274 | **79.06** |
| | GLCM045 | 77.00 | 77.00 | 77.00 | 0.806 | 0.139 | 0.348 | 76.74 |
| | GLCM-90 | 66.00 | 67.00 | 69.00 | 0.859 | 0.094 | 0.079 | 66.66 |
| | GLCM-135 | 72.00 | 70.00 | 71.00 | 0.817 | 0.105 | 0.052 | 69.69 |
| | SC | 65.00 | 65.00 | 64.00 | 0.853 | 0.116 | 0.090 | 65.11 |
| RF | GLCM-0 | 74.00 | 72.00 | 72.00 | 0.777 | 0.158 | 0.288 | 72.09 |
| | GLCM045 | 70.00 | 70.00 | 69.00 | 0.761 | 0.127 | 0.275 | 69.77 |
| | GLCM-90 | 69.00 | 65.00 | 65.00 | 0.798 | 0.106 | 0.182 | 65.11 |
| | GLCM-135 | 79.00 | 79.00 | 79.00 | 0.805 | 0.126 | 0.186 | **79.06** |
| | SC | 67.00 | 67.00 | 67.00 | 0.472 | 0.131 | 0.342 | 67.42 |
| DT | GLCM-0 | 66.00 | 70.00 | 66.00 | 0.865 | 0.073 | 0.192 | 69.76 |
| | GLCM045 | 80.00 | 79.00 | 76.00 | 0.549 | 0.093 | 0.101 | 79.06 |
| | GLCM-90 | 71.00 | 70.00 | 67.00 | 0.664 | 0.118 | 0.250 | 69.79 |
| | GLCM-135 | 72.00 | 72.00 | 71.00 | 0.852 | 0.118 | 0.250 | **72.09** |
| | SC | 72.00 | 70.00 | 71.00 | 0.817 | 0.105 | 0.052 | 69.69 |
| | | | **Average Overall Accuracy** | | | | | **69%** |

**Table 4.** Performance analysis of FCM clustering.

| ML Algorithms | Dataset | P | R | F1 | AUC | MAE | R^2 | A |
|---|---|---|---|---|---|---|---|---|
| LR | GLCM-0 | 79.00 | 79.00 | 76.00 | 0.802 | 0.089 | 0.098 | 79.06 |
| | GLCM045 | 89.00 | 88.00 | 89.00 | 0.950 | 0.080 | 0.401 | **88.37** |
| | GLCM-90 | 71.00 | 72.00 | 71.00 | 0.816 | 0.105 | 0.185 | 72.09 |
| | GLCM-135 | 88.00 | 86.00 | 82.00 | 0.792 | 0.058 | 0.156 | 86.04 |
| | SC | 81.00 | 77.00 | 78.00 | 0.821 | 0.134 | 0.195 | 76.74 |
| NB | GLCM-0 | 75.00 | 60.00 | 62.00 | 0.767 | 0.076 | 0.135 | 60.64 |
| | GLCM045 | 60.00 | 60.00 | 60.00 | 0.716 | 0.113 | 0.143 | 60.45 |
| | GLCM-90 | 63.00 | 63.00 | 63.00 | 0.787 | 0.135 | 0.162 | 62.79 |
| | GLCM-135 | 67.00 | 67.00 | 67.00 | 0.926 | 0.112 | 0.135 | 67.44 |
| | SC | 84.00 | 81.00 | 81.00 | 0.825 | 0.145 | 0.132 | **81.39** |

**Table 4.** *Cont.*

| ML Algorithms | Dataset | P | R | F1 | AUC | MAE | R^2 | A |
|---|---|---|---|---|---|---|---|---|
| SVM | GLCM-0 | 77.00 | 74.00 | 71.00 | 0.805 | 0.073 | 0.106 | 74.41 |
| | GLCM045 | 73.00 | 72.00 | 72.00 | 0.655 | 0.195 | 0.269 | 72.09 |
| | GLCM-90 | 75.00 | 74.00 | 73.00 | 0.822 | 0.176 | 0.265 | 74.41 |
| | GLCM-135 | 72.00 | 72.00 | 72.00 | 0.766 | 0.128 | 0.161 | 72.09 |
| | SC | 83.00 | 84.00 | 83.00 | 0.849 | 0.053 | 0.167 | **83.72** |
| KNN | GLCM-0 | 79.00 | 79.00 | 79.00 | 0.821 | 0.077 | 0.274 | 79.06 |
| | GLCM045 | 76.00 | 74.00 | 74.00 | 0.812 | 0.151 | 0.048 | 74.41 |
| | GLCM-90 | 83.00 | 83.00 | 84.00 | 0.893 | 0.122 | 0.368 | 83.72 |
| | GLCM-135 | 85.00 | 84.00 | 85.00 | 0.866 | 0.098 | 0.312 | **85.31** |
| | SC | 79.00 | 80.00 | 79.00 | 0.910 | 0.079 | 0.171 | 79.07 |
| NN | GLCM-0 | 84.00 | 84.00 | 84.00 | 0.745 | 0.125 | 0.349 | 83.72 |
| | GLCM045 | 87.00 | 85.00 | 82.00 | 0.773 | 0.148 | 0.238 | **84.84** |
| | GLCM-90 | 76.00 | 74.00 | 75.00 | 0.805 | 0.115 | 0.152 | 74.42 |
| | GLCM-135 | 79.00 | 79.00 | 79.00 | 0.805 | 0.126 | 0.186 | 79.07 |
| | SC | 80.00 | 77.00 | 77.00 | 0.771 | 0.101 | 0.156 | 77.18 |
| RF | GLCM-0 | 77.00 | 77.00 | 75.00 | 0.785 | 0.080 | 0.186 | 76.74 |
| | GLCM045 | 81.00 | 86.00 | 71.00 | 0.852 | 0.158 | 0.437 | 68.76 |
| | GLCM-90 | 80.00 | 77.00 | 77.00 | 0.839 | 0.155 | 0.248 | 76.74 |
| | GLCM-135 | 88.00 | 88.00 | 88.00 | 0.899 | 0.073 | 0.114 | **88.37** |
| | SC | 86.00 | 79.00 | 78.00 | 0.795 | 0.086 | 0.090 | 79.06 |
| DT | GLCM-0 | 84.00 | 83.00 | 83.00 | 0.929 | 0.159 | 0.265 | 82.75 |
| | GLCM045 | 88.00 | 88.00 | 88.00 | 0.953 | 0.050 | 0.138 | **88.37** |
| | GLCM-90 | 81.00 | 81.00 | 81.00 | 0.793 | 0.115 | 0.049 | 81.39 |
| | GLCM-135 | 87.00 | 86.00 | 86.00 | 0.938 | 0.064 | 0.053 | 86.04 |
| | SC | 85.00 | 81.00 | 76.00 | 0.813 | 0.131 | 0.095 | 81.39 |
| | | | **Average Overall Accuracy** | | | | | **77%** |

Table 5 shows the efficiency of the algorithm for PSO-based clustering. In this table, it is noted that the NN method attains 90% accuracy. The LR, SVM, KNN, and RF methods give above 80% of the classification accuracy. The NB algorithm again provides the minimum accuracy of 67%. The overall classification accuracy of PSO-based clustering is 78%.

**Table 5.** Performance analysis of PSO-based clustering.

| ML Algorithms | Dataset | P | R | F1 | AUC | MAE | $R^2$ | A |
|---|---|---|---|---|---|---|---|---|
| LR | GLCM-0 | 86.00 | 81.00 | 82.00 | 0.717 | 0.141 | 0.279 | 81.39 |
| | GLCM045 | 88.00 | 86.00 | 85.00 | 0.741 | 0.150 | 0.060 | **86.04** |
| | GLCM-90 | 84.00 | 79.00 | 76.00 | 0.739 | 0.143 | 0.095 | 79.06 |
| | GLCM-135 | 90.00 | 86.00 | 86.00 | 0.963 | 0.065 | 0.093 | **86.04** |
| | SC | 86.00 | 81.00 | 82.00 | 0.793 | 0.092 | 0.334 | 81.39 |
| NB | GLCM-0 | 69.00 | 67.00 | 68.00 | 0.833 | 0.082 | 0.098 | **67.44** |
| | GLCM045 | 60.00 | 64.00 | 66.00 | 0.713 | 0.118 | 0.129 | 63.63 |
| | GLCM-90 | 56.00 | 61.00 | 58.00 | 0.880 | 0.093 | 0.068 | 60.61 |
| | GLCM-135 | 64.00 | 64.00 | 65.00 | 0.764 | 0.012 | 0.165 | 63.63 |
| | SC | 61.00 | 62.00 | 62.00 | 0.876 | 0.118 | 0.148 | 62.69 |
| SVM | GLCM-0 | 84.00 | 79.00 | 76.00 | 0.739 | 0.143 | 0.095 | 79.07 |
| | GLCM045 | 79.00 | 79.00 | 78.00 | 0.827 | 0.085 | 0.142 | 79.06 |
| | GLCM-90 | 71.00 | 72.00 | 71.00 | 0.816 | 0.105 | 0.185 | 72.09 |
| | GLCM-135 | 76.00 | 77.00 | 72.00 | 0.807 | 0.086 | 0.192 | 76.74 |
| | SC | 81.00 | 81.00 | 79.00 | 0.801 | 0.120 | 0.167 | **81.39** |

**Table 5.** *Cont.*

| ML Algorithms | Dataset | P | R | F1 | AUC | MAE | $R^2$ | A |
|---|---|---|---|---|---|---|---|---|
| KNN | GLCM-0 | 82.00 | 79.00 | 80.00 | 0.811 | 0.123 | 0.017 | 79.06 |
| | GLCM045 | 71.00 | 73.00 | 71.00 | 0.864 | 0.082 | 0.108 | 72.72 |
| | GLCM-90 | 70.00 | 67.00 | 68.00 | 0.816 | 0.141 | 0.526 | 67.44 |
| | GLCM-135 | 75.00 | 74.00 | 73.00 | 0.822 | 0.176 | 0.265 | 74.41 |
| | SC | 82.00 | 81.00 | 81.00 | 0.788 | 0.118 | 0.147 | **80.66** |
| NN | GLCM-0 | 62.00 | 76.00 | 68.00 | 0.726 | 0.075 | 0.448 | 75.44 |
| | GLCM045 | 61.00 | 73.00 | 66.00 | 0.848 | 0.123 | 0.261 | 72.12 |
| | GLCM-90 | 88.00 | 84.00 | 83.00 | 0.849 | 0.053 | 0.167 | 83.72 |
| | GLCM-135 | 91.00 | 91.00 | 91.00 | 0.929 | 0.062 | 0.210 | **90.67** |
| | SC | 86.00 | 86.00 | 86.00 | 0.950 | 0.070 | 0.070 | 86.12 |
| RF | GLCM-0 | 84.00 | 81.00 | 81.00 | 0.825 | 0.145 | 0.135 | **81.39** |
| | GLCM045 | 74.00 | 79.00 | 74.00 | 0.885 | 0.114 | 0.264 | 78.77 |
| | GLCM-90 | 79.00 | 70.00 | 79.00 | 0.747 | 0.139 | 0.102 | 79.65 |
| | GLCM-135 | 78.00 | 78.00 | 77.00 | 0.917 | 0.082 | 0.538 | 77.47 |
| | SC | 81.00 | 81.00 | 81.00 | 0.841 | 0.097 | 0.056 | **81.39** |
| DT | GLCM-0 | 87.00 | 84.00 | 80.00 | 0.717 | 0.115 | 0.207 | 83.72 |
| | GLCM045 | 89.00 | 88.00 | 89.00 | 0.929 | 0.081 | 0.229 | **88.37** |
| | GLCM-90 | 87.00 | 85.00 | 82.00 | 0.662 | 0.086 | 0.125 | 84.84 |
| | GLCM-135 | 82.00 | 82.00 | 82.00 | 0.950 | 0.102 | 0.214 | 81.82 |
| | SC | 90.00 | 88.00 | 88.00 | 0.926 | 0.103 | 0.221 | 88.37 |
| | | | **Average Overall Accuracy** | | | | | **78%** |

The performance analysis of the HSCRKM algorithm is shown in Table 6. The LR, NN, and DT algorithms achieve 93% classification accuracy. NB, KNN, and RF give accuracy values of 84%, 85%, and 86%, respectively. It is also interesting to note that the SVM gives the minimum accuracy, i.e., 84%. The overall accuracy of the HSCRKM algorithm is 82%. The proposed method leads the accuracy of 13% for k-means clustering, 5% for FCM, and 4% for PSO-based clustering. It means that the accurate segmentation produces the best performance. The experimental results show that the HSCRKM algorithm accurately segments the nucleus. From the literature review report, the various authors produce above 90% accuracy. However, they are using a very small number of images for the experiments. In this research, around 350 images are used to evaluate the performance of the proposed HSCRKM algorithm.

**Table 6.** Performance analysis of the HSCRKM algorithm.

| ML Algorithms | Dataset | P | R | F1 | AUC | MAE | $R^2$ | A |
|---|---|---|---|---|---|---|---|---|
| LR | GLCM-0 | 84.00 | 84.00 | 85.00 | 0.848 | 0.017 | 0.214 | 84.72 |
| | GLCM045 | 93.00 | 93.00 | 93.00 | 0.944 | 0.072 | 0.584 | **93.02** |
| | GLCM-90 | 87.00 | 86.00 | 86.00 | 0.825 | 0.032 | 0.219 | 87.65 |
| | GLCM-135 | 89.00 | 88.00 | 88.00 | 0.899 | 0.112 | 0.427 | 88.37 |
| | SC | 86.00 | 85.00 | 85.00 | 0.965 | 0.047 | 0.138 | 85.65 |
| NB | GLCM-0 | 70.00 | 70.00 | 70.00 | 0.848 | 0.190 | 0.133 | 69.76 |
| | GLCM045 | 67.00 | 65.00 | 65.00 | 0.782 | 0.128 | 0.171 | 65.11 |
| | GLCM-90 | 67.00 | 65.00 | 65.00 | 0.782 | 0.128 | 0.171 | 65.11 |
| | GLCM-135 | 61.00 | 58.00 | 56.00 | 0.750 | 0.152 | 0.131 | 58.13 |
| | SC | 84.00 | 84.00 | 85.00 | 0.848 | 0.017 | 0.214 | **84.72** |
| SVM | GLCM-0 | 84.00 | 81.00 | 81.00 | 0.760 | 0.140 | 0.206 | 81.39 |
| | GLCM045 | 84.00 | 81.00 | 81.00 | 0.760 | 0.140 | 0.206 | 81.36 |
| | GLCM-90 | 79.00 | 79.00 | 79.00 | 0.768 | 0.321 | 0.341 | 79.06 |
| | GLCM-135 | 80.00 | 74.00 | 73.00 | 0.780 | 0.132 | 0.122 | 74.41 |
| | SC | 86.00 | 84.00 | 84.00 | 0.967 | 0.089 | 0.312 | **83.92** |

**Table 6.** *Cont.*

| ML Algorithms | Dataset | P | R | F1 | AUC | MAE | $R^2$ | A |
|---|---|---|---|---|---|---|---|---|
| KNN | GLCM-0 | 86.00 | 84.00 | 84.00 | 0.967 | 0.072 | 0.309 | 83.92 |
| | GLCM045 | 82.00 | 81.00 | 81.00 | 0.952 | 0.097 | 0.291 | 81.39 |
| | GLCM-90 | 75.00 | 72.00 | 71.00 | 0.727 | 0.127 | 0.102 | 72.09 |
| | GLCM-135 | 77.00 | 77.00 | 76.00 | 0.911 | 0.101 | 0.151 | 76.74 |
| | SC | 86.00 | 85.00 | 85.00 | 0965 | 0.047 | 0.138 | **85.65** |
| NN | GLCM-0 | 86.00 | 86.00 | 86.00 | 0.982 | 0.070 | 0.135 | 86.04 |
| | GLCM045 | 91.00 | 91.00 | 90.00 | 0.950 | 0.054 | 0.274 | 90.69 |
| | GLCM-90 | 84.00 | 84.00 | 85.00 | 0.848 | 0.017 | 0.138 | 84.72 |
| | GLCM-135 | 93.00 | 93.00 | 93.00 | 0.939 | 0.074 | 0.526 | **93.02** |
| | SC | 86.00 | 87.00 | 86.00 | 0.965 | 0.047 | 0.138 | 85.65 |
| RF | GLCM-0 | 82.00 | 81.00 | 81.00 | 0.860 | 0.174 | 0.331 | 81.39 |
| | GLCM045 | 86.00 | 85.00 | 85.00 | 0.965 | 0.047 | 0.138 | 85.65 |
| | GLCM-90 | 82.00 | 81.00 | 81.00 | 0.890 | 0.441 | 0.321 | 81.39 |
| | GLCM-135 | 84.00 | 84.00 | 85.00 | 0.848 | 0.017 | 0.214 | 84.72 |
| | SC | 86.00 | 87.00 | 86.00 | 0.913 | 0.144 | 0.225 | **86.05** |
| DT | GLCM-0 | 84.00 | 84.00 | 85.00 | 0.848 | 0.017 | 0.214 | 84.72 |
| | GLCM045 | 93.00 | 93.00 | 93.00 | 0.944 | 0.072 | 0.584 | **93.02** |
| | GLCM-90 | 86.00 | 84.00 | 84.00 | 0.967 | 0.072 | 0.309 | 83.72 |
| | GLCM-135 | 89.00 | 88.00 | 88.00 | 0.899 | 0.112 | 0.427 | 88.72 |
| | SC | 91.00 | 91.00 | 90.00 | 0.930 | 0.072 | 0.297 | 90.69 |
| **Average Overall Accuracy** | | | | | | | | **82%** |

Figure 5 shows the overall prediction accuracy for various machine learning algorithms. With respect to k-means clustering, all the machine learning algorithms produce the lowest prediction accuracy i.e., below 80%. It is noted that with respect to PSO and FCM, some of the ML methods (i.e., logistic regression, random forest, and decision tree) attain above 80% prediction accuracy. With respect to the HSCRKM clustering algorithm, most of the ML methods (except naive Bayes) achieve above 80% prediction accuracy. It can also be inferred that the proposed HSCRKM clustering algorithm efficiently segment the nucleus, and the extracted features (based on the segments) probably increase the prediction accuracy. To interpret the experimental results, we are manually preserving the best accuracy range as above 80%.

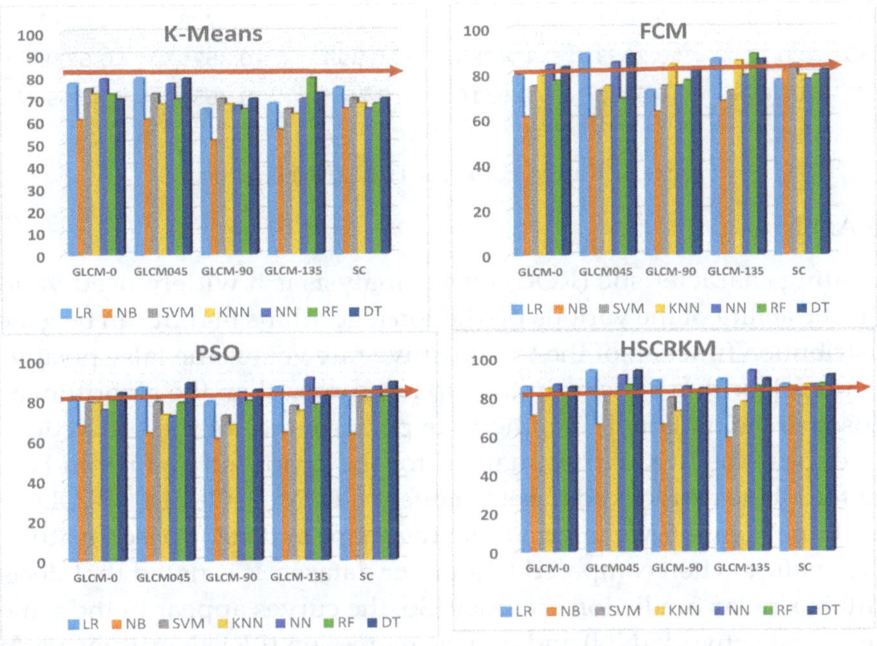


**Figure 5.** Overall prediction accuracy.

### *4.4. Performance Assessments of Machine Learning Algorithms*

#### 4.4.1. Kappa Statistics

Figure 6 shows a comparison of the performances for various prediction algorithms and the proposed HSCRKM algorithm in terms of Cohen's kappa value [42], which is a statistical measure used to evaluate the inter-rater reliability of the classifier. The reliability rate lies on a 0 to 1 scale, where "1" means perfect agreement and less than "1" means less than perfect agreement. With respect to the shape and color-based feature dataset, the proposed algorithm produces a substantial agreement range [43] (i.e., 0.61 to 0.80) amidst all the existing prediction algorithms taken up for study. Compared with other machine learning algorithms, neural networks have the capability to learn and model nonlinear and complex relationships. It also has the ability to perceive all possible interactions between predictor variables and the availability of multiple training algorithms. From the figure, it is noted that the neural network algorithm produces the highest kappa value (i.e., 0.67 to 0.85), which means perfect agreement for prediction. It also produces the highest classification accuracy when compared with other machine learning algorithms.

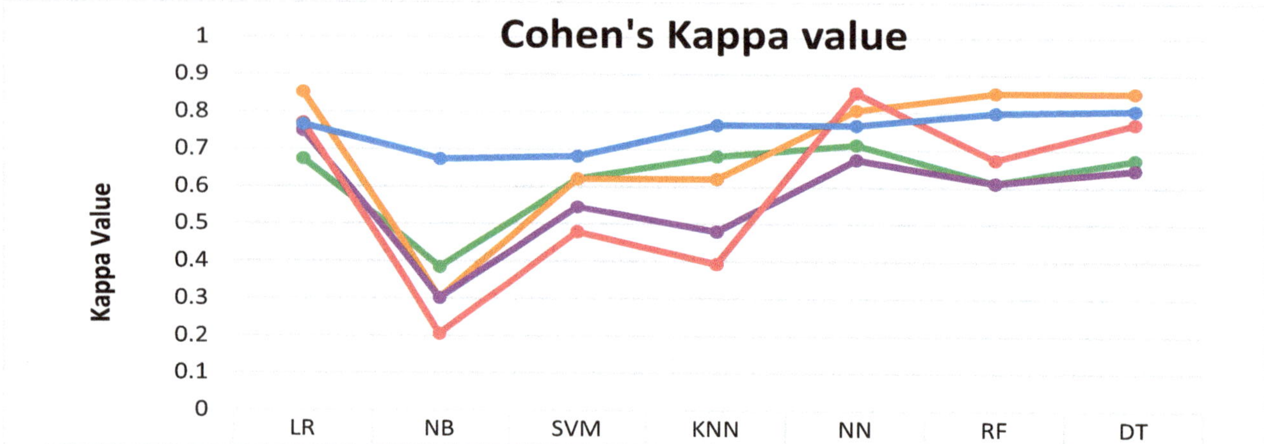


| | LR | NB | SVM | KNN | NN | RF | DT |
|---|---|---|---|---|---|---|---|
| GLCM-0 | 0.6738 | 0.3836 | 0.6211 | 0.6814 | 0.7139 | 0.6117 | 0.6738 |
| GLCM-45 | 0.8525 | 0.3011 | 0.6211 | 0.6211 | 0.8058 | 0.8525 | 0.8525 |
| GLCM-902 | 0.7492 | 0.3011 | 0.5452 | 0.4798 | 0.6738 | 0.6117 | 0.6472 |
| GLCM-135 | 0.77 | 0.2053 | 0.4785 | 0.393 | 0.8525 | 0.6738 | 0.77 |
| SC | 0.7655 | 0.6738 | 0.6814 | 0.7655 | 0.7655 | 0.799 | 0.8058 |

**Figure 6.** Kappa value for HSCRKM clustering.

#### 4.4.2. ROC Curve Analysis

Receiver operating characteristic (ROC) curve analysis is a widely used validation method to evaluate the diagnostic ability of the various prediction algorithms [44]. It can be generated by plotting the cumulative distribution function of the true positive rate versus the false positive rate. If the ROC curve of the prediction algorithm appears in the top left corner, then the algorithm accurately predicts disease. If it is closer to the diagonal line, then the performance of the prediction algorithm is less accurate. Figure 7 depicts the ROC curve analysis for the proposed algorithm HSCRKM. The ROC curve is generated for all the extracted datasets, namely GLCM_0, GLCM_45, GLCM_90, GLCM_135, and Shape_Colour. From Figure 6, we inferred that the shape and color-based feature datasets produce the highest accuracy values when compared to another dataset. It is noted that decision tree, random forest, and SVM attain similar prediction accuracy. So, the curves appear in the same orientation. It is also noted that the neural network (NN) and logistic regression (LR) algorithms performed better than the other machine learning algorithms. Those algorithms curve lines almost appeared in the top left corner of the graph. The naive Bayes algorithm curve line is executed near the diagonal line. So, this method probably attains minimum accuracy compared to the other ML algorithms.

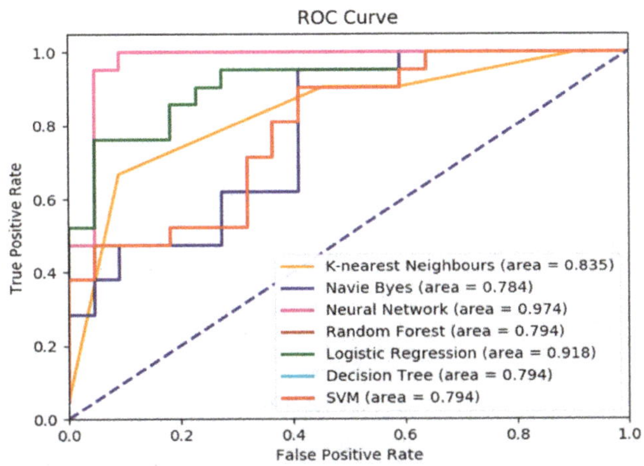


**(a)** GLCM_0

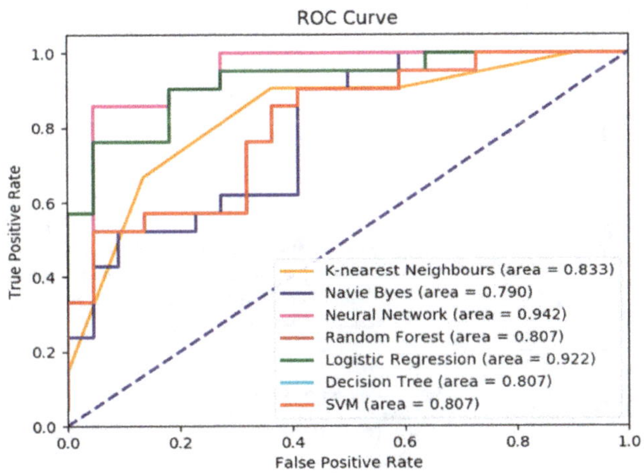


**(b)** GLCM_45

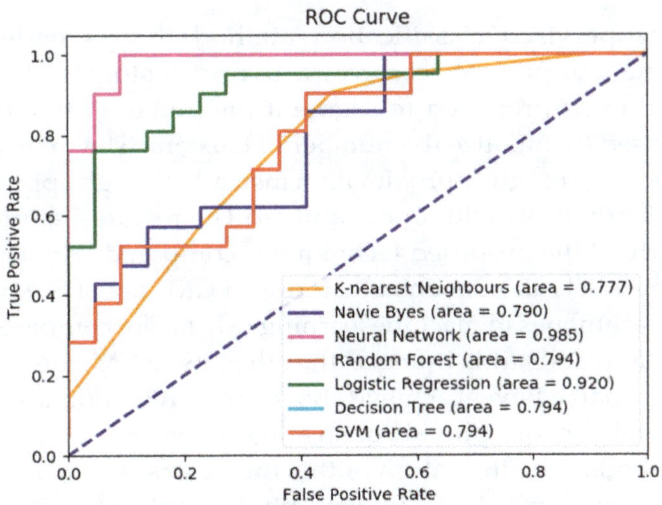


**(c)** GLCM_90

**Figure 7.** *Cont.*

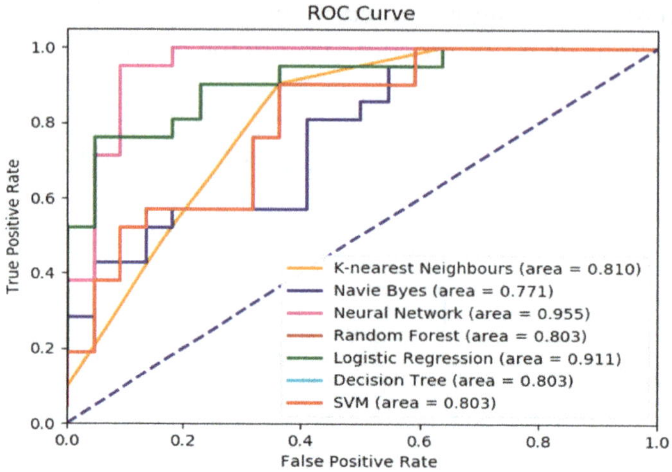


(**d**) GLCM_135

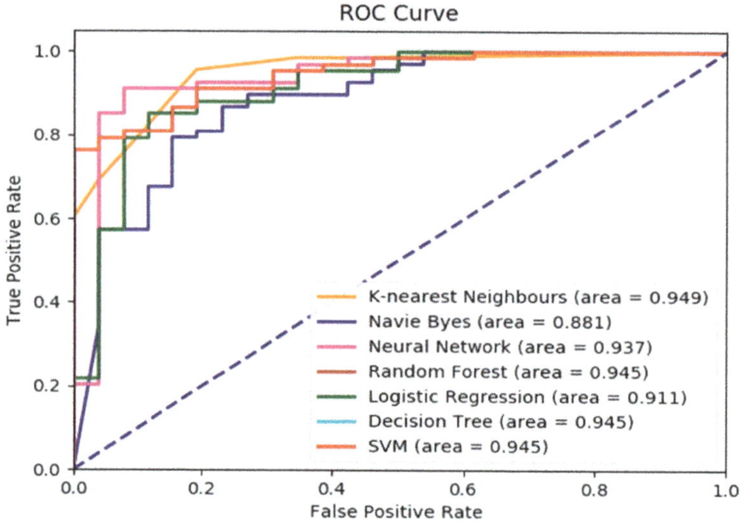


(**e**) Shape

**Figure 7.** ROC curve analysis for HSCRKM clustering.

## 5. Conclusions and Future Work

Clustering is an unsupervised classification method that is widely employed for image segmentation. Throughout the present research, a hybrid histogram-based soft covering rough k-means clustering algorithm is proposed to segment the image of the leukemia nucleus. In this method, the histogram is used to initialize the number of clusters. The main advantage of this method is that it applies the soft covering rough approximation instead of rough approximation. It is a new kind of soft rough set that efficiently deals with uncertainties. The results are interpreted in the following two ways. (1) The efficiency of the proposed technique is compared with the popular and frequently used clustering algorithms such as k-means clustering, FCM, and PSO-based clustering. (2) The state-of-the-art prediction techniques in machine learning (ML) were compared using evolution metrics.

From the experimental results, it is inferred that the HSCRKM clustering algorithm and all of the ML methods (except for naive Bayes) achieve above 80% prediction accuracy. It is also noted that logistic regression and neural network provide on average above 90% accuracy, which performs better than other prediction methods. The limitation of this method is that when we go for multiple color images such as satellite images, agricultural images, photographs etc., the number of peak values in the histogram is increased, and consequently the processing time is also increased. This method is more suitable for the segmentation of medical images and the extraction of specific portions with high clarity (for deep study). In the future, bio-inspired algorithms could be used to optimize the number of clusters.

**Author Contributions:** Conceptualization, J.G., A.T.A., and H.I.H.; methodology, J.G., A.T.A.; software, J.G.; validation, J.G., A.T.A., and H.I.H.; formal analysis, A.T.A. and H.I.H.; investigation, H.I.H.; resources, H.I.H.; data curation, J.G.; writing—original draft preparation, J.G., A.T.A., and H.I.H.; writing—review and editing, A.T.A. and H.I.H.; visualization, J.G.; funding acquisition, A.T.A. All authors have read and agreed to the published version of the manuscript.

**Acknowledgments:** The authors would like to thank Prince Sultan University, Riyadh, Saudi Arabia for supporting and funding this work. Special acknowledgment to Robotics and Internet-of-Things Lab (RIOTU) at Prince Sultan University, Riyadh, SA. In addition, the authors wish to acknowledge the editor and anonymous reviewers for their insightful comments, which have improved the quality of this publication.

## References

1. Surveillance, Epidemiology, and End Results (SEER). Cancer Stat Facts: Leukemia. Available online: https://seer.cancer.gov/statfacts/html/leuks.html (accessed on 3 January 2020).
2. Arora, R.S.; Arora, B. Acute leukemia in children: A review of the current Indian data. *South Asian J. Cancer* **2016**, *5*, 155. [CrossRef] [PubMed]
3. National Centre for Disease Informatics and Research. Available online: http://ncdirindia.org/ (accessed on 3 January 2020).
4. Pawlak, Z. Rough sets. *Int. J. Comput. Inf. Sci.* **1982**, *11*, 341–356. [CrossRef]
5. Zhu, W.; Wang, F. On three types of covering-based rough sets. *IEEE Trans. Knowl. Data Eng.* **2007**, *19*, 1131–1143. [CrossRef]
6. Zhu, W. Topological approaches to covering rough sets. *Inf. Sci.* **2007**, *177*, 1499–1508. [CrossRef]
7. Kumar, S.S.; Inbarani, H.H.; Azar, A.T.; Polat, K. Covering-based rough set classification system. *Neural Comput. Appl.* **2017**, *28*, 2879–2888. [CrossRef]
8. Molodtsov, D. Soft set theory—first results. *Comput. Math. Appl.* **1999**, *37*, 19–31. [CrossRef]
9. Maji, P.K.; Biswas, R.; Roy, A. Softset theory. *Comput. Math. Appl.* **2003**, *45*, 555–562. [CrossRef]
10. Yüksel, Ş.; Güzel Ergül, Z.; Tozlu, N. Soft covering based rough sets and their application. *Sci. World J.* **2014**. [CrossRef]
11. Jothi, G.; Hannah Inbarani, H. Leukemia Nucleus Image Segmentation Using Covering-Based Rough K-Means Clustering Algorithm. In Proceedings of the International Conference on Intelligent Computing Systems, Tamilnadu, India, 15–16 December 2017; pp. 373–385.
12. Zhang, G.P. Neural networks for classification: A survey. *IEEE Trans. Syst. Man Cybern. Part C* **2000**, *30*, 451–462. [CrossRef]
13. Mitchell, T.M. *Machine Learning*; McGraw Hill: Burr Ridge, IL, USA, 1997; Volume 45, pp. 870–877.
14. Cortes, C.; Vapnik, V. Support-vector networks. *Mach. Learn.* **1995**, *20*, 273–297. [CrossRef]
15. Friedman, N.; Geiger, D.; Goldszmidt, M. Bayesian network classifiers. *Mach. Learn.* **1997**, *29*, 131–163. [CrossRef]
16. Liaw, A.; Matthew, W. Classification and regression by random Forest. *R News* **2002**, *2*, 18–22.
17. Patel, N.; Mishra, A. Automated Leukaemia Detection Using Microscopic Images. *Procedia Comput. Sci.* **2015**, *58*, 635–642. [CrossRef]
18. Srisukkham, W.; Zhang, L.; Neoh, S.C.; Todryk, S.; Lim, C.P. Intelligent leukaemia diagnosis with bare-bones PSO based feature optimization. *Appl. Soft Comput.* **2017**, *56*, 405–419. [CrossRef]
19. Su, J.; Liu, S.; Song, J. A segmentation method based on HMRF for the aided diagnosis of acute myeloid leukemia. *Comput. Methods Programs Biomed.* **2017**, *152*, 115–123. [CrossRef] [PubMed]
20. Kaya, I.E.; Pehlivanlı, A.Ç.; Sekizkardeş, E.G.; Ibrikci, T. PCA based clustering for brain tumor segmentation of T1w MRI images. *Comput. Methods Programs Biomed.* **2017**, *140*, 19–28. [CrossRef]
21. Cabria, I.; Gondra, I. MRI segmentation fusion for brain tumor detection. *Inf. Fusion* **2017**, *36*, 1–9. [CrossRef]
22. Küçükkülahlı, E.; Erdoğmuş, P.; Polat, K. Histogram-based automatic segmentation of images. *Neural Comput. Appl.* **2016**, *27*, 1445–1450. [CrossRef]

23. Namburu, A.; kumar Samay, S.; Edara, S.R. Soft fuzzy rough set-based MR brain image segmentation. *Appl. Soft Comput.* **2017**, *54*, 456–466. [CrossRef]
24. Ali, M.; Khan, M.; Tung, N.T. Segmentation of Dental X-ray Images in Medical Imaging using Neutrosophic Orthogonal Matrices. *Expert Syst. Appl.* **2018**, *91*, 434–441. [CrossRef]
25. Rundo, L.; Militello, C.; Russo, G.; D'Urso, D.; Valastro, L.M.; Garufi, A.; Gilardi, M.C. Fully Automatic Multispectral MR Image Segmentation of Prostate Gland Based on the Fuzzy C-Means Clustering Algorithm. In *Multidisciplinary Approaches to Neural Computing. Smart Innovation, Systems and Technologies*; Esposito, A., Faudez-Zanuy, M., Eds.; Springer: Cham, Switzerland, 2017; Volume 69, pp. 23–37.
26. Zhang, P.; Lu, S.; Li, J.; Zhang, P.; Xie, L.; Xue, H.; Zhang, J. Multi-component segmentation of X-ray computed tomography (CT) image using multi-Otsu thresholding algorithm and scanning electron microscopy. *Energy Explor. Exploit.* **2017**, *35*, 281–294. [CrossRef]
27. Ganesh, M.; Naresh, M.; Arvind, C. MRI Brain Image Segmentation Using Enhanced Adaptive Fuzzy K-Means Algorithm. *Intell. Autom. Soft Comput.* **2017**, *23*, 325–330. [CrossRef]
28. Kaur, P. Intuitionistic fuzzy sets based credibilistic fuzzy C-means clustering for medical image segmentation. *Int. J. Inf. Technol.* **2017**. [CrossRef]
29. Dhane, D.M.; Maity, M.; Mungle, T.; Bar, C.; Achar, A.; Kolekar, M.; Chakraborty, C. Fuzzy spectral clustering for automated delineation of chronic wound region using digital images. *Comput. Biol. Med.* **2017**, *89*, 551–560.
30. Ahmed, N.; Yigit, A.; Isik, Z.; Alpkocak, A. Identification of Leukemia Subtypes from Microscopic Images Using Convolutional Neural Network. *Diagnostics* **2019**, *9*, 104. [CrossRef]
31. Yüksel, Ş.; Tozlu, N.; Dizman, T.H. An application of multicriteria group decision making by soft covering based rough sets. *Filomat* **2015**, *29*, 209–219. [CrossRef]
32. Peters, G. Some refinements of rough k-means clustering. *Pattern Recognit.* **2006**, *39*, 1481–1491. [CrossRef]
33. Labati, R.D.; Piuri, V.; Scotti, F. ALL-IDB: The Acute Lymphoblastic Leukemia Image Database for Image Processing. In Proceedings of the IEEE International Conference on Image Processing (ICIP), Brussels, Belgium, 11–14 September 2011.
34. Scotti, F. Robust Segmentation and Measurements Techniques of White Cells in Blood Microscope Images. In Proceedings of the IEEE Instrumentation and Measurement Technology Conference, Sorrento, Italy, 24–27 April 2006; pp. 43–48.
35. Scotti, F. Automatic morphological analysis for acute leukemia identification in peripheral blood microscope images. In Proceedings of the IEEE International Conference on Computational Intelligence for Measurement Systems and Applications, Giardini Naxos, Italy, 20–22 July 2005; pp. 96–101.
36. Piuri, V.; Scotti, F. Morphological classification of blood leucocytes by microscope images. In Proceedings of the IEEE International Conference on Computational Intelligence for Measurement Systems and Applications, Boston, MA, USA, 14–16 July 2004; pp. 103–108.
37. Jothi, G.; Inbarani, H.H. Hybrid Tolerance Rough Set–Firefly based supervised feature selection for MRI brain tumor image classification. *Appl. Soft Comput.* **2016**, *46*, 639–651.
38. Jothi, G.; Inbarani, H.H.; Azar, A.T. Hybrid Tolerance Rough Set: PSO Based Supervised Feature Selection for Digital Mammogram Images. *Int. J. Fuzzy Syst. Appl.* **2013**, *3*, 15–30. [CrossRef]
39. Jothi, G.; Inbarani, H.H. Soft set based feature selection approach for lung cancer images. *arXiv* **2012**, arXiv:1212.5391.
40. Inbarani, H.H.; Azar, A.T.; Jothi, G. Supervised hybrid feature selection based on PSO and rough sets for medical diagnosis. *Comput. Methods Programs Biomed.* **2014**, *113*, 175–185. [CrossRef] [PubMed]
41. Ganesan, J.; Inbarani, H.H.; Azar, A.T.; Polat, K. Tolerance rough set firefly-based quick reduct. *Neural Comput. Appl.* **2017**, *28*, 2995–3008. [CrossRef]
42. Landis, J.R.; Koch, G.G. The measurement of observer agreement for categorical data. *Biometrics* **1977**, *33*, 159–174. [CrossRef] [PubMed]
43. Viera, A.J.; Garrett, J.M. Understanding interobserver agreement: The kappa statistic. *Fam. Med.* **2005**, *37*, 360–363.
44. Fawcett, T. An introduction to ROC analysis. *Pattern Recognit. Lett.* **2006**, *27*, 861–874. [CrossRef]

# 13

# Using the Importance–Satisfaction Model and Service Quality Performance Matrix to Improve Long-Term Care Service Quality in Taiwan

**Shun-Hsing Chen [1], Fan-Yun Pai [2,*] and Tsu-Ming Yeh [3,*]**

1 Department of Marketing and Distribution Management, Oriental Institute of Technology, New Taipei City 220, Taiwan; chen88@mail.oit.edu.tw
2 Department of Business Administration, National Changhua University of Education, Changhua 500, Taiwan
3 Department of Industrial Engineering and Management, National Quemoy University, Kinmen 892, Taiwan
* Correspondence: fypai@cc.ncue.edu.tw (F.-Y.P.); tmyeh@nqu.edu.tw (T.-M.Y.);

**Abstract:** The present study integrates the importance–satisfaction (I-S) model and service quality performance matrix (SQPM) to examine long-term care (LTC) service demands and satisfaction improvement. Many scholars have used a single model to explore project improvement. Each model has advantages, but we think they are too subjective and suggest that it is best to integrate models to determine what should be improved. We established quality attributes of service demands based on more than two sessions of discussions and expert consultations with LTC service users (older adults). The final questionnaire was divided into three parts: a demand survey, satisfaction survey, and demographics survey, and 292 valid questionnaires were collected. The questionnaire items were summarized with means and standard deviations. In this study, if only the I-S model was used to examine LTC in Taiwan, then seven service elements of the system would need to be improved. However, if only the SQPM method was used, then 16 service elements would need to be improved. Only seven service elements were identified by both methods. When time and resources are limited, it is not feasible to take comprehensiveness into account. When many projects must be improved and it is impossible to implement them at the same time, improvement priorities need to be developed. Taiwan lacks sufficient LTC resources, so it is impossible to provide enough resources for all those who need care. To use resources efficiently, the I-S model and SQPM were integrated in this study to identify areas for improvement.

**Keywords:** Long-term care (LTC); importance-satisfaction (I-S) model; performance evaluation matrix (PEM); service quality performance matrix (SQPM); voice of customer (VOC)

---

## 1. Introduction

An aging population and changes in population structure directly impact social systems, such as the labor market, retirement planning, and the medical care system, and can lead to an economic crisis, such as a recession or government bankruptcy [1]. Therefore, population factors have become closely watched important issues in developed countries [2]. Taiwan's population of older adults exceeded 7% in 1993, making it an aging society [3], exceeded 14% in 2018, categorizing it as an aged society [4], and will exceed 20% in 2025, making Taiwan a super-aged society [5].

Long-term care (LTC) involves a variety of services designed to meet people's health or personal care needs during a short or long period of time. These services help people live as independently and safely as possible when they can no longer perform everyday activities on their own [6]. LTC is a very important issue for everyone in an aging society [5]. With the advancement of technology and medical treatments, the global average age has been extended to 75 years [7]. Taiwan is no exception. The continuous extension of life has resulted in changes in population structures [8]. The aging phenomenon is a problem that developed countries must face, along with related problems regarding the care of older adults [9]. In recent years, late marriage, bachelorism, and infertility have continued to intensify. Coupled with extended average life expectancy, low fertility, and population aging, they have also become concerning and unavoidable issues [10].

The implementation of LTC policies is based on the manager perspective rather than the user or customer point of view. In other words, LTC implementation ignores the voice of the customer (VOC). In the present study, the user point of view was used to explore service demands in LTC in Taiwan. Those who require LTC were divided into two groups: healthy older people, who are only interested in living happily, and older people with disabilities or dementia, who require medical interventions [11]. As the demands of these two groups are different, a service demand design would be ineffective, and could even affect national life, if it was viewed from an official perspective. Furthermore, the Taiwanese government has limited resources, and the needed resources would not necessarily be utilized at the same time. To address these issues and prioritize the efficient use of LTC resources, the importance-satisfaction (I-S) model and the revised performance evaluation matrix (PEM) can be used. Such a practice could fulfill LTC service demands by building a complete set of service design measurement methods.

Yang [12] developed the I-S model with reference to the importance performance analysis (IPA) method. The I-S model is the best tool for quality improvement [12,13]. Lambert and Sharma [14] proposed the performance evaluation matrix (PEM) to determine the importance of logistical service quality factors and the performance of companies based on these factors. PEM-related applications have been used in the machinery industry and in education; few applications have been used in long-term care. The PEM can help industries find service items that need improvement. The present study found no analyses on combining the I-S model and the PEM method for LTC service demands in the relevant literature. Due to insufficient studies and that the fact that currently LTC service demand policies are considered to be very important and urgent, the I-S model and PEM are introduced in the present study. It is hoped that this will provide more accurate quality service design and improve the essentials of LTC services to better meet the needs and expectations of the older adult population in Taiwan.

We conducted in-depth interviews in more than two sessions of discussions with experts and scholars through a focused discussion method to understand the LTC demands of the public and further confirm the service demands of caregivers, and we distributed 350 questionnaires. We also used the I-S model and the revised PEM method to find LTC users of corresponding management strategies to serve as a transmission basis for decision makers to adjust their services. This was to ensure that user service demands could be fully satisfied. In general, the purposes of this study can be summarized as follows:

1. To perform in-depth interviews with experts and scholars in focused discussions to confirm user service demands and service resources.
2. To use the I-S model and the revised PEM method to confirm the importance and priority levels of various service demands in order to serve as a basis for decision makers to adjust LTC service quality design and improve care for older adults.

The rest of this study is organized as follows: Section 2 reviews the literature related to long-term care in Taiwan, long-term care service demands of older adults, the service quality evaluation model, the I-S model, the service quality evaluation model, and related research methods. Section 3 presents the research process, methodology, questionnaire design, data collection method, and statistical analysis methods. The results of the analysis and discussion are given in Section 4. Finally, the conclusions of this study and suggestions are presented in Section 5.

## 2. Literature Review

### 2.1. Long-Term Care Act 2.0 of Taiwan

The advent of an aging society has brought about new challenges [11]. In the past, people around the world looked upon older adults as vulnerable and in need of care [8]. Through solutions provided by social welfare programs, we have gradually changed the traditional image that older adults are dependent towards a more positive image [15]. In addition to providing social benefits, such as nursing and medical care, we assist older adults in matters of self-reliance and self-esteem. Therefore, older adults do not become a social burden but instead can share their wisdom and contribute to national competitiveness [16].

Taiwan's LTC industry has taken a significant step forward due to assistance from the government. We must take further preventative measures to cope with the expected rise in the number of older people in Taiwan in the next 10 years. To ease the burden on young people, the Long-Term Care Act 2.0 (LTCA 2.0) is imperative [17]. The overall goal of LTCA 2.0 is to establish a high-quality, affordable, and universal LTC service system that has a community-based spirit, provides disabled people with basic care services, helps older adults to enjoy old age comfortably in familiar environments, and eases the burden of family care [18]. Therefore, a budget of NT$20.079 billion (0.11% of gross domestic product (GDP)) is expected to be allocated to LTCA 2.0, which is over four times the size of the NT$5.126 billion budget in 2016. The LTC Management Center has indicated that the linking of social resources such as medical treatment, LTC, and life support can be carried out through an overall community care model by connecting various service systems to provide needed care, while also saving LTC resources [19]. According to the long-term care policy blueprint proposed by Taiwan's Ministry of Health and Welfare [20], older adults who live at home and get sick and need to see a doctor can go through the medical system, older adults who are healthy and able to live on their own can go through the life support system, and older adults who are unhealthy or even disabled can go through the long-term system. The medical/long-term/life support care model can be seen in Figure 1.

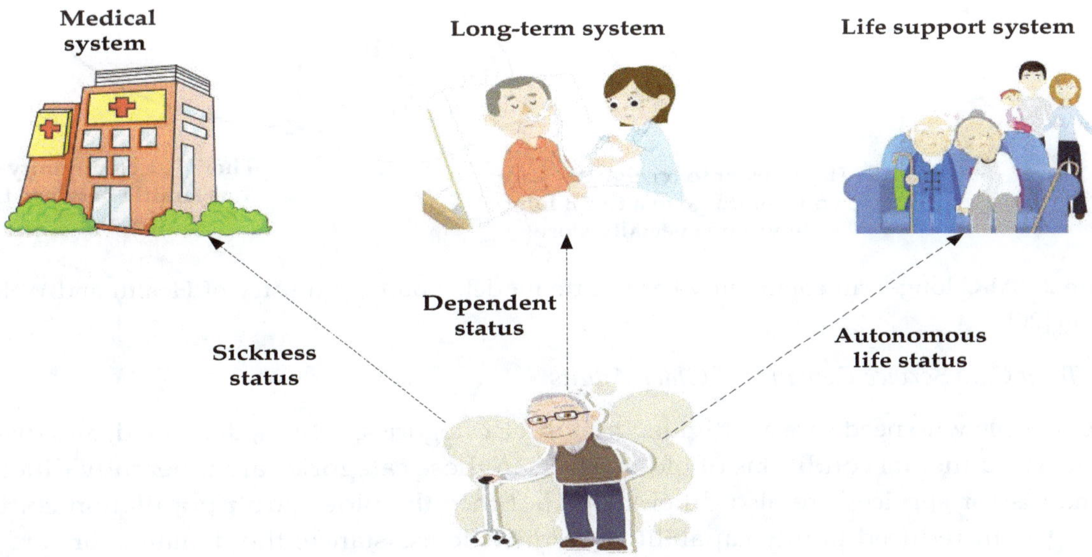


**Figure 1.** Medical/long-term/life support care model. Source: Ministry of Health and Welfare, Taiwan [20].

LTCA 2.0 is an extension of Taiwan's LTC political views. To address Taiwan's increasingly aging society, LTCA 2.0 proposes improving the strategies of three projects [20].

2.1.1. Widen Service Targets

Besides widening the care level of existing service targets, LTCA 2.0 also covers the following targets: (1) older people over 50 years old with dementia and disabled lowland aboriginals over 55 years old, and (2) disabled people younger than 49 years old and frail older people over 65 years old.

2.1.2. Provide Easily Accessible Service Units for the Public

For older people who could not find ways to get help in the past, the government introduced an innovative system by proposing an "ABC" long-term community-based care model (see Figure 2). It is described as follows: Tier A is referred to as the LTC flagship store, tier B as the LTC specialty store, and tier C as the LTC corner store. These "stores" are located within small communities, local neighborhoods, counties, and townships, and the different levels provide different services. For example, if you want to chat with someone, you should go to a tier C LTC corner store. If you want to receive day care, you should go to a tier B LTC specialty store. Finally, if you want to receive complete services, you should go to a tier A LTC flagship store.

2.1.3. Relax Subsidy Approval Regulations

In the past, the LTC Center paid subsidies in advance before asking for payment. This practice often affected service quality due to long processing times. However, under LTCA 2.0, the subsidy approval regulations have been relaxed to allow more institutions to invest in LTC services.

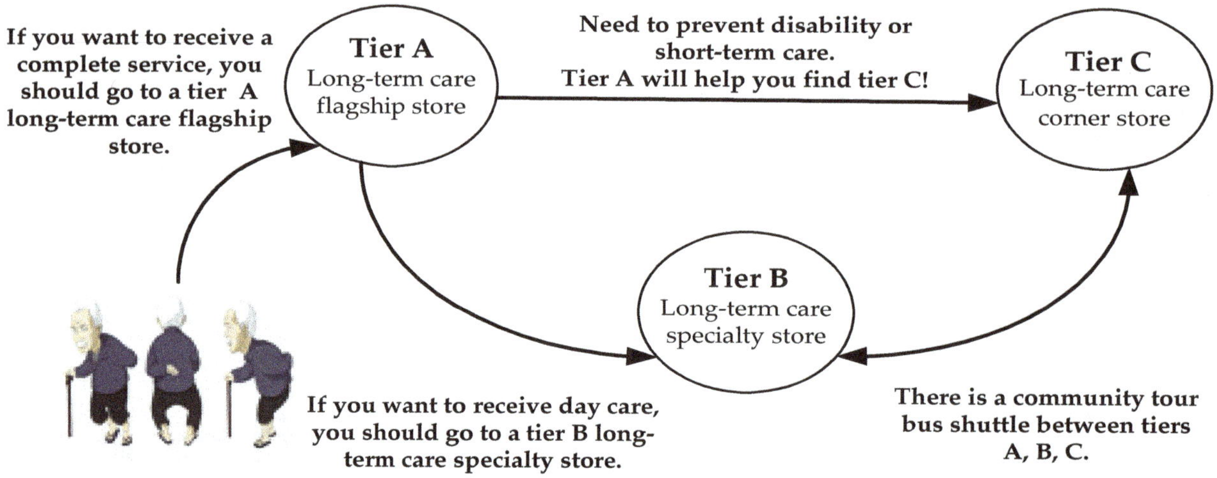


**Figure 2.** ABC long-term community-based care model. Source: Ministry of Health and Welfare, Taiwan [20].

2.2. *Long-Term Care Service Demands of Older Adults*

Older people who need care are divided into three categories: retired, demented, and disabled [8]. The physical and mental conditions of older adults in these categories are inherently different, and their demands for services are also different [11]. Since the older adult population continues to grow, along with reduced family capabilities to provide assistance, the demand for care services continues to rise [21]. Furthermore, although physiological differences between older adults are predictable, their mental, psychological, and behavioral conditions are not. The basic demands of older adults include economic, living, safety, health, leisure, and other types of support [22]. Lin and Chen [23] pointed out that the service demands of older adults include medical treatment, economic support, retirement, and reemployment, social participation, family care, interpersonal relationships, psychological adjustment, LTC, housing arrangements, annuity insurance, transportation, education and learning, leisure and entertainment, and other types of support. Shih et al. [24] divided older adult care services into home-based, community-based, and institution-style. The first two are for older adults living in communities. Home-based services include the following 10 services: health care, rehabilitation, physical care, housework, care visits, telephone-based care, catering, emergency rescue, home environment improvement, and other. Community-based services include the following 15 services: health care, medical care, rehabilitation, psychological counseling, day care, catering, family care, education, legal, transportation, retirement preparation, leisure, provision of information, referrals, and other.

### *2.3. Service Quality Evaluation Model*

#### 2.3.1. Importance Performance Analysis

Martilla and James [25] proposed importance performance analysis (IPA) (see Figure 3). IPA is a technique that prioritizes the relevant attributes of a particular service product by measuring its importance and degree of performance [26]. The IPA framework was first put forward in an attribution study on the motorcycle industry by plotting the average scores of importance and degree of performance in a 2D matrix and proposing different manufacturing/service strategies, depending on the position of each element, to resolve the production process faced by the enterprise [27].

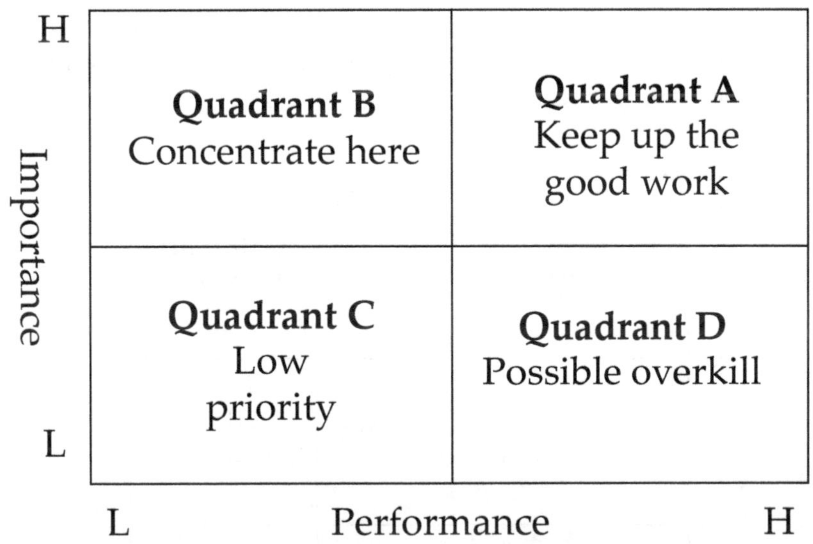


**Figure 3.** Importance performance analysis. Source: Martilla and James [25].

#### 2.3.2. Importance-Satisfaction Model

Businesses generally determine enhancement priorities based on attributes with low satisfaction rather than considering actual customer requirements [28,29]. Although this approach has removed some unsatisfactory quality attributes, these attributes are not the main areas that customers focus on [30]. Yang [12] considered that low-quality attributes should not be the only consideration when designing an improvement plan. In accordance with this rationale, Yang [12] developed the importance–satisfaction (I-S) model, with reference to the IPA method. This model is illustrated in Figure 4. The quadrants are designated as excellent (high importance, high satisfaction), to be improved (high importance, low satisfaction), surplus (low importance, high satisfaction), and unimportant (low importance, low satisfaction). Improvement strategies are based on the area in which each quality attribute is placed.

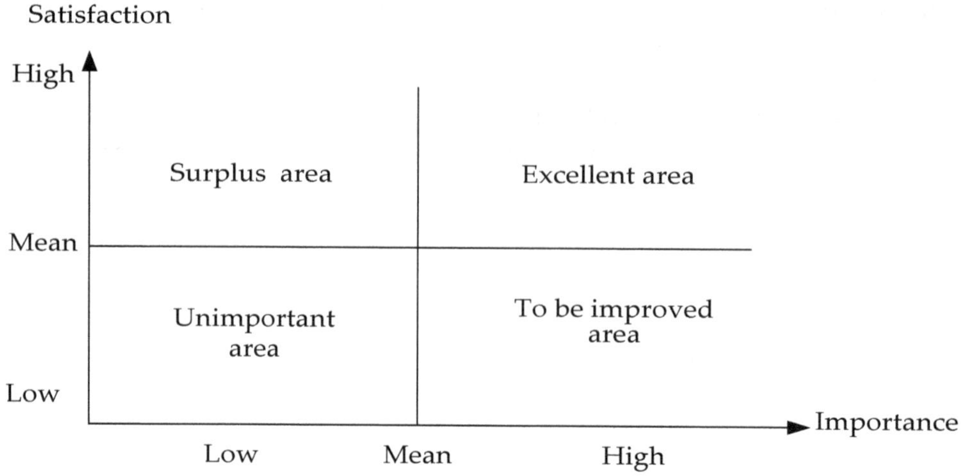


**Figure 4.** Importance–satisfaction model. Source: Yang [31].

2.3.3. Performance Evaluation Matrix

Lambert and Sharma [14] proposed the performance evaluation matrix (PEM) to determine the importance of logistical service quality factors and the performance of companies based on these factors. Performance variables are placed on the horizontal axis, and importance variables on the vertical axis [31]. Improvement strategies are then suggested based on evaluating these two factors in response to different positions (see Figure 5).

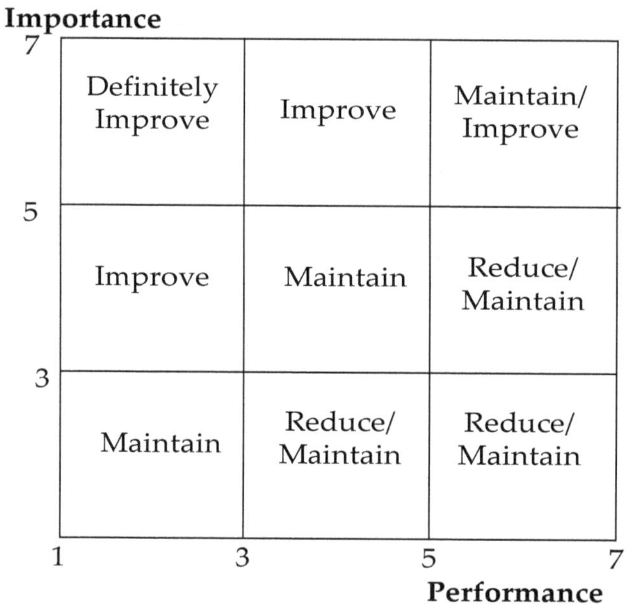


**Figure 5.** Performance evaluation matrix. Source: Lambert and Sharma [32].

From this matrix analysis, the current performance and competition status of the examined organizations can serve as directions for future development. PEM provides a reference for whether or not business owners should adjust their performance and response strategies [32]. Due to different perspectives explored by scholars, the viewpoints vary. Chen and Yeh [13] proposed amending the variables by placing importance variables on the horizontal axis and satisfaction variables on the vertical axis. The revised PEM was developed from these changes (see Figure 6).

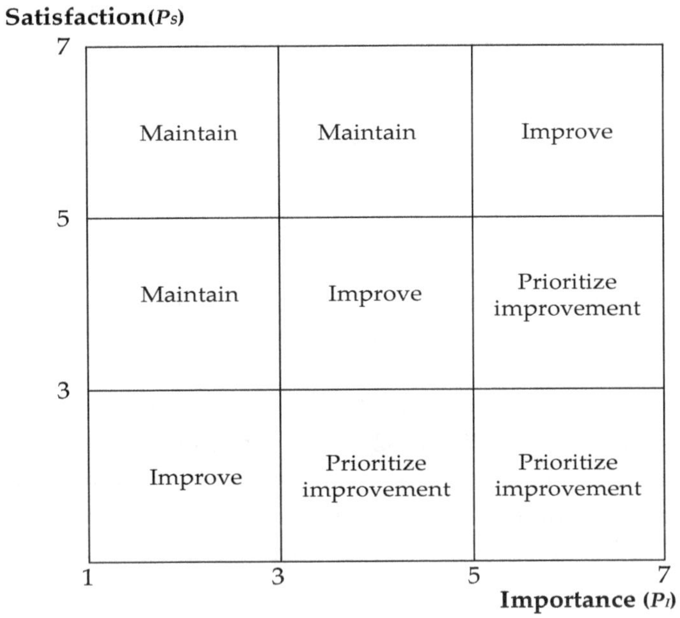


**Figure 6.** Revised performance evaluation matrix. Sources: Chen and Yeh [13].

2.3.4. Establishment of Service Quality Performance Matrix

Lambert and Sharma [14] proposed the PEM as a reference for quality improvement, but this matrix lacks generalization and standardization and is limited to a 7-point Likert scale [33]. Many subsequent scholars, such as Lin et al. [34] and Chen [28], proposed a revised PEM and applied it to the management method of quality improvement in enterprises. Scholars have not implemented this model as a basis for quality improvement in the LTC industry. In light of the views of previous scholars, this study applied a revised PEM to the quality management strategy of the LTC industry (see Figure 7). To generalize and standardize this model, a 5-point Likert scale, which is considered to be the most reliable scaling tool in the literature and widely used by scholars, was adopted in this study [35].

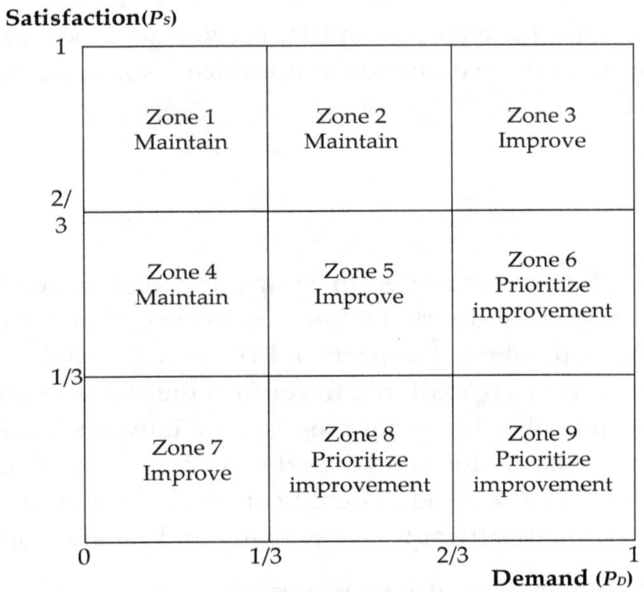


**Figure 7.** The service quality performance matrix.

Below, according to the theory of Hung et al. [33], the random variable $D$ denotes demand, and $S$ denotes satisfaction. A 5-point scale was adopted to evaluate the demand and satisfaction of each item. The indices of demand and satisfaction are defined as follows:

$$P_D = \frac{\mu_D - \min}{R} \quad (1)$$

$$P_S = \frac{\mu_S - \min}{R} \quad (2)$$

where $P_D$ is the index of demand, $P_S$ is index of satisfaction, min is the minimum value of scale k, and $R$ is the full range of scale k. Furthermore, $\mu_D$ and $\mu_S$ are the means of demand *(D)* and satisfaction *(S)*, respectively, min = 1 represents the minimum of scale k, and $R = \mathrm{k} - 1$ is the full range of scale k.

Based on the literature review, we know that PEM has been used extensively in recent years and can be applied to decision-making practices [32]. This method is mostly used in logistics and in the semiconductor, financial, and service industries, and its application in relevant studies of LTC is still rare. Hence, we chose PEM as one of the research methods. In this study, the resource allocation for the LTC concept was used as the basis to explore service satisfaction levels for older people who require care. The corresponding strategies of maintenance, improvement, and priority improvement of the revised PEM put forward by Chen and Yeh [13] were re-proposed. This matrix is called the service quality performance matrix (SQPM). Zones 1, 2, and 4 are areas where older adults' cognitive satisfaction exceeds demand. Therefore, service resources should be maintained at their current status, and the strategy is to maintain service quality. Zones 3, 5, and 7 are areas where satisfaction is equal to demand, indicating that the service does not exceed user expectations; therefore, organizations must improve their existing service quality by investing in more resources, and the proposed strategy is to improve. Zones 6, 8, and 9 are areas where demand exceeds satisfaction, indicating that older adults are well aware of service projects, but they are not satisfied with the services provided. As a result, governments and organizations must actively make improvements to correct these issues, and the response strategy is to prioritize improvement. All factors that prioritize improvement are the response strategies that this study puts forward and are regarded as factors that should be prioritized.

In the relevant literature, most PEM-related applications were in the machinery industry [34] and education [36], and few were applied in the service industry, and PEM was not formally applied to LTC service demand and resource allocation at all. In this study, the literature and relevant practical experience were used to identify the elements of LTC service demands, and the SQPM method was used to determine the priority of these demands to optimize resource allocation and implement care for older adults' retirement.

## 3. Research Methods

### *3.1. Research Process*

This study aimed to explore issues related to aging and long-term care services in Taiwan. First, the relevant literature was analyzed and sorted to serve as a conceptual framework for the construction of LTC service demands. Second, relevant impacts of LTC on national development, politics, culture, and the quality of the population were explored to confirm the status of and problems faced by LTC. According to the long-term care policy blueprint proposed by Taiwan's Ministry of Health and Welfare and more than two sessions of discussions and expert consultations with LTC users (older adults) to ensure the service elements of LTCA 2.0, the 20 quality attributes of service demands were established as follows. We used these 20 quality attributes for demand and satisfaction surveys.

1. Retirement pension or living allowance subsidies
2. Health-promoting physical fitness activities
3. Visits or telephone care services by social welfare agencies
4. Catering delivery services

5. Emergency medical care and rescue services
6. Transportation services
7. Older people eating meals together
8. Retirement planning
9. Employment services
10. Day care center services
11. Family companionship
12. Financial planning
13. Hospice care
14. Prices charged (older people eating meals together or class fees)
15. Service staff attitudes
16. Institutional accessibility
17. Community/residential institution environmental cleanliness
18. Community/institution activity planning
19. Community/institution dining comfort
20. Community/institution emergency response.

### *3.2. Design and Size of the Questionnaire*

The questionnaire was based on: (i) a review of the literature [22,23,37] and (ii) discussions with experts (including LTC consultants and scholars) and older adults. The final questionnaire included 40 items (20 quality attributes for demand and satisfaction surveys) and was divided into three parts:

1. Demand survey: included 20 quality attributes, responses requested on a 5-point Likert-type scale, with 1 representing extremely low demand and 5 representing extremely high demand; we used a mean value of these items.
2. Satisfaction survey: included 20 quality attributes, responses requested on a 5-point Likert-type scale, with 1 representing extremely dissatisfied and 5 representing extremely satisfied; we also used a mean value of these items.
3. Demographics survey: gender, marital status, age, living status, education degree, and occupation prior to retirement.

The samples for this research were people older than 55 years (service targets of LTC) who lived in a long-term institution or attended a senior citizens' learning camp. Taiwanese older people residing in Taipei and New Taipei were the participants in this study. In addition, in the process of questionnaire distribution, some older people were found to be much older or illiterate. In these cases, the questionnaire was administered verbally to make the questions more comprehensive.

### *3.3. Data Analysis*

In this study, we first reported the frequency and percentage distributions of the participants' basic characteristics (such as gender, marital status, age, living status, education and occupation before retirement). Descriptive statistics were used to summarize the respondents' profiles and then the mean and standard deviation of service demand and satisfaction. Cronbach's alpha was calculated for the sums of demand items and satisfaction items surveys as an estimate of the reliability of a psychometric test. Finally, we put all 20 service elements into the Importance–satisfaction (I-S) model and Service Quality Performance Matrix to determine the items that need to improve. Improvement strategies are then suggested based on evaluating these two factors in response to different positions. We used SPSS version 18 (SPSS, Chicago, IL, USA) to execute all analyses.

## 4. Research Results

### 4.1. Sample Narrative Statistical Analysis

The samples of this research were people older than 55 years (service targets of LTC) who lived in a long-term institution or attended a senior citizens' learning camp. Out of the 350 questionnaires distributed from January to May 2018, 315 were collected, for a recovery rate of 90.0%. A total of 23 questionnaires were found to be invalid, making the total valid responses 292. The results of the questionnaire indicated that 267 respondents were married (91.44%); 189 were female (64.73%); 115 lived in residential institutions (39.38%); 84 had a university education background (28.77%); 87 were in the military, government employees, or teachers before retirement (29.79%); and 87 were in the age range 65–70 years old (29.79%), as shown in Table 1.

**Table 1.** Descriptive statistics of the sample population.

| Category | Items | No. | % | Category | Items | No. | % |
|---|---|---|---|---|---|---|---|
| Gender | Male | 103 | 35.27% | Education degree | Illiterate | 17 | 5.82% |
| | Female | 189 | 64.73% | | Elementary school | 60 | 20.55% |
| Marital status | Unmarried (divorced) | 25 | 8.56% | | Junior high school | 51 | 17.47% |
| | Married | 267 | 91.44% | | High school | 78 | 26.71% |
| Age | 55–64 | 52 | 17.81% | | College/university | 84 | 28.77% |
| | 65–70 | 87 | 29.79% | | Above master | 2 | 0.68% |
| | 71–75 | 51 | 17.47% | Occupation before retirement | Office holder | 87 | 29.79% |
| | 76–80 | 80 | 27.40% | | Service industry | 61 | 20.89% |
| | Above 80 | 22 | 7.53% | | Industry | 49 | 16.78% |
| Living status | Living with children/couples | 106 | 36.30% | | High-tech industry | 12 | 4.11% |
| | Living with relatives | 51 | 17.47% | | Agriculture industry | 7 | 2.40% |
| | Living in a residential institution | 115 | 39.38% | | Household | 61 | 20.89% |
| | Living alone | 20 | 6.85% | | Self-employed | 15 | 5.14% |

A service needs survey was conducted to examine the demand level of older adults for essential elements. The higher the demand level, the more important these elements are to older adults; therefore, the government should pay attention to them in its administrative measures. The results are shown in Table 2. The average value of the demand survey was found to be 4.16, with a standard deviation of 0.99, showing that older adults have a very high awareness of all the elements, and each element is vital to them. The three items with the highest demand were retirement pension or living allowance subsidies, emergency medical care and rescue services, and retirement planning.

The survey was meant to understand the service demands of older adults and confirm whether their demands were satisfied. The lower the satisfaction level, the higher the dissatisfaction with services provided by the government and service providers, indicating that these items should be improved. The average value of the satisfaction survey was found to be 2.93, with a standard deviation of 0.78, indicating that older adults are less satisfied with all elements. The three items with the lowest satisfaction levels were retirement pension or living allowance subsidies, emergency medical care and rescue services, and family companionship. These elements must be listed in the improvement priorities.

**Table 2.** The mean and standard deviation of service demand and the satisfaction survey (N = 292).

| Item | | Demand | | Satisfaction | |
|---|---|---|---|---|---|
| | | ME | S.D. | ME | S.D. |
| 1. | Retirement pension or living allowance subsidies | 4.89 | 0.95 | 2.19 | 0.49 |
| 2. | Health-promoting physical fitness activities | 4.67 | 0.81 | 2.67 | 0.65 |
| 3. | Visits or telephone care services by social welfare agencies | 4.01 | 1.01 | 2.70 | 0.68 |
| 4. | Catering delivery services | 4.10 | 1.11 | 2.68 | 1.12 |
| 5. | Emergency medical care and rescue services | 4.79 | 0.91 | 2.48 | 0.54 |
| 6. | Transportation services | 4.33 | 1.05 | 2.61 | 0.91 |
| 7. | Older people eating meals together | 4.61 | 0.99 | 2.72 | 0.56 |
| 8. | Retirement planning | 4.72 | 1.08 | 2.97 | 0.54 |
| 9. | Employment services | 4.06 | 1.11 | 2.66 | 0.83 |
| 10. | Day care center services | 3.91 | 1.18 | 2.64 | 1.13 |
| 11. | Family companionship | 4.24 | 0.91 | 2.56 | 0.75 |
| 12. | Financial planning | 3.99 | 1.04 | 2.65 | 0.82 |
| 13. | Hospice care | 4.34 | 1.10 | 2.64 | 1.03 |
| 14. | Prices charged (older people eating meals together or class fees) | 4.69 | 1.02 | 3.05 | 1.07 |
| 15. | Service staff attitudes | 3.51 | 0.98 | 3.92 | 0.71 |
| 16. | Institutional accessibility | 4.18 | 0.87 | 3.46 | 0.93 |
| 17. | Community/residential institution environmental cleanliness | 3.58 | 0.75 | 3.37 | 0.87 |
| 18. | Community/institution activity planning | 3.32 | 0.91 | 3.86 | 0.77 |
| 19. | Community/institution dining comfort | 3.28 | 0.85 | 3.40 | 0.69 |
| 20. | Community/institution emergency response | 4.01 | 1.07 | 3.32 | 0.59 |
| | Total of all 20 items | 4.16 | 0.99 | 2.93 | 0.78 |

Note: ME = mean; S.D. = standard deviation.

### *4.2. Reliability Analysis*

A reliability test is used to measure whether a tool is consistent and reliable, and Cronbach's alpha is generally used as a benchmark to measure the reliability of a questionnaire. If Cronbach's alpha is greater than 0.7, it has high reliability, while if it falls between 0.35 and 0.7, the reliability is barely acceptable [38,39]. In this study, Cronbach's alpha for service demand was 0.82, and for satisfaction was 0.89. As the overall reliability value of 0.91 is greater than 0.7, it shows high reliability and indicates that the scale has good consistency and reliability.

### *4.3. Importance-Satisfaction Model Results*

When all the service elements were placed in the I-S model, as shown in Figure 8, those in the excellent area were items 8, 14, and 16. Service demand and service satisfaction are above the average, which indicates that customers need these services, and older adults feel satisfied about services provided by the government or service providers. This also shows that the resources can be used effectively.

The service elements in the to be improved area were items 1, 2, 5, 6, 7, 11, and 13, indicating that service demand is above the average, and satisfaction is below the average. This indicates that customers highly need these services, but they are not offered by service providers or have not been provided at a level found to be satisfactory by older adults. Given the low level of satisfaction, it is recommended that service providers should improve these services first.

The service elements in the surplus area were items 15, 17, 18, 19, and 20, indicating that service demand is below the average, and customers are not concerned with these services. Service satisfaction is higher than the average, indicating that resources are being misplaced or wasted. Therefore, surplus resources should be reallocated to service items with high demand and low satisfaction.

The service elements in the unimportant area were items 3, 4, 9, 10, and 12, indicating that service demand and satisfaction are lower than the average. Customers do not value these services but accept the performance of service providers. Therefore, as long as these elements are provided appropriately, it is not necessary to enhance the service quality. In fact, increasing resources in this area could be considered a waste.

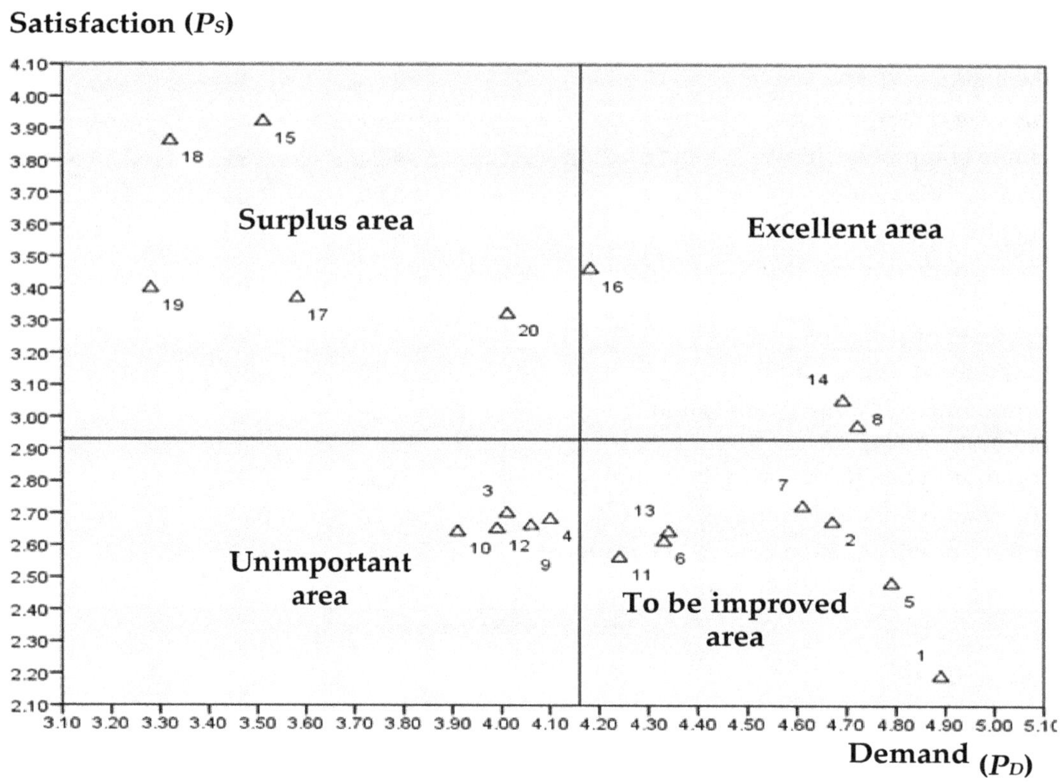


**Figure 8.** Importance–satisfaction (I-S) model results.

## 4.4. Service Quality Performance Matrix Results

The average value and index of each question were calculated through Formulas (1) and (2), as shown in Table 3, and the relevant values were introduced into the SQPM, as shown in Figure 9. The service elements in the priority improvement area were items 1–16 and 20, indicating that the demand for these services exceeds satisfaction, and older adults are unsatisfied with them. Therefore, they need to be improved. The service elements in the improvement area were items 17 and 19, indicating that the demand for these services is equal to the satisfaction, and they are accepted by older adults. Therefore, service providers can list surplus resources as secondary improvement items. The service elements in the maintenance area were items 15 and 18, indicating that satisfaction for these services is higher than the demand, and older adults are happy about them and highly satisfied. Therefore, service providers can maintain the current service quality.

**Table 3.** Relative values for I-S model and service quality performance matrix (SQPM).

| No. | $\mu_D$ | $\mu_P$ | $P_D$ | $P_P$ | I-S Model | SQPM |
|---|---|---|---|---|---|---|
| 1 | 4.89 | 2.19 | 0.97 | 0.30 | To be improved | Prioritize improvement |
| 2 | 4.67 | 2.67 | 0.92 | 0.42 | To be improved | Prioritize improvement |
| 3 | 4.01 | 2.70 | 0.75 | 0.43 | Unimportant | Prioritize improvement |
| 4 | 4.10 | 2.68 | 0.78 | 0.42 | Unimportant | Prioritize improvement |
| 5 | 4.79 | 2.48 | 0.95 | 0.37 | To be improved | Prioritize improvement |
| 6 | 4.33 | 2.61 | 0.83 | 0.40 | To be improved | Prioritize improvement |
| 7 | 4.61 | 2.72 | 0.90 | 0.43 | To be improved | Prioritize improvement |
| 8 | 4.72 | 2.97 | 0.93 | 0.49 | Excellent | Prioritize improvement |
| 9 | 4.06 | 2.66 | 0.77 | 0.42 | Unimportant | Prioritize improvement |
| 10 | 3.91 | 2.64 | 0.73 | 0.41 | Unimportant | Prioritize improvement |
| 11 | 4.24 | 2.56 | 0.81 | 0.39 | To be improved | Prioritize improvement |
| 12 | 3.99 | 2.65 | 0.75 | 0.41 | Unimportant | Prioritize improvement |
| 13 | 4.34 | 2.64 | 0.84 | 0.41 | To be improved | Prioritize improvement |
| 14 | 4.69 | 3.05 | 0.92 | 0.51 | Excellent | Prioritize improvement |
| 15 | 3.51 | 3.92 | 0.63 | 0.73 | Surplus | Maintain |
| 16 | 4.18 | 3.46 | 0.80 | 0.61 | Excellent | Prioritize improvement |
| 17 | 3.58 | 3.37 | 0.65 | 0.59 | Surplus | Improve |
| 18 | 3.32 | 3.86 | 0.58 | 0.71 | Surplus | Maintain |
| 19 | 3.28 | 3.40 | 0.57 | 0.60 | Surplus | Improve |
| 20 | 4.01 | 3.32 | 0.75 | 0.58 | Surplus | Prioritize improvement |

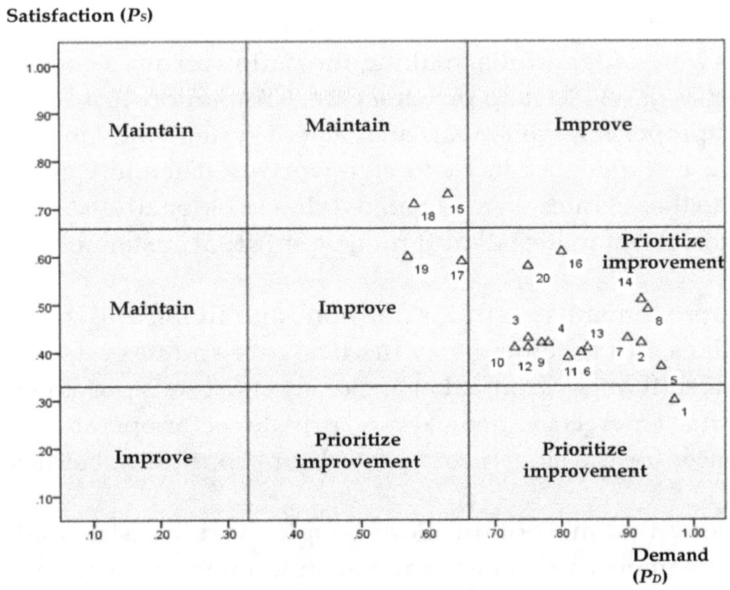


**Figure 9.** SQPM results.

*4.5. Discussion*

Many scholars have used a single model or tool, such as IPA, the I-S model, or the PEM, to explore projects that organizations need to improve. Each model has its advantages, but we think they are too subjective. Instead, it is best to use several models to repeatedly determine the areas that need to be improved before proposing an improvement strategy. The present study integrates the importance-satisfaction (I-S) model and service quality performance matrix (SQPM) to examine long-term care (LTC) service demands and satisfaction improvement.

Japan's LTC system was established in 2000 to support older people with LTC demands and alleviate the burden of caregiving on family members [40]. People choosing to use LTC services, including in-home, facility, and community services, reduce their financial expenses and improve their quality of care [41]. Taiwan established LTCA 1.0 in 1998, and amended it to develop LTCA 2.0 in 2018. The implementation schedule in Taiwan was earlier than in Japan, but its effectiveness has not been high. Therefore, the Taiwanese government and service providers must actively emphasize implementing the LTC system and making improvements regarding older adults' demands.

Generally speaking, when time and resources are limited, it is not feasible to take comprehensiveness into account. When many projects must be improved and it is impossible to implement them at the same time, improvement priorities are developed [42]. In this study, if only the I-S model was used to examine LTC in Taiwan, then seven elements of the system would need to be improved: items 1, 2, 5, 6, 7, 11, and 13. However, if only SQPM were used, 16 elements would need to be improved: items 1–16 and 20. In other words, the outcomes are different when using different models.

As mentioned earlier, Taiwan lacks sufficient LTC resources, so it is impossible to provide enough resources for all those who need care. To use resources efficiently, the I-S model and SQPM were integrated in this study to identify areas for improvement, and items 1, 2, 5, 6, 7, 11, and 13 were identified by both methods.

From the empirical analysis, it was found that the average demand score is approximately 4 and the average satisfaction score is approximately 3, showing that older adults have a very high demand level, but their tendency for satisfaction is low. Regarding improvements, it was found that older adults are most dissatisfied with pensions and living allowances. Therefore, the results of this study are consistent with the viewpoints of other scholars [22,43]. After all, adequate pensions or government subsidies would allow older adult retirees without income and/or in poor health to feel more assured.

Taiwan's declining birthrate and aging population have become more severe. In 2018, more than 14% of the populations were older adults, making the nation an aged society. This has forced some people to rely on foreign workers to help provide care, companionship, and other support for older adults. However, the improper foreign labor management system and language barriers have caused frequent incidents of abuse of older adults by foreign workers. Therefore, four service elements (items 5, 6, 11, and 13) related to these issues were generated due to older adults' helplessness and loneliness. In addition to satisfaction about materials and money, spiritual sustenance and care for older adults are equally crucial.

Items that need improvement, except for pensions and living allowances, cannot be improved due to financial difficulties, but for emergency medical care and rescue services and transportation services, it is recommended that government agencies and hospitals provide transportation resources for the elderly. For travel to emergency medical care, private sector operators should be encouraged to invest in transport services for the elderly and provide appropriate subsidies to enhance emergency medical services.

The results also shows that most of the older people lived in residential institutions were male, their education level were mainly university, their economic status were better, and their work were mainly in the military, government employees, or teachers before retirement. In a Chinese society, many older people were unwilling to live in residential institutions. In addition to considering financial planning factors, they were also afraid of giving others a feeling that they have been abandoned by their children. Therefore, the proportions of living with their families were also high. The interview found that the older people living families alone have poor financial support, their need government subsidies, and transportation services. The older people lived in residential institutions have a stable pension or their children provide financial assistance therefore, the needs were family companionship and health-promoting physical fitness activities.

Finally, this study attempts to analyze the differences from the sample background information, such as gender, age, education, occupation, living status, marital status, etc., to compare the differences in the needs of different people for LTC. After analysis of I-S model and SQPM, the research results show that there is no significant difference between different background samples and the overall sample. It is speculated that the reason for this might be that the samples for this research were Taiwanese older people residing in Taipei and New Taipei who lived in a long-term institution or attended a senior citizens' learning camp. And Taipei and New Taipei City are the two largest Taiwanese Cities, the population is evenly distributed, and older adults' views are also converging, which were also likely to be factors in the results.

## 5. Conclusions and Suggestions

### 5.1. Conclusions

The advancement of medical science and technology has extended the average life expectancy and brought about changes in social structure and values and, together with the declining birthrate, has accelerated the advent of aged societies. To cope with the current global aging population, LTC for older adults is an essential goal of government administrations. To meet older people's needs, it is unwise to construct aid devices or service needs from a managerial perspective instead of listening to them and customizing relevant services based on a user perspective. It is also important to encourage healthy older people to continue being active, such as by performing volunteer work, participating in community services, and acting as guides, to enrich their retirement lives and simultaneously increase their contribution to society. Older adults who are in poor health, suffering from illnesses such as dementia, or facing disabilities can be provided with medical care to reduce their pains, ensuring that all older people receive proper care. The government is responsible for appropriately allocating the necessary resources.

During the implementation process, the I-S model and SQPM were mainly used to evaluate resource allocation, followed by a secondary consideration of service quality improvement. Seven services were found to be in urgent need of improvement by this study after integrating the I-S model and SQPM. This research results can serve as a basis for quality improvement for the Taiwanese government and service providers investing in resources. If government resources are limited and cannot be allocated simultaneously, it is suggested to prioritize the improvement projects in order.

### 5.2. Suggestions and Research Limitations

Rapid population aging has made the burden of caring for older adults relatively heavy. Following an extension of the average life expectancy of older adults, their demand for care services has also intensified. Advances in medical technology have led to the control of many diseases, but such advances still cannot fully restore the original state of health, and many older people suffer from physical and mental disabilities. With the continuous growth of the older adult population and the decline of family function, the demand for care services continues to rise, along with the need to rely on foreign workers to handle these jobs. Therefore, it is imperative to strengthen professional training for foreign workers.

There are significant differences in physical and mental health among older people who need care, and the nonuniformity of care resources has created a high variance in care needs. Therefore, healthy older people who could move freely in the community or institutions were chosen as the objects of this study, and those with physical and mental disabilities were excluded. Based on the empirical research, the study proposes the following suggestions:

1. Although the government has established the ABC LTC model, the new system has not properly implemented departmental linkages and integrated resources. Therefore, it is recommended that the government, nongovernment organizations, and social welfare groups coordinate and integrate their communications as soon as possible.

2. From the outside, the LTC industry has the impression of being low-paid, humble work focused on helping older adults with their toileting routines. As a result, young people are not very interested in entering this field. As an alternative, it is suggested to hire foreign workers for this kind of work. It is also the government's responsibility to urgently encourage young people to join and manage this industry, making it into a respectful and dignified profession.

The samples for this research were Taiwanese older people residing in Taipei and New Taipei who lived in a long-term institution or attended a senior citizens' learning camp. The follow-up researchers can expand the sample size to compare the LTC needs. They may find significant differences between different background samples.

**Author Contributions:** S.-H.C. and T.-M.Y. developed the idea, motivation, and question of the paper and contributed to the discussion. F.-Y.P. outlined and revised the manuscript and made substantial contributions to the design of this study. All authors have read and agreed to the published version of the manuscript.

**Acknowledgments:** The authors would like to express their sincere gratitude to the editor and the anonymous reviewers for their insightful and constructive comments.

## References

1. Lin, C.S.; Jeng, M.Y.; Yeh, T.M. The elderly perceived meanings and values of virtual reality leisure activities: A means-end chain approach. *Int. J. Environ. Res. Public Health* **2018**, *15*, 663. [CrossRef] [PubMed]
2. Wang, Z.H.; Yang, Z.H.; Dong, T. A review of wearable technologies for elderly care that can accurately track indoor position.recognize physical activities and monitor vital signs in real time. *Sensors* **2017**, *17*, 341. [CrossRef] [PubMed]
3. Jeng, M.Y.; Pai, F.Y.; Yeh, T.M. The virtual reality leisure activities experience on elderly people. *Appl. Res. Qual. Life* **2017**, *12*, 49–65. [CrossRef]
4. Lin, T.C. Discussion on the Health Promotion Management and the Demand of Life Support in Senior Citizen: A Case study with Taiwan. *CSR Summit Entrep. Cross Strait Coop.* **2019**, *4*, 36–52.
5. Lee, I.; Chiou, C.J.; Su, H.S. Comparison of Caring Status and Needs between Elderly and Non-Elderly Family Caregivers. *J. Long-term Care* **2017**, *21*, 149–164.
6. Lehnert, T.; Heuchert, M.; Hussain, K.; König, H. Stated preferences for long-term care: A literature review. *Ageing Soc.* **2019**, *39*, 1873–1913. [CrossRef]
7. Huang, F.S. The Rise, Trends and Recent Developments of Elder Education in Taiwan. *J. Adult Lifelong Educ.* **2012**, *43*, 2–14.
8. Lin, Y.Y. Strategies of enhancing capacity of long-term care policy by government: A case study of taichung city government. *J. Long-Term Care* **2017**, *21*, 19–25.
9. Kim, J.; Han, W. Improving Service Quality in Long-term Care Hospitals: National Evaluation on Long-term Care Hospitals and Employees Perception of Quality Dimensions. *Osong Public Health Res. Perspect.* **2012**, *3*, 94–99. [CrossRef]
10. Chen, S.H. Determining the service demands of an aging population by integrating QFD and FMEA method. *Qual. Quant.* **2016**, *50*, 283–298. [CrossRef]
11. Chen, S.F.; Teng, S.W. The Development of the Long-Term Care Service System in Taiwan. *J. Nurs.* **2010**, *57*, 5–10.
12. Yang, C.C. Improvement actions based on the customers' satisfaction survey. *Total Qual. Manag. Bus. Excell.* **2003**, *14*, 919–930. [CrossRef]
13. Chen, S.H.; Yeh, T.M. Integration PEM and AHP methods to determine service quality improvement strategy for the medical industry. *Appl. Math. Inf. Sci.* **2015**, *9*, 3073–3082.
14. Lambert, D.M.; Sharma, A. A customer-based competitive analysis for logistics decisions. *Int. J. Phys. Distrib. Logist. Manag.* **1990**, *20*, 17–24. [CrossRef]
15. Shieh, M.D.; Hsiao, H.C.; Lin, Y.H.; Lin, J.Y. A study of the elderly people's perception of wearable device forms. *J. Interdiscip. Math.* **2017**, *20*, 789–804. [CrossRef]
16. Helbostad, J.L.; Vereijken, B.; Becker, C.; Todd, C.; Taraldsen, K.; Pijnappels, M.; Aminian, K.; Mellone, S. Mobile health applications to promote active and healthy ageing. *Sensors* **2017**, *17*, 622. [CrossRef]
17. Huang, Y.C.; Chang, T.Y. A Study of Long-term Care Policy 2.0 Edition: An Example for Pingtung County. *J. Manag. Syst.* **2019**, *26*, 241–269.
18. Chung, C.C. Reflect on for long-term care 2.0 from the view point of quality of medical life. *Qual. Mag.* **2017**, *53*, 5–11.

19. Lee, M.C.; Kuo, T.C.; Ueng, W.N. Perspectives on Long-Term Care in Taiwan-Integration of Health Care and Welfare services. *HOSPITAL* **2019**, *52*, 1–5.
20. Ministry of Health and Welfare. *Long Term Care Plan for Ten Years 2.0 Report*; Ministry of Health and Welfare: Taiwan, China.
21. Sun, W.J.; Chu, D.C.; Huang, S.J. Medical Home Care and National Long-Term Care Integration. *J. Med.* **2018**, *22*, 278–282.
22. Liu, Y.H. Older clinical psychology lecture (1). *Consult. Couns.* **2010**, *289*, 56–60.
23. Lin, Y.G.; Chen, P.W. The application of community consultation model in the service of the elderly. *Couns. Q.* **2009**, *45*, 49–60.
24. Shih, Y.; Lo, H.T.; Chen, C.Y. Study on Quality of Services and Satisfaction for Elderly Day Care Centers: A Case Study of a Hospital in Southern Taiwan. *J. Gerontechnol. Serv. Manag.* **2018**, *6*, 121–136.
25. Martilla, J.A.; James, J.C. Importance-Performance Analysis. *J. Mark.* **1997**, *41*, 77–79. [CrossRef]
26. Sampson, S.E.; Showalter, M.J. The performance-importance response function: Observations and implications. *Serv. Ind. J.* **1999**, *19*, 1–25. [CrossRef]
27. Guo, D.S.; Su, S.C. An IPA Analysis of Customer Value. *Manag. Sci. Res.* **2016**, *10*, 83–96.
28. Chen, S.H. A performance matrix for strategies to improve satisfaction among faculty members in higher education. *Qual. Quant.* **2011**, *45*, 75–89. [CrossRef]
29. Cheng, C.C.; Tsai, M.C.; Lin, S.P. Developing strategies for improving the service quality of casual-dining restaurants: New insights from integrating IPGA and QFD analysis. *Total Qual. Manag. Bus. Excell.* **2015**, *26*, 415–429. [CrossRef]
30. Wong, K.; Tunku, U.; Rahman, A. Constructing a survey questionnaire to collect data on service quality of business academics. *Eur. J. Soc. Sci.* **2012**, *29*, 209–221.
31. Yeh, T.M.; Lai, H.P. Evaluating the effectiveness of implementing quality management practices in the medical industry. *J. Nutr. Health Aging* **2015**, *19*, 102–112. [CrossRef]
32. Chen, S.H.; Liu, A.C.; Chen, F.Y. Using the PEM method to determine service quality improvement strategies of medical industry. *Int. J. Manag. Stud. Res.* **2014**, *2*, 41–46.
33. Hung, Y.H.; Huang, M.L.; Chen, K.S. Service quality evaluation by service quality performance matrix. *Total Qual. Manag. Bus. Excell.* **2003**, *14*, 79–89. [CrossRef]
34. Lin, W.T.; Chen, S.C.; Chen, K.S. Evaluation of performance in introducing CE marking on the European market to the machinery industry in Taiwan. *Int. J. Qual. Reliab. Manag.* **2005**, *22*, 503–517. [CrossRef]
35. Wu, M.L. *Paper Writing and Quantitative Research*; Wu-Nan Publishing Company: Taipei, Taiwan, 2018.
36. YuCMChang, H.T.; Chen, K.S. Developing a performance evaluation matrix to enhance the learner satisfaction of an e-learning system. *Total Qual. Manag. Bus. Excell.* **2018**, *29*, 727–745.
37. Kim, S.H.; Kim, D.H.; Kim, W.S. Long-Term Care Needs of the Elderly in Korea and Elderly Long-Term Care Insurance. *Soc. Work Public Health* **2010**, *25*, 176–184. [CrossRef] [PubMed]
38. Nunnally, J.C. *Psychometric Theory*; McGraw-Hill: New York, NY, USA, 1987.
39. Cuieford, J.P. *Fundamental Statistics in Psychology and Education*, 4th ed.; McGraw Hill: New York, NY, USA, 1965.
40. Iwagami, M.; Tamiya, N. The Long-Term Care Insurance System in Japan: Past, Present 2019, and Future. *JMA J.* **1965**, *2*, 67–69.
41. Araia, A.; Ozakib, T.; Katsumatac, Y. Behavioral and psychological symptoms of dementia in older residents in long term care facilities in Japan: A cross-sectional study. *Aging Ment. Health* **2017**, *21*, 1099–1105. [CrossRef]
42. Chen, S.H.; Yang, C.C.; Shiau, J.Y.; Wang, H.H. The development of an employee satisfaction model for higher education. *TQM Mag.* **2006**, *18*, 484–500. [CrossRef]
43. Liao, W.C.; Chiu, L.A.; Yueh, H.P. A study of rural elderly's health information needs and seeking behavior. *J. Libr. Inf. Stud.* **2012**, *10*, 155–204.

# 14

# A Deep Learning Approach to EMG-Based Classification of Gait Phases during Level Ground Walking

**Christian Morbidoni *, Alessandro Cucchiarelli, Sandro Fioretti and Francesco Di Nardo ***

Department of Information Engineering, Università Politecnica delle Marche, 60100 Ancona, Italy
* Correspondence: c.morbidoni@univpm.it (C.M.); f.dinardo@staff.univpm.it (F.D.N.);

**Abstract:** Correctly identifying gait phases is a prerequisite to achieve a spatial/temporal characterization of muscular recruitment during walking. Recent approaches have addressed this issue by applying machine learning techniques to treadmill-walking data. We propose a deep learning approach for surface electromyographic (sEMG)-based classification of stance/swing phases and prediction of the foot–floor-contact signal in more natural walking conditions (similar to everyday walking ones), overcoming constraints of a controlled environment, such as treadmill walking. To this aim, sEMG signals were acquired from eight lower-limb muscles in about 10.000 strides from 23 healthy adults during level ground walking, following an eight-shaped path including natural deceleration, reversing, curve, and acceleration. By means of an extensive evaluation, we show that using a multi layer perceptron to learn hidden features provides state of the art performances while avoiding features engineering. Results, indeed, showed an average classification accuracy of 94.9 for learned subjects and 93.4 for unlearned ones, while mean absolute difference ($\pm SD$) between phase transitions timing predictions and footswitch data was 21.6 ms and 38.1 ms for heel-strike and toe off, respectively. The suitable performance achieved by the proposed method suggests that it could be successfully used to automatically classify gait phases and predict foot–floor-contact signal from sEMG signals during level ground walking.

**Keywords:** sEMG; deep learning; neural networks; gait phase; classification; everyday walking

---

## 1. Introduction

Electromyography is a widely-accepted tool able to provide an essential and original contribution to the characterization of the neuromuscular system [1]. In particular, surface electromyography (sEMG) is acknowledged as a non-invasive approach, specifically suitable to monitor muscle activity during dynamic tasks, such as walking [2–4]. In order to achieve a spatial/temporal characterization of muscular recruitment during walking, gait events, such as the instant of foot-floor contact and ground clearance, need to be assessed. This process starts from the identification of the two main gait phases, stance and swing. The stance phase designates the entire period during which the foot is on the ground, while the swing phase is characterized by the time the foot is in the air for limb advancement. The transitions between a swing and the subsequent stance phase is commonly referred to as heel-strike (HS), while the transition between a stance and the subsequent swing phases is referred to as toe-off (TO). Stance and swing identify the functional subdivisions of total limb activity within the gait cycle [2], thus precisely identifying HS and TO events is important to analyze the gait activity. For this reason, sEMG signals are typically coupled with signals able to provide the synchronization of the gait cycle, such as signals from foot-switch sensors [5], pressure mats [6], stereo-photogrammetric systems [7], and inertial measurements units (accelerometers and gyroscopes) [8].

Stereo–photogrammetric systems and pressure mats are affected by different relevant issues: high costs of the instrumentation, limited number of cycles observed, and/or invasiveness of experimental set-up. The use of wearable sensors seems to mitigate the impact of the costs and to allow the identification of gait events in a suitable number of cycles. Even so, the problems of encumbrance and time-consuming experimental set-up are still relevant, especially for applications in pathology. Moreover, wearable sensors can require particular care for the correct placement and the need of specific calibration procedures, not consistent with the timing of clinical practice. Thus, the idea of overcoming all these limitations developing novel techniques able to detect and classify gait events from sEMG signal alone is indeed starting to catch on. This kind of approach may involve machine learning and deep learning techniques.

### 1.1. *Aim of the Study*

Classifying gait events is a typical task which could be addressed by machine learning and deep learning techniques. Many examples were reported in literature [9–12]. However, only few reports addressed the issue of gait-phase classification from sEMG signal only [13–15]. These very recent approaches were based on hand-crafted features extracted from sEMG signals during treadmill walking and were evaluated on a relatively small number of subjects (up to eight). Walking on a treadmill is known to affect gait performance, resulting in increased number of steps and cadence, decreased preferred walking speed, stride and stance-phase length, slightly decreased joint range of motion, and changes in EMG activation with respect to level ground walking [16–19]. Thus, the reliability of the above mentioned EMG-based classifiers of stance and swing phases [13–15] is limited to treadmill data and is not tested on ground-walking data. In addition, treadmill walking occurs in very controlled conditions, characterized by a high repeatability of spatial/temporal parameters (including stance and swing duration). In contrast, everyday walking is characterized by a wider variability of spatial/temporal parameters and sEMG signals introduced by deceleration, reversing, curves and acceleration [16–19]. This variability is expected to affect the performance of a possible stance/swing classification and the consequent prediction of temporal parameters, such as heel-strike and toe-off timing.

Therefore, the aim of the present study is to propose an artificial neural network (ANN)-based approach to classify gait events (proper stance and swing phases) and to predict foot-floor-contact signal from sEMG signals, in conditions similar to everyday walking. With "conditions similar to everyday walking" we mean that, differently from previous study where gait phases were classified in the very controlled conditions of treadmill walking [13–15], in the present study each subject walked on level ground following an eight-shaped path (Figure 1) which includes natural deceleration, reversing, curve, and acceleration.

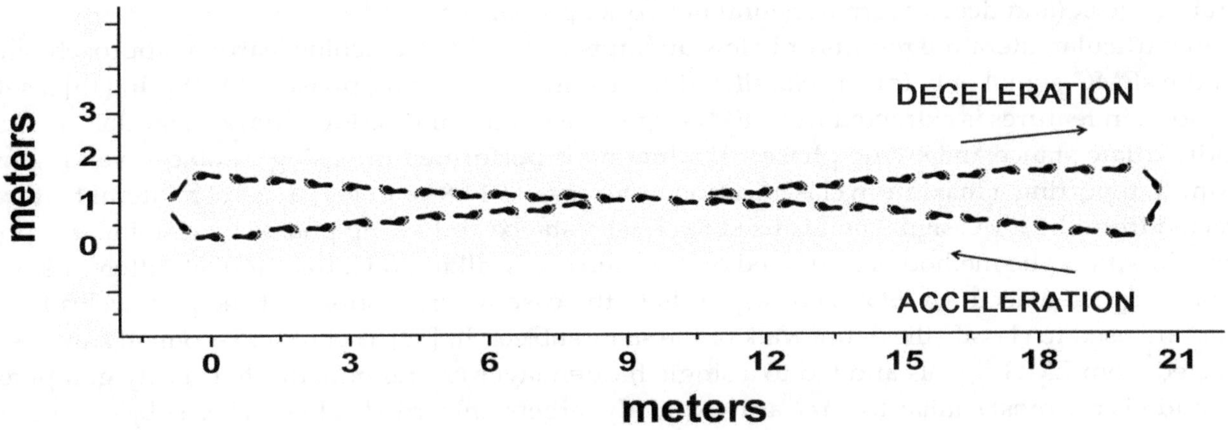


**Figure 1.** Illustration of the eight-shaped path used in our experiments.

*1.2. Contributions*

The main contributions of the present study are three:

- first, providing a classification of stance and swing phases and the prediction of foot-floor-contact signal in more natural walking conditions (similar to everyday walking), overcoming the limitations and the constraints of a controlled environment, such as treadmill walking;
- second, proposing a different approach to process the sEMG signal used to train deep neural networks: while previous studies [13–15] processed sEMG signals to extract time/frequency domain features which were used to feed the neural networks, the present study directly used the envelopes of the EMG signal to train the networks, attempting to automatically learn relevant higher level (hidden) features;
- third, improving the reliability of the prediction of gait events (HS and TO) in unseen subjects reported in literature [13], despite the challenging condition of everyday walking. This has been achieved by both enlarging the testing data (four-minute ground walking of 23 different subjects) and decreasing the average error in the prediction of HS and TO timing.

The remainder of this paper is organized as follows. Section 2 reports a brief review of the related works. Section 3 describes the dataset, the acquisition and the pre-processing of the signals, and the gait- phase classification by deep learning. Section 4 reports and discusses the results. Section 5 concludes the present study.

## 2. Related Works

Machine learning techniques, such as ANNs, are typically used for analyzing and classifying large amount of data and complex signals. Many applications of machine learning approaches in health care were reported [20–22]. Similar approaches were proven to be reliable also in classifying EMG signals during different tasks. Wavelet neural network and multi-layer perceptrons were used to handle EMG signals in order to identify neuromuscular disorders [23,24]. Learning vector quantization, support vector machine, and Levenberg–Marquardt-based networks were applied to EMG signals for classifying hand-motion patterns [25–27]. EMG-based unsupervised competitive learning techniques were employed for the identification of the muscle activity during pregnancy [28]. Efforts have been made to adapt these techniques for walking-task characterization: different machine learning approaches were applied to gait analysis data by Joyseeree et al. for disease identification [9]. Kaczmarczyk et al. [11] applied ANNs for gait classification in post stroke patients. Wang and Zieliska [12] designed an EMG-based method for detecting the variability in gait features depending on footwear, by applying vector quantization classifying networks and clustering competitive networks. Zou et al. [10] performed gait recognition analyzing inertial sensor data by means of deep convolutional neural network (and deep recurrent neural network approaches

In particular, literature reports only few attempts to provide a machine learning approach which used the sEMG signal only for the classification of stance and swing phases [13–15]. In [15] a set of time-domain features is extracted from EMG signal segments and hidden Markov models are used to individuate stance and swing phases. Evaluation is performed on a single subject walking on a treadmill, reporting a maximum classification accuracy of 91.08%. In [14] a novel bilateral feature is extracted from the EMG signal and is used to classify stance and swing phases by training a support vector classifier. The method is evaluated on two subjects walking on a treadmill at different speeds. The best reported accuracy (96%) corresponds to the case where a subset of the gait cycles from a subject are used to classify the entire walk of the same subject. In [13] a set of time-domain features are extracted from EMG signals and fed to a single hidden layer neural network to classify gait phases. This study is the most similar to ours, as it explicitly targets unlearned subjects, i.e., subjects not used as inputs during the training phase and attempts to predict timing of phase transitions. However, the data used is derived from 8 subjects walking on a treadmill and the evaluation of phase transition detection is performed on only 5 s of the walking of a single unlearned subject, reporting a mean average error of 35 ± 25 ms for HS and 49 ± 15 ms for TO. All these recent approaches were based on hand-crafted features extracted from sEMG signals during treadmill walking and were evaluated on relatively small populations of subjects (up to eight).

## 3. Materials and Methods

### 3.1. Dataset

The dataset included signals recorded from 23 healthy adults (12 females and 11 males), acquired in the Movement Analysis Laboratory of Università Politecnica delle Marche, Ancona, Italy. Mean (±SD) characteristics were: age = 23.8 ± 1.9 years; height = 173 ± 10 cm; mass = 63.3 ± 12.4 kg; body mass index (BMI) = 20.8 ± 2.1 kg/m$^2$. None of the subjects presented any pathological condition or had undergone orthopedic surgery that might have affected lower limb mechanics. Therefore, subjects with joint pain, neurological pathologies, orthopedic surgery, abnormal gait or a body mass index (BMI) higher than 25 (overweight and obese) were not recruited. The research was undertaken in compliance with the ethical principles of the Helsinki Declaration and was approved by an institutional expert committee. Participants signed informed consent prior to the beginning of the test.

### 3.2. Signal Acquisition

The multichannel recording system, Step 32 (Medical Technology, Italy, Version PCI-32 ch2.0.1. DV, resolution: 12 bit; sampling rate: 2 kHz) was used to acquire surface electromyographic (sEMG) and basographic signals (i.e., the signals from footswitches). Each lower limb was instrumented with three foot-switches and four sEMG probes. Foot-switches (surface: 1.21 cm$^2$, activation force: 3 N), were pasted beneath the heel, the first and the fifth metatarsal heads of the foot. Single differential sEMG probes with fixed geometry (Ag/Ag-Cl disk; electrode diameter: 0.4 cm; inter-electrode distance: 0.8 cm; gain: 1000; high-pass filter: 10 Hz; input impedance: 1.5 G; CMRR > 126 dB; input referred noise: 1 Vrms) and with variable geometry (Ag/Ag-Cl disks; minimum inter-electrode distance: 12 mm, gain: 1000, high-pass filter: 10 Hz, input impedance >1.5 G, CMRR >126 dB, input referred noise 200 nVrms) were placed on the belly muscle to detect the sEMG signals. Skin was shaved, cleansed with abrasive paste and wet with a damp cloth. Probes were placed over tibialis anterior, gastrocnemius lateralis, hamstrings, and vastus lateralis, following the recommendations provided by the European concerted action SENIAM (surface EMG for a non-invasive assessment of muscles) for electrodes location with respect to tendons, motor points and fiber orientation [29]. Each volunteer walked barefoot on the floor at her/his own chosen pace for about 5 min, following an eight-shaped path [30], which includes natural deceleration, reversing, curve and acceleration (Figure 1).

### 3.3. Pre-Processing

Footswitch signals were converted and processed so as to identify the different gait cycles and phases (stance and swing), according to the approach discussed in details in [31].

Electromyographic signals were processed by a high-pass, linear-phase FIR filter (cut-off frequency: 20 Hz), in order to avoid phase distortion effects and by a low-pass, linear-phase FIR filter (cut-off frequency: 450 Hz). Then, sEMG signals were full-wave rectified and the envelope was extracted (second-order Butterworth low-pass filter, cut-off frequency: 5 Hz). Figures 2 and 3 showed, respectively, the raw EMG signals recorded for the right leg and the envelope obtained as a result of the pre-processing step.

The sEMG and basographic data analyzed in the present study are going to be published in a public dataset, and are currently available for research purposes by contacting the authors.

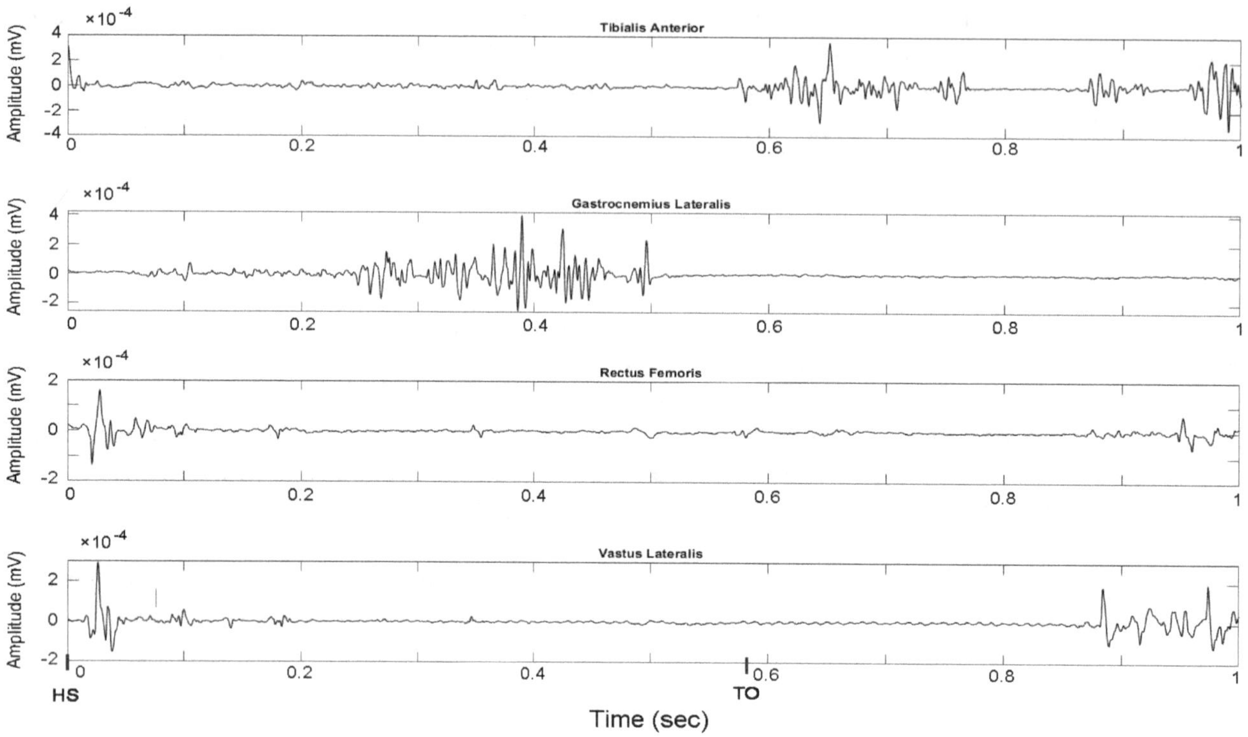


**Figure 2.** Raw electromyographic (EMG) signals recorded from the four muscles of the right leg. Corresponding heel-strike (HS) and toe-off (TO) timing are highlighted.

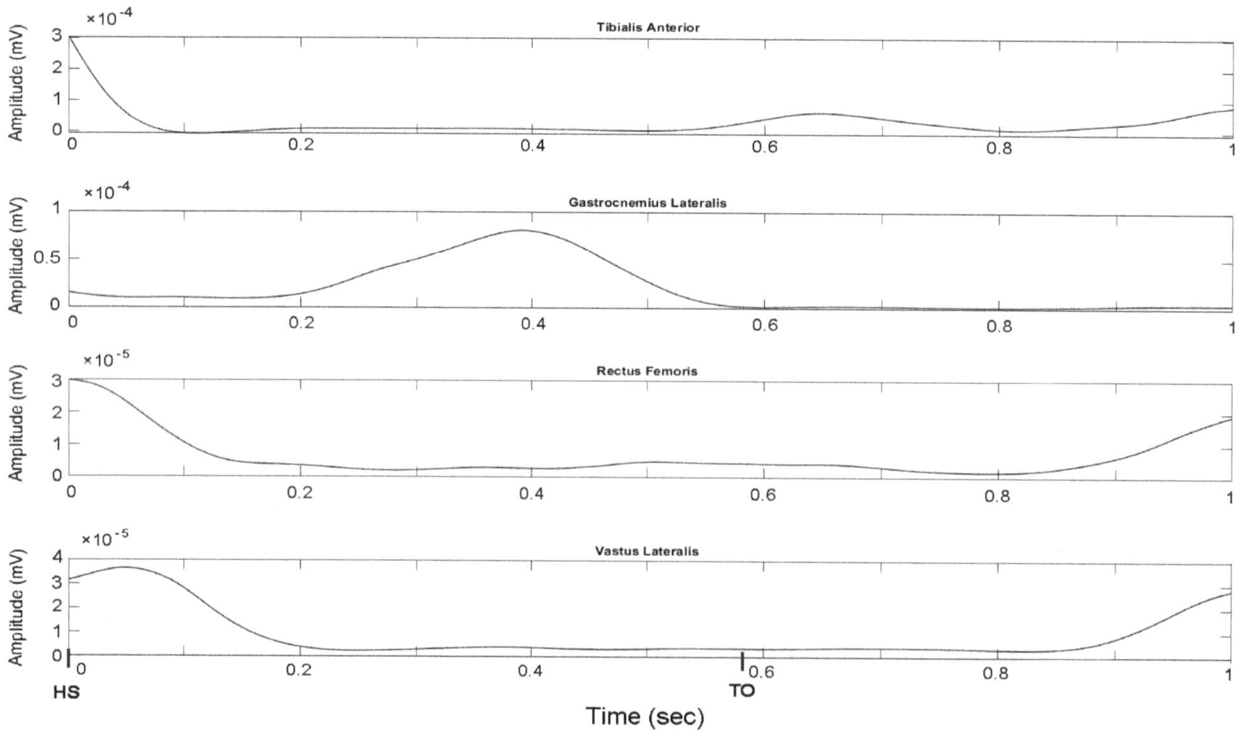


**Figure 3.** The envelope resulting from the pre-processing of the raw EMG signals recorded from the four muscles of the right leg. Corresponding HS and TO timing are highlighted.

### 3.4. Gait Phase Classification

#### 3.4.1. Data Preparation

Before feeding data into the classifier, a min-max normalization of each muscle signal was performed within each subject, thus mapping the values in the [0–1] interval. In order to train the classifier, we split the signals into 20 data samples windows (corresponding to 10 milliseconds) for both stance and swing phases.

We then aggregated the synchronized EMG-signal segments corresponding to the eight muscles (four for each leg) into a single vector of 160 elements. Each EMG vector was composed of 20 sequences of eight elements. Each element represents the EMG-signal values of the eight muscles in that single time-sample. Thus, the first eight elements of the vector were the EMG signal values of the eight muscles computed in the first sample of the segment. The following eight elements of the vector are the EMG signal values of the eight muscles computed in the second sample of the segment, and so on up to the twentieth sample. The structure of the input vector is illustrated in Figure 4. $L1_i$, $L2_i$, $L3_i$, and $L4_i$ were the values of EMG signals in the sample $i$ corresponding to the muscles of the left leg, respectively: tibialis anterior, gastrocnemius lateralis, hamstring, vastus lateralis. $R1_i$, $R2_i$, $R3_i$, and $R4_i$ represented the correspondent for the right leg. Each input vector was assigned to the label 0 if the corresponding signals belong to a stance phase, and to 1 if the corresponding signals belong to a swing phase. After removing the segments before the first swing phase, to avoid considering muscle activation recorded in non-walking conditions, we obtained 522.936 labelled segments from the 23 subjects.

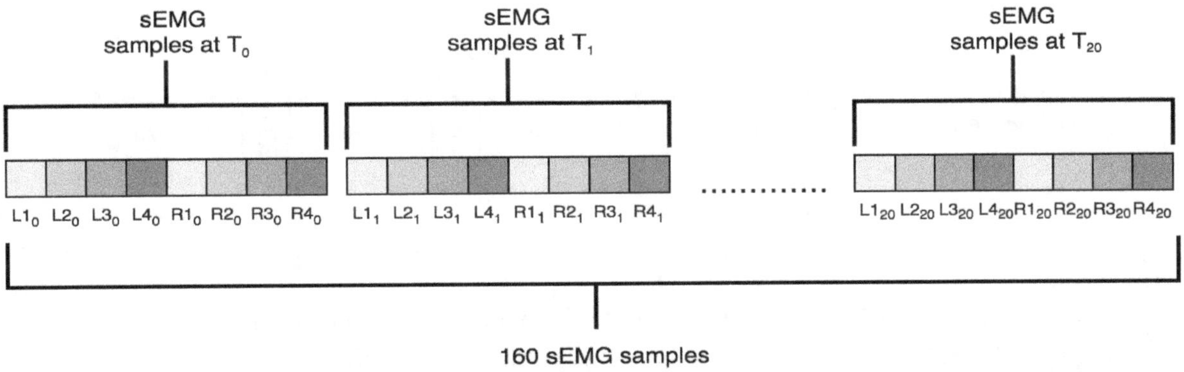


**Figure 4.** The structure of EMG vectors fed as input to the artificial neural networks (ANNs).

In our study we attempted to classify gait phases and to detect the timing of phase transitions (HS and TO events). In particular we are targeting previously unseen subjects, i.e., subjects whose gait recordings were not used in the training phase.

Accordingly, we performed a cross-validation using 23 folds, each of which uses data from 22 subjects (LS set) in training and 1 in test (US set). At each fold, a different subject is used as the test subject (unseen). In order to measure the phase classification performances also for learned subjects, we further split the LS set into training set (LS-train) and test set (LS-test). More precisely, LS-train includes the first 90% of the each subject strands (approximately 3 min and 30 s, 180 gait cycles) and LS-test the remaining 10% (approximately 30 s, 20 gait cycles).

#### 3.4.2. Neural Networks

We experimented with different multi layer perceptron (MLP) architectures. In Table 1 we summarize the different architectures for which we report the results in the following section. The first model ($MLP_1$) was a shallow network with one single hidden layer composed of 128 units (neurons) and had a one-dimensional output. The output was fed to a sigmoid function and a 0.5 threshold is used to obtain a binary output: when the output of the sigmoid was >0.5 we assigned the label

1, otherwise we assigned the label 0. We then experimented with deeper networks, composed of 2–5 hidden layers (Table 1). In all the architectures we used rectified linear units (ReLU) to provide non-linearity between hidden layers. As an example, in Figure 5 we illustrate the structure of the $MLP_4$ architecture.

In our experiments, we used stochastic gradient descent (SGD) as the optimization algorithm and binary cross entropy as the loss function (BCE).

The value 0.1 was experimentally identified as the optimal learning rate for all the tested models and thus adopted in all the experiments. Finally, all ANN models were trained using an early stop technique, according to the following procedure. The networks were trained for a maximum of 100 epochs, stopping when the accuracy on the validation set did not increase for 10 consecutive epochs. The best-performing learned parameters were adopted to evaluate the model performances over LS-test and US sets and the basographic signal was used as ground truth.

**Table 1.** Overview of the multi layer perceptron (MLP) architectures.

| Model Name | Model Structure |
|---|---|
| $MLP_1$ | mlp(128) |
| $MLP_2$ | mlp(256, 128) |
| $MLP_3$ | mlp(512, 256, 128) |
| $MLP_4$ | mlp(1024, 512, 256 ,128) |
| $MLP_5$ | mlp(1024, 1024, 512, 256 ,128) |

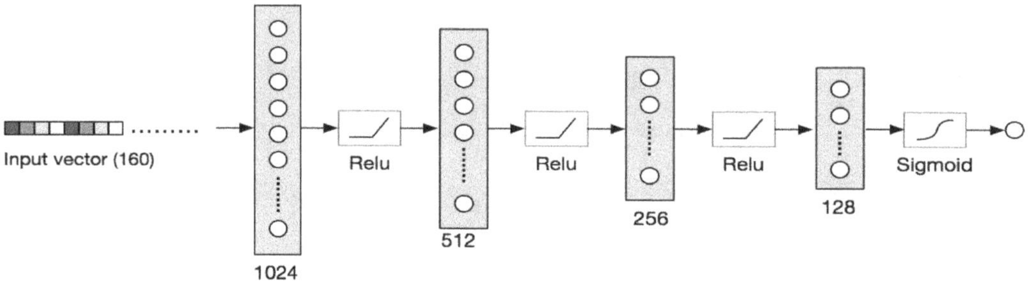


**Figure 5.** The architecture of multi layer perceptron (MLP)$_4$.

### *3.5. Gait Events Timing Detection*

The predicted foot–floor-contact signal was reconstructed by chronologically arranging the binary output of the network. Thus, a vector was obtained, composed of sequences of 0 (stance phase) alternating with sequences of 1 (swing phase). This vector was chronologically scanned in order to detect the transitions between gait phases: from swing to stance phase (HS) and from stance to swing phase (TO). HS was identified as the sample where the transition from 1 to 0 occurred. TO was identified as the sample where the transition from 0 to 1 occurred.

Then, the predicted signal was cleaned by removing those phases that were too short according to physiological constraints, probably due to classification errors. We adopted the following procedure. Starting from the first HS, the following 500 samples (250 ms) were scanned to find out and remove those having a value of 1. Then, the following HS was identified, the process was repeated and so on. In the same way, starting from the first TO, the following 500 samples were scanned to find out and remove the samples which assumed the value of 0. Then, the following TO was identified, the process was repeated and so on. Eventually, the cleaned vector was chronologically scanned again in order to detect the transitions between gait phases (from 0 to 1 and from 1 to 0) and thus the timing of the gait events.

### 3.6. Evaluation Measures

In this work, a EMG signal's segment classifier is ultimately used to predict a biographic signal, that is predicting the precise timing of gait phase transition. We first evaluate the performance of the classifier in assigning the correct label (0 for stance and 1 for swing) to single EMG segments. This is done using standard classification metrics, by calculating accuracy, precision, recall and $F_1$ score, as the harmonic average of the precision and recall. However, this measure does not provide enough information to evaluate the performances of the basographic signal prediction. In fact, even a high accuracy, if errors are concentrated in proximity of transitions, may lead to unsatisfactory results in terms of time error of transition instants. Furthermore, we apply a post processing to the classifier output, to remove false prediction and improve performances, thus we need to explicitly evaluate the predicted basographic.

For that purpose, we adopt the following procedure, used in literature to evaluate gait events prediction, e.g., in [32,33]. We first chose a temporal tolerance $T$, which we set to 600 milliseconds. Then we consider as true positive each predicted TO or HS event at time $tp$ if an event of the same type exists in the ground truth signal at time $tg$ such that $|tg - tp| < T$. Otherwise we consider the predicted event a False Positive. We then measure the precision, recall and $F_1$ score and, for all the true positives, we calculate the mean average error (MAE) as the average time distance between the predicted event and the one, of the same type, in the ground truth signal.

We adopted this evaluation strategy to measure the performances of our approach and comparing it with a feature-based one.

## 4. Results and Discussion

To the best of our knowledge, this study is the first attempt to provide a reliable binary classification of level ground walking into stance and swing phases, by means of the application of deep learning techniques to sEMG signal. Starting from gait-phase classification, the study achieves also a prediction of foot-floor-contact signal and a consequent identification of heel-strike and toe-off timing.

### 4.1. Gait-Phase Classification

Mean classification accuracy (±SD) obtained over the 23 folds with different MLP architectures for both learned subjects (LS-test set) and unlearned ones (US set) is shown in Table 2, where the best results are in bold. The same convention is used in all the tables.

**Table 2.** Gait phase classification accuracy (± standard deviation (SD)) averaged over the 23 folds for each considered network.

| | **Accuracy on US** | **Accuracy on LS-Test** |
|---|---|---|
| $MLP_1$ | 92.62 ± 2.3 | 93.83 ± 0.28 |
| $MLP_2$ | 93.01 ± 2.1 | 94.41 ± 0.23 |
| $MLP_3$ | **93.41** ± 2.3 | 94.83 ± 0.2 |
| $MLP_4$ | 93.25 ± 2.9 | **94.94** ± 0.3 |
| $MLP_5$ | 93.03 ± 2.8 | 94.93 ± 0.2 |

As expected, classification accuracy for learned subjects was higher than for unseen ones. However, the limited gap (around 1–2 percent) suggests that all the networks succeed in learning signal patterns that generalize well to unseen subjects. The best accuracy on unlearned subjects was obtained with $MLP_3$. By looking at the standard deviation reported in Table 2, one can notice that, while for learned subjects the accuracy was uniform across the different folders, there was a higher variability when considering unseen subjects. This is partially due to the fact that there were 22 unlearned subjects in the LS-test in each folder, while the US set was composed of a single subject. Such a variability also suggests that walking patterns might be very different from subject to subject, especially in everyday walking conditions, making the classification harder if a subject had never been seen before. However, looking at results on US sets over the 23 folds, as shown in Figure 6, the accuracy does not fall below 87.6% (subject 13) and reaches the highest value of 97.3% (subject 20). Such results are, in our opinion, promising and suggest that the variability could be reduced, and mean accuracy increased, by considering a larger number of subjects to learn from. Tables 3 and 4 report precision, recall and $F_1$ score of the classification of Stance and Swing phases for, respectively, unlearned (US set) and learned (LS-test set) subjects. Results are averaged over the 23 folds. It is worth noticing that, in line with what was reported in literature [2], the segments belonging to a stance phase were more frequent (around 60%) than those belonging to a swing phase. This is because in normal walking the stance phase duration was 60% of the gait cycle (while the swing phase duration was the remaining 40%) on average. Despite this, results obtained for swing labelled segments are better than those obtained for stance labeled ones, both in unlearned and learned data.

**Table 3.** Gait phase classification performances for stance and swing phases in unlearned subjects (set US). Precision, recall and $F_1$ scores are averaged over the 23 folds.

| | **Stance Phase** | | |
|---|---|---|---|
| | **Precision** | **Recall** | **$F_1$ Score** |
| $MLP_1$ | 92.99 ± 4.5 | 90.50 ± 5.9 | 91.49 ± 2.9 |
| $MLP_2$ | 93.15 ± 4.4 | 91.22 ± 4.9 | 91.99 ± 2.4 |
| $MLP_3$ | **93.68** ± 3.9 | 91.57 ± 5.0 | **92.46** ± 2.7 |
| $MLP_4$ | 93.29 ± 2.9 | **91.78** ± 5.3 | 92.35 ± 3.2 |
| $MLP_5$ | 92.89 ± 4.7 | 91.53 ± 5.2 | 92.04 ± 3.4 |
| | **Swing Phase** | | |
| | **Precision** | **Recall** | **$F_1$ Score** |
| $MLP_1$ | 92.49 ± 4.8 | 94.74 ± 3.2 | 93.45 ± 2.0 |
| $MLP_2$ | 92.97 ± 4.3 | 94.84 ± 3.1 | 93.77 ± 1.9 |
| $MLP_3$ | 93.24 ± 4.3 | **95.21** ± 2.9 | **94.11** ± 2.1 |
| $MLP_4$ | **93.32** ± 4.7 | 94.80 ± 3.6 | 93.93 ± 2.7 |
| $MLP_5$ | 93.29 ± 4.0 | 94.47 ± 3.7 | 93.77 ± 2.5 |

**Table 4.** Gait phase classification performances for stance and swing phases in learned subjects (set LS-test). Precision, recall and $F_1$ scores are averaged over the 23 folds.

| | **Stance Phase** | | |
|---|---|---|---|
| | **Precision** | **Recall** | **$F_1$ Score** |
| $MLP_1$ | 94.15 ± 0.3 | 91.72 ± 0.8 | 92.92 ± 0.3 |
| $MLP_2$ | 94.48 ± 0.6 | 92.75 ± 0.8 | 93.60 ± 0.3 |
| $MLP_3$ | 94.63 ± 0.5 | 93.59 ± 0.5 | 94.11 ± 0.2 |
| $MLP_4$ | **94.80** ± 0.5 | 93.67 ± 0.9 | 94.22 ± 0.4 |
| $MLP_5$ | 94.50 ± 0.5 | **93.99** ± 0.6 | **94.24** ± 0.3 |
| | **Swing phase** | | |
| | **Precision** | **Recall** | **$F_1$ Score** |
| $MLP_1$ | 93.60 ± 0.5 | 95.50 ± 0.3 | 94.54 ± 0.2 |
| $MLP_2$ | 94.37 ± 0.5 | 95.72 ± 0.6 | 95.04 ± 0.2 |
| $MLP_3$ | 94.99 ± 0.3 | 95.81 ± 0.4 | 95.40 ± 0.2 |
| $MLP_4$ | 95.06 ± 0.7 | **95.94** ± 0.4 | **95.50** ± 0.2 |
| $MLP_5$ | **95.28** ± 0.5 | 95.68 ± 0.4 | 95.48 ± 0.2 |

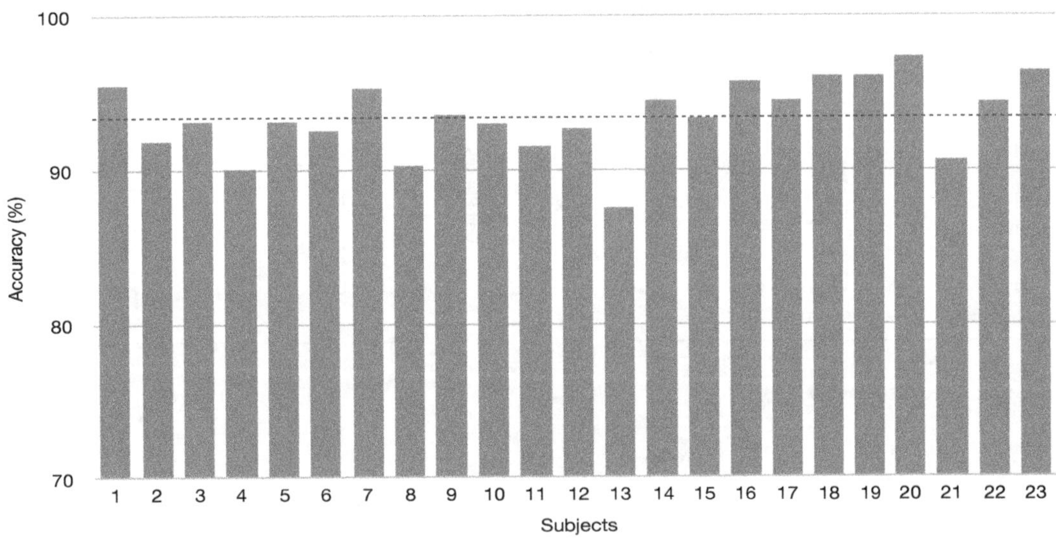


**Figure 6.** Classification accuracy over the 23 folds for the unlearned subjects (US set).

### *4.2. Comparison with Feature-Based Approach*

Classification of EMG signals from lower-limb muscles is usually based on time/frequency domain features extraction [34]. In order to provide a comparison with a feature-based method, we implemented a classifier following the approach described in [13]. We used a window size of 200 samples and for each sEMG signal we calculated the following features: standard deviation (SD), root mean square (RMS), mean absolute value (MAV), integrated EMG (IEMG) and waveform length (WL). They correspond to the group 2 features used in [13], which provide the best classification accuracy. We then concatenated the features obtaining a 40 length input vector (five features for each of the eight muscles). This was fed into a multi layer perceptron to train a gait phase classifier. A single hidden layer with 10 units is used in [13], where the input vector length was 10. We ran classification experiments over the 23 folds training a single layer network with 10 units, a single layer network with 40 units (corresponding to the size of our input vector) and all the networks in Table 1. The best average classification accuracy of $87.69 \pm 5.9$ for unlearned subjects was achieved with $MLP_3$, while accuracy for LS was $88.03 \pm 2.7$, thus we used $MLP_3$ for predicting HS an TO timing, adopting the same procedure applied to our approach and described in Section 3.5. In the following sections we refer to such a feature based method as *FB*.

### *4.3. Gait Events Detection*

The analysis of the results identified $MLP_3$ as the best model for the classification of unlearned data, obtaining an accuracy of 93.41% (Table 2), a $F_1$ score of 92.46% for stance phases and of 94.11% for swing phases (Tables 3 and 4). Thus, $MLP_3$ has been adopted to predict foot-floor-contact signal and identify HS and TO timing in unlearned subjects, following the procedure described in Section 3.5. The prediction was tested by comparing HS and TO timing provided by the present approach vs. heel-strike and toe-off timing measured from the basographic signal. Examples of prediction of foot–floor-contact signal provided by the present approach in US subjects (blue line) vs. the ground truth (red line) are depicted in Figure 7. As one can see, our method provides good predictions also in the presence of an irregular walking activity, i.e., non uniform gait phases duration, due to the everyday walking conditions addressed in this study.

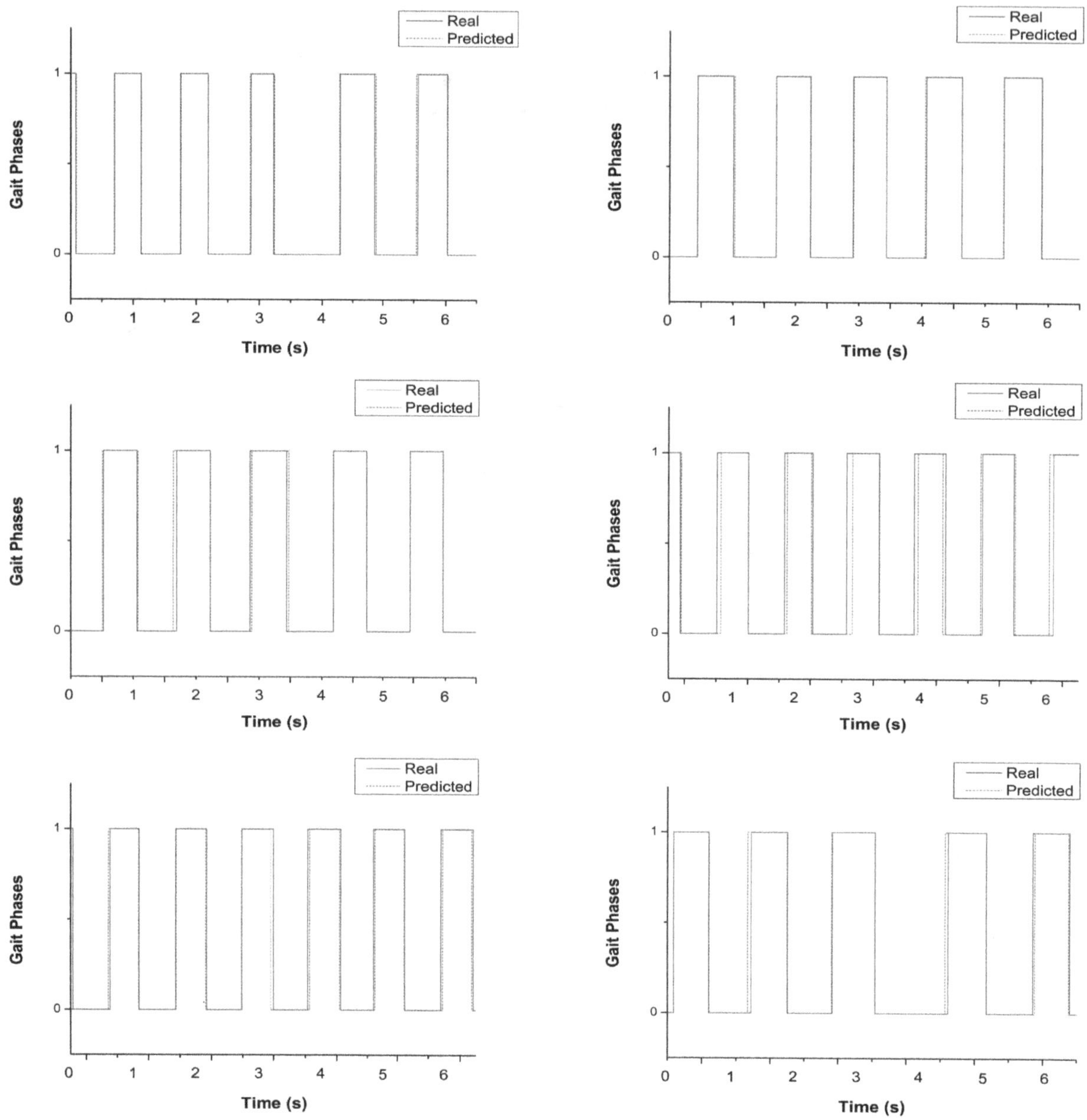


**Figure 7.** Examples of TO and HS predictions on six random subjects.

Purely data-driven approaches for gait-phase identification have been shown to achieve lower performance in less controlled scenarios, such as conditions similar to everyday walking [32]. Adapting to the larger variability of sEMG signals collected from dynamic environments and activities is more challenging for the classifiers. This could be due to the reported differences [16–19] between treadmill and straight ground walking (i.e., increased number of steps and cadence, decreased preferred walking speed, stride and stance-phase length and changes in sEMG activation) and to the further variability of spatial and temporal parameters and sEMG signals introduced by deceleration, reversing, curve and acceleration typical of everyday walking [16]. Despite this, the accuracy of $MLP_3$ classification is good for both LS-test subjects and US subjects (93.41%). The high classification accuracy and the effective post-processing of model output allowed to achieve an average absolute prediction error over unlearned subjects of $21.42 \pm 7.0$ ms for HS and $38.1 \pm 15.2$ ms for TO (Table 5). Both HS and TO predictions may be considered reasonably suitable, since they show an average absolute error <1% and <2% of a gait cycle duration, respectively. The present approach shows better performance in detecting heel-strikes rather than toe-offs. This result matches previous EMG-based and accelerometer-based reports [13,32].

**Table 5.** Performance of toe-off (TO) and heel-strike (HS) detection for unlearend subjects over 23 folds.

| | HS | | | |
|---|---|---|---|---|
| | **MAE** | **Precision** | **Recall** | $F_1$ |
| $MLP_3$ | **21.6** ± 7.0 | **99.67** ± 0.5 | **99.50** ± 2.9 | **99.04** ± 2.6 |
| *FB* | 56.7 ± 31.9 | 99.19 ± 1.5 | 96.40 ± 9.4 | 97.56 ± 2.6 |
| | **TO** | | | |
| | **MAE** | **Precision** | **Recall** | $F_1$ |
| $MLP_3$ | **38.1** ± 15.2 | **99.07** ± 1.5 | **97.90** ± 3.5 | **98.40** ± 2.4 |
| *FB* | 64.4 ± 42.7 | 98.45 ± 2.6 | 95.67 ± 9.9 | 96.84 ± 6.9 |

To test the reliability of HS and TO prediction, results provided by our approach have been compared with the results achieved by feature-based (FB) approach. Comparison is reported in Table 5. Our approach outperformed the FB one, suggesting that the neural network succeeded in learning latent features that are better suited for the task at hand if compared to the ones used in previous studies [13]. Besides the above reported direct comparison with the FB approach in the same population, an idea of the quality of the present results could be given also through the analysis of the results reported in [13] in their own population, during treadmill walking. The classification accuracy reported in [13] was 87.5% on learned subjects and 77% for unlearned ones. The associated average prediction error computed in unlearned subjects was 35 ± 25 ms for HS and 49 ± 15 ms for TO. Compared with those performances, results provided by the present study are encouraging, despite the challenging conditions of everyday walking. Besides the different approach (different neural network and different processing of the input signal), the elevated classification-accuracy values and the satisfactory HS/TO-prediction achieved here are supposed to be due also to the characteristics of the experimental set-up: high number of strides acquired per subject (about 500) associated with quite a large number of subjects (23); four different muscles per leg for every subject involved in training process. Moreover, foot-switches [31,35] represent the gold standard in gait segmentation since each gait phase can be associated with a specific value of the sensor output [36]. Finally, in the present study, data from three foot-switches was considered, in line with what reported in literature [31]. Using three foot-switches, instead of the two used in [13], probably improved the reliability of basographic signals as ground truth as well as the reliability of performance evaluation.

## 5. Conclusions

The present study proposed a suitable approach for classifying stance vs. swing and predicting the occurrence of the transition between phases, such as heel strike and toe off. The main contribution of the study is to provide reliable performances in gait-phase classification and gait-event prediction in natural walking conditions (similar to everyday walking), overcoming the constraints associated to the controlled environment (such as treadmill walking) used by previous studies to address this kind of task. A further methodological contribution consists of proposing a different pre-processing of sEMG-signal in order to better train the neural networks; the direct use of linear envelopes proposed here allows the network to automatically learn relevant higher level (hidden) features, avoiding hand crafting ad-hoc features and contributing to improve the performances.

From the clinical point of view, a relevant contribution is the fact that the present approach is based on sEMG signals only. This could considerably help reduce the number of sensors necessary for a complete gait protocol, limiting the clinical encumbrance, time-consumption, and cost. Thus, one of the main application domains of the present methodology should be in the field of neuromuscular diseases, such as spastic cerebral palsy, where the acquisition and then the analysis of sEMG signals are essential and special care should be exercised in the treatment of the patients.

Moreover, the present classifier may also support the process of gait phase detection in EMG-driven assistive devices [37], such as hip–knee, ankle–foot, and knee–ankle–foot orthoses and exoskeletons, as the identification of gait events is a continuing concern in the use of these devices. Evaluating the performance of the classifier after reducing the complexity of experimental protocol (i.e., the number of monitored muscles) could also be valuable. At the time of writing, all these applications are beyond the goals of the present work. However, future efforts will point in that direction.

**Author Contributions:** conceptualization, F.D.N., C.M., S.F. and A.C.; methodology, F.D.N. and C.M.; software, C.M.; investigation, C.M. and F.D.N.; validation, C.M.; resources, F.D.N. and S.F. ; data curation, F.D.N. and C.M.; writing—original draft preparation, F.D.N. and C.M.; writing—review and editing, A.C. and S.F.; visualization, F.D.N. and C.M.; supervision, A.C. and S.F.

**Acknowledgments:** Thanks to Guido Mascia and Lorenzo Principi for the support provided in preparing the experiments.

## References

1. Loeb, G.E.; Gans, C. *Electromyography for Experimentalists*; University of Chicago Press: Chicago, IL, USA, 1986.
2. Perry, J. *Gait Analysis: Normal and Pathological Function*; Slack Inc.: Thorofare, NJ, USA, 1992.
3. Špulák, D.; Čmejla, R.; Bačáková, R.; Kračmar, B.; Satrapová, L.; Novotný, P. Muscle activity detection in electromyograms recorded during periodic movements. *Comput. Biol. Med.* **2014**, *47*, 93–103. [CrossRef] [PubMed]
4. Wang, W.; Stefano, A.; Allen, R. A simulation model of the surface EMG signal for analysis of muscle activity during the gait cycle. *Comput. Biol. Med.* **2006**, *36*, 601–618. [CrossRef] [PubMed]
5. Mengarelli, A.; Maranesi, E.; Burattini, L.; Fioretti, S.; Di Nardo, F. Co-contraction activity of ankle muscles during walking: A gender comparison. *Biomed. Signal Process. Control* **2017**, *33*, 1–9. [CrossRef]
6. Gurney, J.; Kersting, U.; Rosenbaum, D. Between-day reliability of repeated plantar pressure distribution measurements in a normal population. *Gait Posture* **2008**, *27*, 706–709. [CrossRef] [PubMed]
7. Bovi, G.; Rabuffetti, M.; Mazzoleni, P.; Ferrarin, M. A multiple-task gait analysis approach: Kinematic, kinetic and EMG reference data for healthy young and adult subjects. *Gait Posture* **2011**, *33*, 6–13. [CrossRef] [PubMed]
8. Caldas, R.; Mundt, M.; Potthast, W.; Buarque de Lima Neto, F.; Markert, B. A systematic review of gait analysis methods based on inertial sensors and adaptive algorithms. *Gait Posture* **2017**, *57*, 204–210. [CrossRef] [PubMed]
9. Joyseeree, R.; Abou Sabha, R.; Mueller, H. Applying Machine Learning to Gait Analysis Data for Disease Identification. *Stud. Health Technol. Inf.* **2015**, *210*, 850–854. [CrossRef]
10. Zou, Q.; Wang, Y.; Zhao, Y.; Wang, Q.; Shen, C.; Li, Q. Deep Learning Based Gait Recognition Using Smartphones in the Wild. *arXiv* **2018**, arXiv:1811.00338.
11. Kaczmarczyk, K.; Wit, A.; Krawczyk, M.; Zaborski, J.; Piłsudskii, J. Artificial Neural Networks (ANN) Applied for Gait Classification and Physiotherapy Monitoring in Post Stroke Patients. In *Artificial Neural Networks*; IntechOpen: Rijeka, Croatia, 2011; Chapter 16.
12. Wang, J.; Zielińska, T. Gait features analysis using artificial neural networks—Testing the footwear effect. *Acta Bioeng. Biomech.* **2017**, *19*, 17–32.
13. Nazmi, N.; Abdul Rahman, M.; Yamamoto, S.I.; Ahmad, S. Walking gait event detection based on electromyography signals using artificial neural network. *Biomed. Signal Process. Control* **2019**, *47*, 334–343. [CrossRef]
14. Ziegier, J.; Gattringer, H.; Mueller, A. Classification of Gait Phases Based on Bilateral EMG Data Using Support Vector Machines. In Proceedings of the IEEE RAS and EMBS International Conference on Biomedical Robotics and Biomechatronics, Enschede, The Netherlands, 26–29 August 2018; Volume 2018, pp. 978–983. [CrossRef]

15. Meng, M.; She, Q.; Gao, Y.; Luo, Z. EMG signals based gait phases recognition using hidden Markov models. In Proceedings of the 2010 IEEE International Conference on Information and Automation, ICIA 2010, Harbin, China, 20–23 June 2010; pp. 852–856. [CrossRef]
16. Stolze, H.; Kuhtz-Buschbeck, J.; Mondwurf, C.; Boczek-Funcke, A.; Jöhnk, K.; Deuschl, G.; Illert, M. Gait analysis during treadmill and overground locomotion in children and adults. *Electroencephalogr. Clin. Neurophysiol. Electromyogr. Mot. Control* **1997**, *105*, 490–497. [CrossRef]
17. Batlkham, B.; Oyunaa, C.; Odongua, N. A Kinematic Comparison of Overground and Treadmill Walking. *Value Health* **2014**, *17*, A774. [CrossRef] [PubMed]
18. Riley, P.O.; Paolini, G.; Della Croce, U.; Paylo, K.W.; Kerrigan, D.C. A kinematic and kinetic comparison of overground and treadmill walking in healthy subjects. *Gait Posture* **2007**, *26*, 17–24. [CrossRef] [PubMed]
19. Song, J.; Hidler, J. Biomechanics of overground vs. treadmill walking in healthy individuals. *J. Appl. Physiol.* **2008**, *104*, 747–755. [CrossRef]
20. Alanazi, H.; Abdullah, A.; Qureshi, K. A Critical Review for Developing Accurate and Dynamic Predictive Models Using Machine Learning Methods in Medicine and Health Care. *J. Med. Syst.* **2017**, *41*, 69. [CrossRef] [PubMed]
21. Abbas, R.; Hussain, A.; Al-Jumeily, D.; Baker, T.; Khattak, A. Classification of Foetal Distress and Hypoxia Using Machine Learning Approaches. *Lect. Notes Comput. Sci.* **2018**, *10956*, 767–776._81. [CrossRef]
22. Aljaaf, A.; Al-Jumeily, D.; Haglan, H.; Alloghani, M.; Baker, T.; Hussain, A.; Mustafina, J. Early Prediction of Chronic Kidney Disease Using Machine Learning Supported by Predictive Analytics. In Proceedings of the 2018 IEEE Congress on Evolutionary Computation (CEC), Rio de Janeiro, Brazil, 8–13 July 2018.
23. Subasi, A.; Yilmaz, M.; Ozcalik, H.R. Classification of EMG signals using wavelet neural network. *J. Neurosci. Methods* **2006**, *156*, 360–367. [CrossRef]
24. Elamvazuthi, I.; Duy, N.; Ali, Z.; Su, S.; Khan, M.; Parasuraman, S. Electromyography (EMG) based Classification of Neuromuscular Disorders using Multi-Layer Perceptron. In Proceedings of the 2015 IEEE International Symposium on Robotics and Intelligent Sensors (IEEE IRIS2015), Langkawi, Malaysia, 18–20 October 2015; Volume 76, pp. 223–228. [CrossRef]
25. Ibrahimy, M.; Ahsan, M.; Khalifa, O. Design and optimization of levenberg-marquardt based neural network classifier for EMG signals to identify hand motions. *Meas. Sci. Rev.* **2013**, *13*, 142–151. [CrossRef]
26. Liu, Z.; Luo, Z. Hand motion pattern classifier based on EMG using wavelet packet transform and LVQ neural networks. In Proceedings of the 2008 IEEE International Symposium on IT in Medicine and Education, ITME 2008, Xiamen, China, 12–14 December 2008; pp. 28–32. [CrossRef]
27. Oskoei, M.; Hu, H. Support vector machine-based classification scheme for myoelectric control applied to upper limb. *IEEE Trans. Biomed. Eng.* **2008**, *55*, 1956–1965. [CrossRef]
28. Moslem, B.; Diab, M.; Khalil, M.; Marque, C. Classification of multichannel uterine EMG signals by using unsupervised competitive learning. In Proceedings of the 2011 IEEE Workshop on Signal Processing Systems, SiPS 2011, Beirut, Lebanon, 4–7 October 2011; pp. 267–272. [CrossRef]
29. Hermens, H.; Freriks, B.; Disselhorst-Klug, C.; Rau, G. Development of recommendations for SEMG sensors and sensor placement procedures. *J. Electromyogr. Kinesiol.* **2000**, *10*, 361–374. [CrossRef]
30. Di Nardo, F.; Mengarelli, A.; Maranesi, E.; Burattini, L.; Fioretti, S. Gender differences in the myoelectric activity of lower limb muscles in young healthy subjects during walking. *Biomed. Signal Process. Control* **2015**, *19*, 14–22. [CrossRef]
31. Agostini, V.; Balestra, G.; Knaflitz, M. Segmentation and classification of gait cycles. *IEEE Trans. Neural Syst. Rehabil. Eng.* **2014**, *22*, 946–952. [CrossRef]
32. Khandelwal, S.; Wickstrasm, N. Evaluation of the performance of accelerometer-based gait event detection algorithms in different real-world scenarios using the MAREA gait database. *Gait Posture* **2017**, *51*, 84–90. [CrossRef]
33. Trojaniello, D.; Cereatti, A.; Della Croce, U. Accuracy, sensitivity and robustness of five different methods for the estimation of gait temporal parameters using a single inertial sensor mounted on the lower trunk. *Gait Posture* **2014**, *40*, 487–492. [CrossRef]
34. Toledo-Pérez, D.; Martínez-Prado, M.; Gómez-Loenzo, R.; Paredes-García, W.; Rodríguez-Reséndiz, J. A study of movement classification of the lower limb based on up to 4-EMG channels. *Electronics* **2019**, *8*, 259. [CrossRef]

35. Taborri, J.; Palermo, E.; Rossi, S.; Cappa, P. Gait partitioning methods: A systematic review. *Sensors* **2016**, *16*, 66. [CrossRef]
36. Winiarski, S.; Rutkowska-Kucharska, A. Estimated ground reaction force in normal and pathological gait. *Acta Bioeng. Biomech.* **2009**, *11*, 53–60.
37. Ma, Y.; Xie, S.; Zhang, Y. A patient-specific EMG-driven neuromuscular model for the potential use of human-inspired gait rehabilitation robots. *Comput. Biol. Med.* **2016**, *70*, 88–98. [CrossRef]

# 15

# Ten Points for High-Quality Statistical Reporting and Data Presentation

**Pentti Nieminen**

Medical Informatics and Data Analysis Research Group, University of Oulu, 90014 Oulu, Finland; pentti.nieminen@oulu.fi

**Featured Application: In this work, an applicable instrument is proposed to quickly evaluate the quality of the statistical reporting and data presentation in research papers.**

**Abstract:** Background: Data analysis methods have become an essential part of empirical research papers, especially in health sciences and medical research. It has previously been reported that a noteworthy percentage of articles have flaws in their statistical reporting. Reporting problems have been a long-term issue, and despite continued efforts to improve the situation, improvements have been far from satisfactory. One explanation is an inadequate assessment of statistical reporting during peer review. This communication proposes a short instrument to assess the quality of data analysis reporting in manuscripts and published papers. Method: A checklist-type instrument was developed by selecting and refining items from previous reports about the quality of statistical reporting in medical journals and from published guidelines for reporting and data presentation. Items were pretested and modified during pilot studies. A total of 160 original medical research articles that were published in 4 journals were evaluated to test the instrument. Interrater and intrarater agreements were examined by comparing quality scores assigned to 40 articles published in a psychiatric journal. Results: The data analysis reporting test consists of nine questions that assess the quality of health research from a reader's perspective. The composed scale has a total score ranging from 0 to 10 and discriminated between journals and study designs. A high score suggested that an article had a good presentation of findings in tables and figures and that the description of analysis methods was helpful to readers. Interrater and intrarater agreements were high. Conclusion: An applicable checklist for quickly testing the statistical reporting quality of manuscripts and published research papers was developed. This instrument aims to improve the quality of empirical research in scientific fields where statistical methods play an important role.

**Keywords:** data analysis; statistics; reporting; data presentation; publications; medicine; health care

---

## 1. Introduction

Statistical reporting plays an important role in medical publications [1]. A high proportion of medical articles are essentially statistical in their presentation. For the reader, the main outward demonstration of a publication consists of statistical expressions that summarize the raw data used in the research. Regardless of the quality of the data and the variables chosen to express the results, the overt evidence of the research is produced as the lists of numbers, tables, plots, graphs, and other displays, i.e., the descriptive statistics. The communication of the descriptive statistics may also be combined with statistical inference procedures, such as test statistics and $p$-values [2].

The accurate communication of research results to the scientific community (i.e., other researchers) is essential providing reliable results [3,4]. Failure to report analysis methods or inadequate data presentation could lead to inaccurate inferences, even if the statistical analyses were performed correctly.

Several findings have demonstrated that a noteworthy percentage of articles, even those published in high-prestige journals, have flaws in their statistical reporting [3–8]. Methodological and reporting problems have been reported over several decades, and despite continued efforts to improve the situation [9], the improvements have been far from satisfactory. One explanation is the inadequate assessment of statistical reporting during peer review [8].

Author instructions and editorials alone have been insufficient to change the quality of statistical reporting. Numerous reporting guidelines offer tools or checklists to evaluate the reporting of health research [10]. The EQUATOR Network listed 424 such guidelines in March 2020 [11]. What is often problematic in these checklists is their extent. They try to evaluate all possible aspects of analysis from study design, settings, participants, description of measurements and variables, sample sizes, data analysis methods, specific methods, descriptive data, outcome data, and ancillary analysis. Often it is impossible to evaluate all these points. When reviewing and editing health care and medical papers, I have noticed that a few points will reveal the quality of reporting of data analysis. There is no need to read the whole manuscript and check all the statistical details to ensure that the manuscript contains all the information that readers need to assess the study's methodology and validity of its findings. Editorial processes of medical manuscripts often fail to identify obvious indicators of good and poor data presentation and reporting of results. Editors, reviewers and readers need new tools to quickly identify studies with inadequate descriptions of statistical methods and poor quality of data presentation.

I took on the challenge of compacting and refining the available quality criteria for statistical reporting and data presentation. I had three guiding starting points for assessing statistical reporting. The first key point was that if the data analysis methods are described with enough details, readers will be able to follow the flow of the analyses and to critically assess whether the data analyses provide reliable results. My second key point was the use of tables and figures in data presentation. Tables and figures are a fundamental means of scientific communications and they are included in most submitted and published medical and health care articles [12]. Most readers browse through tables and illustrations, but few read the whole article. Well-prepared tables and figures with proper titles, clear labeling, and optimally presented data will empower readers to scrutinize the data. I presume that the quality of tables and figures indicates the overall quality of data presentation. My third starting key point was that the new tool should be easy to use. I wanted to develop a short evaluation form with a low number of items.

In short, my objective was to develop a handy and reliable instrument to assess the quality of statistical reporting and data presentation that was applicable for a wide variety of medical and health care research forums, including both clinical and basic sciences. In this article, I define nine items for the proposed quality test. In addition, I report findings from an initial evaluation of its functionality and reliability.

## 2. Materials and Methods

### 2.1. Prework

My intention was to develop a test or checklist that would complement and not replicate other checklists. The construction of my quality evaluation tool began with a literature search. It included the following steps:

- Search for papers evaluating the use and misuse of statistics in medical articles.
- Search for papers evaluating statistical reporting and data presentation.
- Review medical statistics textbooks.
- Review statistical reporting guidelines, including journal guidelines for authors.
- Assess my experience as a handling editor and referee for medical and medicine-related journals.

After reading and reviewing the existing body of evidence, I discovered that including an assessment of statistical errors into a quality instrument would be very difficult. Several studies have reviewed medical papers and tried to find errors in the selection of statistical procedures [5,8,13]. Most of the statistical problems in medical journals reported in these reviews are related to elementary statistical techniques [14]. The errors in medical papers are probably more a matter of judgment. There is no general agreement on what constitutes a statistical error [6,15,16]. The recommended methods for a particular type of question may not be the only feasible methods, and may not be universally agreed upon as the best methods [17]. In addition, I decided to avoid any judgment of the content, such as the originality, ethics, or scientific relevance.

I found hundreds of journal guidelines for statistical reporting. I observed strong heterogeneity among the guidelines. Some journals have kept these guidelines to the minimum required for a decent manuscript presentation, whereas a large number of journals displayed too many instructions and journal-specific recommendations. Some recommendations regarding the test statistics (reporting of values, degrees of freedom and p-values) or the contents of tables were even contradictory (between journals). Most reporting guidelines said more about the presentation of methods than about the reporting of results. In addition, medical statistics textbooks did not cover the topic of statistical reporting.

By the end of the prework process, I had identified and formulated 20 items phrased as questions and grouped them into two domains (description of methods and data presentation). The draft questions were as follows:

Statistical analysis (or Data analysis) subsection in the Material and Methods section:

- Was Statistical analysis subsection included?
- Was there a sample size justification before the study?
- Did authors state how variables were described and summarized?
- Did authors state which methods were used to evaluate the statistical significances?
- Did authors identify the variables for each analysis and mentioned all the statistical methods used?
- Was extended description of some specific procedures provided?
- Did authors verify how data conformed to assumptions of the methods used?
- Was statistical software reported?
- Was missing data addressed?
- Were references to statistical literature provided?
- Was subject attrition or exclusion addressed?
- How any outlying data were treated in the analysis?

Data presentation:

- Was a table included where the basic characteristics of the study subjects were summarized with descriptive statistics?
- Were total and group sample sizes reported for each analysis in all tables and figures?
- Did all tables and figures have a clear and self-explanatory title?
- Were statistical abbreviations explained in all tables and figures?
- Were summary statistics, tests or methods identified and named in all tables and figures?
- Were *p*-values reported properly (e.g., no expressions like NS, $p < 0.05$, $p = 0.000$)
- Was the total number of reported *p*-values and confidence intervals in tables and figures less than 100?
- Were all tables and figures appropriate?

In line with my original key principles, the evaluation form should include two sections: (1) Material and Methods section and (2) tables and figures in Results section. In addition, the test form should be only one page long. I developed several pilot versions to structure the assessment of the quality of statistical reporting in an article or manuscript. Within these frames I reviewed the 20 draft questions for their importance and uniqueness with my health care students, who tested the instrument drafts during their studies. Further testing of the instrument, a review of the literature related to the topic and expert opinions from my colleagues resulted in the generation of 9 items pertaining to the description of statistical and data management procedures and the reporting of results in tables and figures. Following the pilot studies, several items were also reworded, rearranged, and consolidated in the test form for clarity. Because tables and figures should be self-explanatory, I decided to place the assessment of tables and figures at the beginning of the evaluation form. Thus, the assessment of the description of the statistical analysis in the Materials and methods section now follows the assessment of the tables and figures. The updated version of the instrument is included in as Table 1. In the evaluation form, questions 1–4 relate to basic guidelines for preparing effective tables and figures. Questions 5–9 evaluate the description of the data analysis methods.

**Table 1.** Statistical reporting and data presentation evaluation form.

| *TABLES AND FIGURES IN RESULTS SECTION:* | **No** | **Yes** |
|---|---|---|
| 1. Was a table included where the basic characteristics of the study participants were summarized with descriptive statistics? | 0 | 1 |
| 2. Was the total number of participants provided in all tables and figures? | 0 | 1 |
| 3. Were summary statistics, tests and methods identified and named in all tables and figures? | 0 | 1 |
| 4. Were tables and figures well prepared? | | |
| 0 = more than 50% of the tables and figures had presentation issues<br>1 = 50% or fewer of the tables and figures had presentation issues<br>2 = no presentation issues in any of the tables and figures | | 0<br>1<br>2 |
| *MATERIALS AND METHODS SECTION:* | | |
| 5. Was the statistical analysis (or data analysis) subsection provided in the Materials and Methods section? | 0 | 1 |
| 6. Did authors identify the variables (and methods) for each analysis done in the study? | 0 | 1 |
| 7. Was it verified that the data conformed to the assumptions and preconditions of the methods used to analyze them? | 0 | 1 |
| 8. Were references to statistical literature provided? | 0 | 1 |
| 9. Was the statistical software reported? | 0 | 1 |
| TOTAL SCORE: | | |

### *2.2. Ten Items to Assess the Quality of Statistical Reporting and Data Presentation*

In the following chapter, I present the items as a sequence of 9 numbered questions and explain some of the reasoning behind the questions.

#### 2.2.1. Item 1: Was a Table Included Where the Basic Characteristics of the Study Subjects Were Summarized with Descriptive Statistics?

Most papers reporting an analysis of health care and medical data will at some point use statistics to describe the sociodemographic characteristics, medical history and main outcome variables of the study participants. An important motive for doing this is to give the reader some idea of the extent to which study findings can be generalized to their own local situation [18]. The production of descriptive statistics is a straightforward matter, but often authors need to decide which statistics to present. The selected statistics should be included in a paper in a manner that is easy for readers to assimilate. When many patient characteristics are being described, the details of the statistics used and the number of participants contributing to analysis are best incorporated in tabular presentation [12,18,19].

I give one point if the main features of important characteristics of the participants were displayed in a table.

#### 2.2.2. Item 2: Was the Total Number of Participants Provided in all Tables and Figures?

The medical literature shows a strong tendency to accentuate significance testing, specifically "statistically significant" outcomes. Most papers published in medical journals contain tables and figures reporting *p*-values [16,20,21]. Finding statistically significant or nonsignificant results depends on the sample size [22,23]. When evaluating the validity of the findings, the reader must know the number of study participants. Sample size is an important consideration for research. A larger sample size leads to a higher level of precision and thus a higher level of power for a given study to detect an effect of a given size. An excessively large number of study participants may lead to statistically significant results even when there is no clinical practicality; an inappropriately small number of study participants can fail to reveal important and clinically significant differences. The total number of participants or sample size of each group should be clearly reported.

I give one point if most of the tables and figures (at least 75%) have provided the total number of participants or number of participants in each subgroup.

#### 2.2.3. Item 3: Were Summary Statistics, Tests, and Methods Identified and Named in all Tables and Figures?

Tables and figures should be able to stand alone [24]. That is, all information necessary for interpretation should be included within the table or figure, legend or footnotes [25]. This means that descriptive statistics, significance tests, and multivariable modeling methods used are named. Many readers will skim an article before reading it closely and identifying data analysis methods in the tables or figure will allow the readers to understand the procedures immediately. It is not necessary to define well known statistical abbreviations, such as SD, SE, OR, RR, HR, CI, r, R2, n, or NA, but the methods producing these statistics should be named.

I give one point if statistical summary statistics, tests, and methods in tables and figures were named.

#### 2.2.4. Item 4: Were Tables and Figures Well Prepared?

High quality tables and figures increase the chance that readers can take advantage of an article's results. In effective scientific writing, it is essential to ensure that the tables and figures are flawless, informative, and attractive. Below is a list of a number of presentation issues that may prevent readers grasping the message quickly and will lower the overall quality of data presentation [12,24,26].

- Messy, inferior, or substandard overall technical presentation of data.
    - A table or a figure did not have a clear title.
    - The formatting of a table resembled a spreadsheet, and the lines of the same size between each row and each column did not help to clarify the different data presented in the table.
    - In a figure, data values were not clearly visible.
    - Data values were not defined.
    - Obvious errors in presented numbers or data elements.
- Tables or figures included unnecessary features:
    - In a figure, nondata elements (gridlines, shading, or three dimensional perspectives) competed with data elements and they did not serve a specific explanatory function in the graph.
    - A table or a figure was unnecessary because the data had too few values. Authors could have presented their results clearly in a sentence or two. For example, a sentence is preferred to a pie char.
- General guiding principles for reporting statistical results were not followed:

- $p$-Values were denoted with asterisks or with a system of letters in tables or figures, and actual $p$-values were not reported. Actual $p$-values should be reported, without false precision, whenever feasible. Providing the actual $p$-values prevents problems of interpretation related to $p$-values close to 0.05 [12,22]. Very small $p$-values do not need exact representation and $p < 0.001$ is usually sufficient.
- Numbers were not reported with an appropriate degree of precision in tables. In interpreting the findings, the reader cannot pay attention to the numbers presented with several decimals.
- The standard error of the mean (SE) was used to indicate the variability of a data set.
- Confidence intervals were not reported with the effect sizes (regression coefficients, ORs, HRs, or IRRs) in regression analyses or meta-analyses. The results of the primary comparisons should always be reported with confidence intervals [27].
- A table included only $p$-values. $p$-value cannot tell readers the strength or size of an effect, change, or relationship. In the end, patients and physicians want to know the magnitude of the benefit, change or association, not the statistical significance of individual studies [23,28].

I give zero points if more than 50% of the tables and figures included presentation issues.

I give one point if 50% or fewer of the tables and figures included presentation issues.

I give two points if all tables and figures were prepared efficiently and accurately, and the presentation issues mentioned above were avoided.

#### 2.2.5. Item 5: Was a Statistical Analysis (or Data Analysis) Subsection Provided in the Methods Section?

Most general reporting guidelines and recommendations require that original research articles include a Methods section [10,24,29]. In these recommendations, it is stated that the Methods section should aim to be sufficiently detailed such that others with access to the data would be able to reproduce the results. This section should include at least the following subsections: Selection and description of participants, technical information about variables (primary and secondary outcomes, explanatory variables, other variables) and statistical methods. To many researchers, it seems quite obvious that a Statistical analysis (or Data analysis) subsection with a clear subheading should be provided in the Materials and Methods section when the manuscript contains some elements of statistical data analysis. However, in my experience, this is not obvious to all biomedical or health science researchers. I have reviewed several biomedical manuscripts for journals wherein the laboratory experiments were described in depth, but nothing was said about how the reported $p$-values were obtained. When statistical methods are described with enough detail in the Statistical analysis subsection, a knowledgeable reader can judge the appropriateness of the methods for the study and verify the reported methods.

I therefore give one point if the Methods section included a subsection headed with Statistical analysis (or Data analysis or Statistical methods).

#### 2.2.6. Item 6: Did Authors Identify the Variables and Methods for Each Analysis?

Authors know their own work so well that some find it difficult to put themselves in the position of a reader encountering the study for the first time. As a reader, I often request more information about some aspect of the data analysis. Within the Statistical analysis section, authors need to explain which statistical methods or tests were used for each analysis, rather than just listing all the statistical methods used in one place [30]. In a well-written statistical analysis subsection, authors should also identify the variables used in each analysis. Readers should be informed which variables were analyzed with each method. Care must be taken to ensure that all methods are listed and that all tests listed are indeed applied in the study [31]. The statistical section should be consistent with the Results section.

I give one point if authors describe the goal (research question), the variables and the method used for each analysis done in the study.

2.2.7. Item 7: Was It Verified that the Data Conformed to the Assumptions and Preconditions of the Methods Used to Analyze Them?

All basic data analysis methods and multivariable techniques depend on assumptions about the characteristics of the data [32]. If an analysis is performed without satisfying the assumptions, incorrect conclusions may be made on the basis of erroneous results. For example, a widely applied analysis of variance depends at least on three assumptions [33]. In actual data analysis it is unlikely that all the assumptions for the analysis of variance will be satisfied. Some statistical assumptions are essential, while some assumptions are quite lenient. A normal distribution of main variables is a strong requirement in a number of statistical techniques and should be verified and reported. On the other hand, the use of a nonparametric significance test instead of a more powerful parametric test should be justified. If a brief justification is provided, readers may better understand why a specific data analysis method has been applied [14]. Regression modeling has several constraints or preconditions, such as linearity, independence between explanatory variables, and number of participants per variable. In an excellent description of multivariable methods, authors should describe possible limitations or preconditions.

I give one point if authors describe how the data satisfactorily fulfill the underlying assumptions and preconditions of the main analysis methods.

2.2.8. Item 8: Were References to Statistical Literature Provided?

The use of all the statistical methods in a study needs to be documented with a relevant description to help the readers to validate the findings described by the authors. References enable others to identify and trace the methods used in the data analyses. Common statistical methods can be described in brief, but some less common or obscure methods should be explained in detail. The International Committee of Medical Journal Editors (ICMJE) also instructs to give references to established methods [29]. Good scientific writing is includes references and brief descriptions for methods that have been published but are not well known or not commonly used, descriptions of new or substantially modified methods, reasons for using uncommon methods, and an evaluation of the method's limitations [34].

I give one point for providing statistical references.

2.2.9. Item 9: Was the Statistical Software Used in the Analysis Reported?

Identifying the statistical software package used in the data analysis is important because all statistical programs do not use the same algorithms or default options to compute the same statistics. As a result, the findings may vary from package to package or from algorithm to algorithm. In addition, privately developed algorithms may not be validated and updated [12].

I give one point for reporting statistical software if the name and version of the statistical program or package (name, version) is provided.

*2.3. Total Score*

Users of this tools can calculate a total score by summing all 9 items. The total score ranges from 0 to 10. I have assigned the following labels to the corresponding ranges of the total score:

9–10 Excellent
7–8 Good
5–6 Acceptable
3–4 Weak
0–2 Poor

Although this division is plain and unsophisticated, it does provide useful interpretation of the scores.

### 2.4. Set of Articles

I used original research articles published between 2017 and 2019 in 4 journals to test the instrument for published studies. I selected two highly visible medical journals (*Lancet* and *JAMA Psychiatry*), one dental journal (*Journal of Dentistry*) (*JD*), and one journal from environmental and public health subfields (*International Journal of Environmental Research and Public Health*) (*IJERPH*) for the evaluation. I chose these journals to cover the range of statistical reporting both in established journals, and in lower visibility journals. I analyzed 40 articles per journal. The starting articles for each journal were chosen randomly from the journal's chronological list of articles, with the only criteria being that there would be at least 39 eligible subsequent articles published that year in the journal in question. The following consecutive 39 articles were also included for the review. Editorials, letters, case reports and review articles were excluded from the evaluation.

### 2.5. Data Analysis

Cross-tabulation was used to report the differences in the study design and sample size of the evaluated articles by the publication journals. For the total score of statistical reporting and data presentation, the mean value with standard deviation and box plots were used to describe the distribution by study design, sample size, and journal. Analysis of variance (ANOVA) was applied to evaluate the statistical significance of possible differences in the mean values of the total score. The quality score was approximately normally distributed, and the normality assumption of the analysis of variance test was met by the data. The chi-squared test was applied to reveal the statistically significant differences in the distributions of the items of the statistical reporting and data presentation instrument across journals. All of the statistical analyses were executed using IBM SPSS Statistics (version 25) software.

When using quality evaluation forms, several methodological aspects can impact accuracy and reliability. For instance, to obtain an appropriate description of statistical methods, the basic statistical methods must be familiar. Additionally, the level of expertise reviewers have about scientific writing can affect their ability to accurately detect shortcomings in reporting. Therefore, it was important to determine the interrater and test-retest reliability of the proposed tool using raters with low (Rater 1) and moderate (Rater 2) medical statistics experience. I recruited a junior medical researcher to serve as an independent rater (Rater 1). I acted as Rater 2 myself. Rater 1 had minimal experience with medical data analysis but had been involved with medical writing for the previous 2 years. Rater 1 received training in the use of the assessment form, and general guidelines were given on the items of the instrument.

The reliability study started in parallel with a pilot study of the evaluation form. The reliability of the evaluation was checked by comparing Rater 1 ratings with the ratings of Rater 2. We independently read and evaluated 40 articles published in *JAMA Psychiatry*. These articles were selected from the previously described set of 160 articles.

First, agreement between the summary scores was assessed using an intraclass correlation coefficient ICC (with agreement definition, single measures, and mixed model) and Pearson correlation coefficient [35]. Generally, good agreement is defined as an ICC > 0.80. To evaluate the test-retest (or intrarater) performance, I read the 40 articles published in *JAMA Psychiatry* twice. The time interval between the scoring sessions was six months.

Second, the percentage agreement and Cohen's kappa coefficient were used to assess the degree of agreement for each item [35]. The simple percentage agreement is an adequate measure of agreement for many purposes, but it does not account for agreement arising from chance alone. Categorical agreement is often measured with the kappa coefficient, which attempts to account for the agreement that may arise from chance alone. A kappa score in the range of 0.81 to 1 was considered to represent high agreement.

## 3. Results

### 3.1. Characteristics of the Evaluated Articles

The articles in the validation sample came from a variety of specialties: general medicine, clinical topics, psychiatry, dentistry, environmental topics, public health, and dentistry. Table 2 shows the basic characteristics of the article set. Observational studies (cross-sectional surveys, longitudinal and case-control studies) were performed at a higher frequency in *JAMA Psychiatry* and *IJERPH*. The proportion of experimental studies (randomized clinical trials, non-randomized intervention studies) was highest in *Lancet* (67.5%). The test article set also included laboratory works that applied data analysis methods scantily and had low intensity of statistical methods. Sample sizes were larger in the more prominent journals.

**Table 2.** Distribution of study design and sample size of the evaluated articles by the publication journal.

| | *Lancet* n (%) | *JAMA Psy* n (%) | *IJERPH* n (%) | *JD* n (%) | All n (%) |
|---|---|---|---|---|---|
| **Study design** | | | | | |
| Observational studies | 11 (27.5) | 27 (67.5) | 27 (67.5) | 13 (32.5) | 78 (48.8) |
| Experimental studies | 27 (67.5) | 9 (22.5) | 6 (15.0) | 6 (15.0) | 48 (30.0) |
| Reliability | 1 (2.5) | 0 | 2 (5.0) | 2 (5.0) | 5 (3.1) |
| Laboratory works | 0 | 0 | 4 (10.0) | 14 (35.0) | 18 (11.3) |
| Meta-analysis | 1 (2.5) | 4 (10.0) | 1 (2.5) | 5 (12.5) | 11 (6.9) |
| **Sample size** | | | | | |
| <99 | 0 | 3 (7.5) | 14 (35.0) | 20 (50.0) | 37 (23.1) |
| 100–499 | 5 (12.5) | 12 (30.0) | 12 (30.0) | 8 (20.0) | 37 (23.1) |
| 500–2999 | 22 (55.0) | 7 (17.5) | 6 (15.0) | 5 (12.5) | 40 (25.0) |
| >3000 | 12 (30.0) | 18 (45.0) | 5 (12.5) | 3 (7.5) | 38 (23.8) |
| Missing | 1 (2.5) | 0 | 3 (7.5) | 4 (10.0) | 8 (5.0) |
| Total number of articles | 40 | 40 | 40 | 40 | 160 |

*JAMA Psy = JAMA Psychiatry, IJERPH = International Journal of Environmental Research and Public Health, and JD = Journal of Dentistry.*

### 3.2. Distribution of the Total Quality Score

The total score assessing quality of statistical reporting ranges from 0 to 10. Figure 1 shows the distribution of the quality score among all 160 articles. A total of 14 (8.8%) articles were poor and 42 (26.3%) articles did not reach up to an acceptable level.

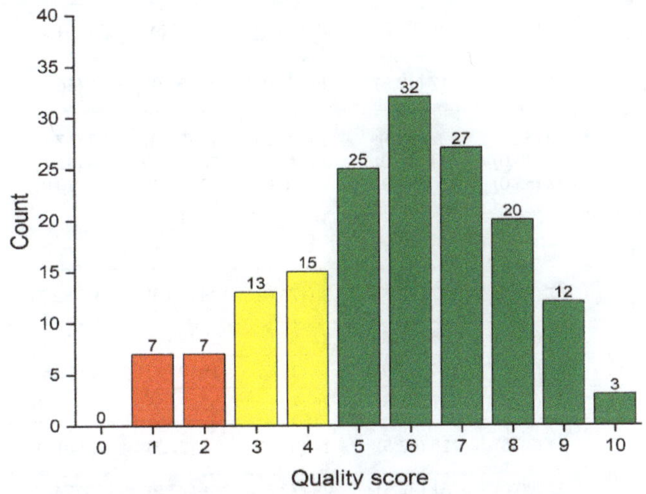


**Figure 1.** Column graph of the data analysis reporting quality score of 160 articles. Articles with poor quality (0–2) are denoted with red column color, those with weak quality (3–4) with yellow color and at least acceptable (5–10) articles with green color.

The distribution of the data analysis reporting score is summarized in Table 3 by article characteristics. The mean (SD) of quality score in all 160 evaluated reports was 5.7 (SD 2.2). The reporting quality was highest in the meta-analyses and lowest in laboratory works. The data analysis reporting quality was associated with the sample size of the evaluated study.

**Table 3.** Mean and standard deviation of the data analysis reporting score from 160 articles by study design and sample size.

| | Number of Articles | Mean | Standard Deviation |
|---|---|---|---|
| Study design | | | |
| • Observational studies | 78 | 5.5 | 2.2 |
| • Experimental studies | 48 | 6.5 | 1.8 |
| • Reliability | 5 | 5.4 | 2.6 |
| • Laboratory works | 18 | 3.9 | 1.9 |
| • Meta-analysis | 11 | 7.4 | 2.2 |
| Sample size | | | |
| • <99 | 37 | 4.7 | 2.2 |
| • 100–499 | 37 | 5.6 | 2.0 |
| • 500–2999 | 40 | 7.2 | 1.5 |
| • >3000 | 38 | 6.0 | 1.9 |
| • Missing | 8 | 2.9 | 1.0 |
| All articles | 160 | 5.7 | 2.2 |

*p*-Value of ANOVA $< 0.001$ for study design and sample size.

### 3.3. *Quality of Statistical Reporting and Data Presentation by the Journal*

Table 4 summarizes the distributions of the data analysis reporting test items in tables and figures by the journals. Neglecting to state the number of participants was the most common defect (65.6%). The quality of tables and figures was related to the journal; the failures to provide data and report findings was less common in the *Lancet*.

**Table 4.** The distributions of the data analysis reporting test items by the journals.

| Item | *Lancet* n (%) | *JAMA Psy* n (%) | *IJERPH* n (%) | *JD* n (%) | All n (%) | *p*-Value of the Chi-Squared Test |
|---|---|---|---|---|---|---|
| **Tables and figures in results section:** | | | | | | |
| Basic characteristics reported in a table | 35 (87.5) | 27 (77.5) | 27 (67.5) | 12 (30.0) | 101 (63.1) | <0.001 |
| Total number of participants provided | 27 (67.5) | 9 (22.5) | 12 (30.0) | 7 (17.5) | 55 (34.4) | <0.001 |
| Statistics, tests and methods identified | 34 (85.0) | 17 (42.5) | 20 (50.0) | 20 (50.0) | 91 (56.9) | <0.001 |
| Presentation issues:<br>• several<br>• 50% or less<br>• no issues | <br>2 (5.0)<br>16 (40.0)<br>22 (55.0) | <br>6 (15.0)<br>14 (35.0)<br>20 (50.0) | <br>10 (25.0)<br>18 (45.0)<br>12 (30.0) | <br>10 (25.0)<br>20 (50.0)<br>10 (25.0) | <br>28 (17.5)<br>68 (42.5)<br>64 (40.0) | 0.029 |
| **Materials and methods section** | | | | | | |
| Statistical analysis subsection provided | 37 (92.5) | 37 (92.5) | 30 (75.0) | 28 (70.0) | 132 (82.5) | 0.011 |
| Variables identified | 23 (57.5) | 35 (87.5) | 22 (55.0) | 22 (55.0) | 102 (63.7) | 0.005 |
| Assumptions verified | 14 (35.0) | 14 (35.0) | 11 (27.5) | 15 (37.5) | 54 (33.8) | 0.858 |
| Software reported | 32 (80.0) | 31 (77.5) | 29 (72.5) | 31 (77.5) | 123 (76.9) | 0.911 |
| References to statistical literature | 14 (35.0) | 25 (62.5) | 14 (35.0) | 11 (27.5) | 64 (40.0) | 0.008 |
| Software reported | 32 (80.0) | 31 (77.5) | 29 (72.5) | 31 (77.5) | 123 (76.9) | 0.911 |
| Total number of articles | 40 | 40 | 40 | 40 | 160 | |

*JAMA Psy = JAMA Psychiatry, IJERPH = International Journal of Environmental Research and Public Health and JD = Journal of Dentistry.*

Table 4 also compares the prevalence of adequate description of methods in the four journals. The failure to verify that the data conformed to the assumptions and preconditions of the methods used was very common (66.2%). A total of 28 articles (17.5%) did not provide a statistical analysis subsection; 60.0% (96 articles) did not provide references to statistical literature; and 23.1% (37 articles) did not report the statistical software.

Figure 2 shows how the quality score varies by journals. The high-impact general medical journal *Lancet* had mean score of 6.9 (SD 1.7) while the mean score in the leading psychiatric journal *JAMA Psy* was 6.1 (SD 1.4). The quality core also identified the journals (*IJERPH* and *JD*) that publish more laboratory studies with smaller sample sizes. Articles published in these journals had lower scores, with a mean score of 5.2 (SD 2.3) in *IJERPH* and a mean score of 5.0 (SD 2.3) in *JD*. The mean values were statistically significantly different ($p$-value of ANOVA $< 0.001$).

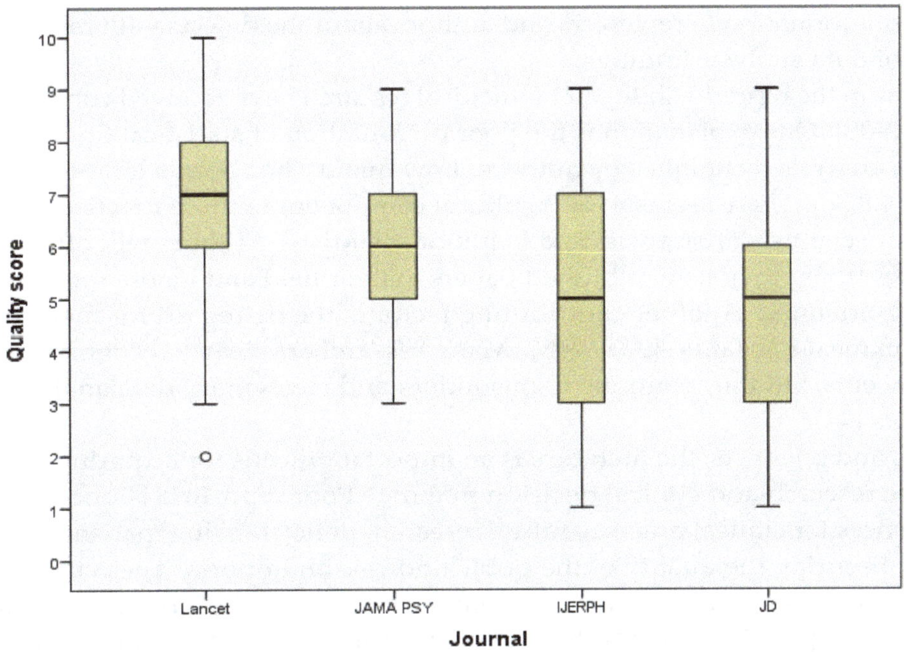


**Figure 2.** Box plot graph of the data analysis reporting quality score of 160 articles published in four journals. There were 40 articles from each journal. *JAMA Psy* = *JAMA Psychiatry*, *IJERPH* = *International Journal of Environmental Research and Public Health*, and *JD* = *Journal of Dentistry*.

### *3.4. Interrater and Test-Retest Reliability*

The interobserver agreement measured by the ICC and Pearson correlation coefficient were 0.88 and 0.89, respectively. The test-retest reliability was excellent with identical mean scores for the first and second evaluations (Pearson's correlation coefficient was 0.95, and the intraclass correlation coefficient was 0.95).

The interrater reliability between Rater 1 and Rater 2 was also analyzed for each item. The overall percentage agreement ranged from 80% to 100% and kappa values ranged from 0.53 to 1. Individual item analyses showed very high agreement (100%) for items 5 (providing a statistical analysis subsection) and 9 (reporting software). The most common disagreement among Raters 1 and 2 was in the description of statistical methods. For Item 6 ("Did authors identify the variables with the methods for each analysis done in the study?"), the agreement was 92.5% and kappa was 0.53. For item 3 ("Were summary statistics, tests and methods identified and named in all tables and figures?") these values were 80% and 0.60, respectively.

The test-retest evaluation showed good agreement for each item: Agreement percentage ranged from 90% to 100% and the kappa coefficients ranged from 0.72 to 1. For items 1, 2, 5, 8, and 9, the reliability measures provided complete agreement. This preliminary intrarater validation analysis revealed that disagreement arose especially for item 6.

**4. Discussion**

My purpose was to help authors, editors, reviewers, and readers to evaluate the quality of statistical reporting and data presentation in research papers when data analysis procedures are invoked to clarify findings and to draw conclusions from raw data. I developed a test for quickly assessing the quality by selecting the checklist items from readers' and reviewers' perspectives. The composed scale from 0 to 10 assessed the selected reporting characteristics in the reviewed articles. A high value suggested that an article had a good presentation of findings in tables and figures and that the description of analysis methods was helpful to readers. This indicates an emphasis on analysis and reporting in the study and indicates that the methodological quality is high and understandable. The items included in the index also gave detailed information to reviewers and authors about the defects with respect to specific parts of the reporting of data analysis findings.

The problems in the reproducibility of biomedical research have received considerable attention in recent years [8,36–38]. One explanation is the poor presentation of statistical findings and inadequate reporting of data analysis techniques by authors. Low quality has been a long-term issue in medical research papers [4,8,36]. There seems to be a cultural component to these practices [39]. The reporting practices of senior scientists are transmitted to junior scientists. Authors will often copy inadequate reporting practices from previously published papers in their field and ignore the recommendations of current general guidelines. Another contributing factor is the disregard for medical biostatistics in biomedical and clinical education [36,40–43]. Many researchers clearly recognize the importance of data analysis concepts, but they continue to misunderstand elementary data analysis techniques and statistical concepts [44].

To clinicians and scientists, the literature is an important means for acquiring new information to guide health care research and clinical decision making. Poor reporting is unethical and may have serious consequences for clinical practice, future research, policy making, patient care, and ultimately for patients [10]. Securing the quality of the publications is an important activity of journals in their editorial policy. Journals need to be more proactive in providing information about the quality of what journals publish [10,45]. Journals should consider strategies and actions to verify that authors realize full responsibility for the statistical reporting quality of their manuscripts. Use of the short checklist proposed in this paper with reporting guidelines would be an important step towards quality-secured research.

Peer review provides the foundation for the scientific publishing system. During the editorial process peer reviewers are required to comment on whether the methods and findings are clearly reported [46]. This approach heavily relies on the statistical expertise of subject reviewers. In general, peer reviewers are competent in a specific range of statistical methods, but they may not necessarily be aware of more general statistical issues and best practices [16,36,47]. It has been claimed that due to the inadequate assessment of statistical reporting and data presentation during peer review and editorial processes, the quality of biomedical articles has not improved [8,36,47–49].

Medical journals often ask their subject reviewers if they are able to assess all statistical aspects of the manuscript themselves or whether they recommend an additional statistical review [47]. Leading medical journals, such as *Lancet*, *BMJ*, *Annals of Medicine* and *JAMA* have adopted statistical review. Despite demonstration of widespread statistical and data presentation errors in medical articles, increasing the use of statistical reviewers has been slow [50]. A recent survey found that only 23% of the top biomedical journals reported that they routinely employed statistical review for all original research articles [51]. Introduction of specialist statisticians to the peer review process has made peer review more specialized. In addition, statistical reviewing is time intensive, limited by both reviewer supply and expense.

In biomedical journals, there is no single model for statistical review in peer review strategies [51–53]. Some journals recruit statistical methodologists to the editorial board, some draw their statistical reviewers from an external pool. If all papers cannot be statistically reviewed, editors have to select which manuscripts should undergo statistical scrutiny. There are also models where subject reviewers are assisted to comment on the statistical aspects of a manuscript [47,48,54]. However, these checklists cover extensively all aspects of data analysis and are not straightforward for non-statistical reviewers to get an overall impression of the statistical quality. Some form of simplified checklist could be handy for editors and reviewers to spot the issues that might indicate more serious problems in the reporting of scientific articles. I hope that editors and reviewers could use the short quality test proposed in this paper for deciding when the presentation in a manuscript is clearly inadequate and they should recommend rejecting the manuscript. I agree with Kyrgidis and Triaridis [48] that if the reviewer cannot find the basic information and description related to the data analysis, the reviewer does not need to read the whole article. After checking tables and figures and reading through the statistical analysis subsection in the methods section, the reviewer can reject the manuscript on good grounds. When the proposed simple quality test shows that the statistical reporting and data presentation are appropriate, the whole article needs to be read and further reviewed.

In recent years, several journals have tried to improve peer review processes [55]. Their efforts have been focused on introducing openness and transparency to the models of peer review [56]. New strategies in peer review might help to address persistent statistical reporting and data presentation issues in the medical literature [55]. Software algorithms and scanners have been developed to assess internal consistency and validity of statistical tests in academic writing [57]. However, their use is still rare and limited to flag specific potential errors. The open peer review, where all peer reviews are made openly available brings into use new models where the quality of a paper may be assessed by the whole scientific community. The pre- and post-publication peer review models include commenting systems for the readership. Readers could use tools, such as proposed in this paper, to give feedback to authors. Subsequently, authors prepare a second version of the manuscript reflecting the comments and suggestions proposed by the scientific community.

My validation set of articles included four journals with different levels of prestige and visibility. The reporting of data analysis information was more detailed and useful for the reader in the more visible journals (*Lancet* and *JAMA Psychiatry*). This is in line with previous studies [5,6]. High-impact journals have more rigorous review process, including extensive statistical reviews. Several researchers in scientific communication have recommended sending out all manuscripts with numerical data for statistical review [8,58,59]. In addition, the strict monitoring of revisions made in manuscripts is important.

The proposed quality test is short. It includes only nine items. These items measure the data presentation quality and the description of data analysis methods. It does not include items about study design, justification of sample size, potential sources of bias, common statistical methodological issues, or interpretation of results. Several reporting guidelines and checklists are available to ensure that authors have paid attention to these other aspects [10,11]. However, these checklists have had little impact on the quality of statistical reporting, and they have not been sufficient for ensuring that issues related to poor statistical reporting and inadequate data presentation are eliminated from manuscripts [3,8,60]. In addition, the general checklists do not include detailed recommendations for reporting how statistical analyses were performed and how to present data.

The article set for pilot testing the proposed instrument included only published studies. Editors and reviewers can use the proposed tool to judge whether manuscripts should be accepted for publication. Educators can utilize it when educating researchers about how to improve statistical reporting and data presentation. A future study is required to apply the instrument at the initial submission of manuscripts to scientific journals and to test how applicable it is in the peer review process. In addition, content and construct validity properties [61] need to be evaluated in future studies.

It should be noted that the instrument was specifically developed for health care, biomedical and clinical studies, and limitations may arise if it is used in nonmedical fields that apply statistical methods.

## 5. Conclusions

In summary, I have developed an applicable checklist for quickly testing the statistical reporting quality of manuscripts and published research papers. One aim of this work was to help authors prepare manuscripts. Good research deserves to be presented well, and good presentation is as much a part of the research as the collection and analysis of the data. With this instrument authors could test the effectiveness of their presentations (tables and figures) for their readers. In addition, they could check that they have not described statistical methods too briefly or superficially.

Competent editors and scientific reviewers should be able to identify errors in basic statistical analysis and reporting. However, there is accumulative evidence that inadequate reporting of basic statistics is a persistent and ubiquitous problem in published medical studies. Editors and reviewers can improve the quality of reporting by identifying submitted manuscripts with poor-quality statistical reporting and data presentation. I hope that the editors and reviewers of scientific journals will incorporate the proposed test instrument in their editorial process. For a manuscript to be considered for full review, its statistical presentation has to be good enough for readers, subject reviewers, and statistical reviewers to understand what statistical methods have been applied and what data are presented in tables and figures. Manuscripts with poor-quality statistical reporting (total score ranges from 0 to 2) should be rejected. Giving detailed comments in review reports to improve the reporting may not be straightforward in those cases.

Readers can use the proposed data analysis reporting test as an initial indicator of research quality. They can easily check whether, based on numerical data analyses, a published research article is readable, understandable and accessible to healthcare professionals who might wish to use similar techniques in their future work or to those who are not experts in a particular subfield. A high score indicates that the authors have focused on reporting and readers should be able to express an opinion about the results after reading the main text.

Further refinement of the data analysis reporting instrument will continue, and I invite feedback.

**Author Contributions:** P.N. has undertaken all the works of this paper.

**Acknowledgments:** I am grateful to Jasleen Kaur who provided useful comments on the draft of the instrument items. I wish to thank all health since students at the University of Oulu who participated in the piloting of the instrument.

## References

1. Sato, Y.; Gosho, M.; Nagashima, K.; Takahashi, S.; Ware, J.H.; Laird, N.M. Statistical Methods in the Journal—An Update. *N. Engl. J. Med.* **2017**, *376*, 1086–1087. [CrossRef] [PubMed]
2. Nieminen, P.; Miettunen, J.; Koponen, H.; Isohanni, M. Statistical methodologies in psychopharmacology: A review. *Hum. Psychopharmacol. Clin. Exp.* **2006**, *21*, 195–203. [CrossRef] [PubMed]
3. Norström, F. Poor quality in the reporting and use of statistical methods in public health—The case of unemployment and health. *Arch. Public Health* **2015**, *73*, 56. [CrossRef] [PubMed]
4. Diong, J.; Butler, A.A.; Gandevia, S.C.; Héroux, M.E. Poor statistical reporting, inadequate data presentation and spin persist despite editorial advice. *PLoS ONE* **2018**, *13*, e202121. [CrossRef] [PubMed]
5. Altman, D.G. Poor-quality medical research: What can journals do? *JAMA* **2002**, *287*, 2765–2767. [CrossRef]
6. Nieminen, P.; Carpenter, J.; Rucker, G.; Schumacher, M. The relationship between quality of research and citation frequency. *BMC Med. Res. Methodol.* **2006**, *6*, 42. [CrossRef]
7. McClean, M.; Silverberg, J. Statistical reporting in randomized controlled trials from the dermatology literature: A review of 44 dermatology journals. *Br. J. Dermatol.* **2015**, *173*, 172–183. [CrossRef]

8. Dexter, F.; Shafer, S.L. Narrative Review of Statistical Reporting Checklists, Mandatory Statistical Editing, and Rectifying Common Problems in the Reporting of Scientific Articles. *Anesth. Analg.* **2017**, *124*, 943–947. [CrossRef]
9. Vandenbroucke, J.P.; Von Elm, E.; Altman, D.G.; Gøtzsche, P.C.; Mulrow, C.D.; Pocock, S.J.; Poole, C.; Schlesselman, J.J.; Egger, M. Strengthening the Reporting of Observational Studies in Epidemiology (STROBE): Explanation and elaboration. *PLoS Med.* **2007**, *4*, 1628–1654. [CrossRef]
10. Moher, D.; Altman, D.G.; Schultz, K.F.; Simera, I.; Wager, E. *Guidelines for Reporting Health Research. User's Manual*; John Wiley & Sons, Ltd.: Chichester, UK, 2014.
11. EQUATOR Network. Available online: https://www.equator-network.org/ (accessed on 30 March 2020).
12. Lang, T.A.; Michelle, S. *How to Report Statistics in Medicine: Annotated Guidelines for Authors, Editors and Reviewers*, 2nd ed.; American College of Physicians: Philadelphia, PA, USA, 2006.
13. Strasak, A.M.; Zaman, Q.; Pfeiffer, K.P.; Gobel, G.; Ulmer, H. Statistical errors in medical research—A review of common pitfalls. *Swiss Med. Wkly.* **2007**, *137*, 44–49.
14. Lee, S. Avoiding negative reviewer comments: Common statistical errors in anesthesia journals. *Korean J. Anesthesiol.* **2016**, *69*, 219–226. [CrossRef] [PubMed]
15. Altman, D.G. Statistical reviewing for medical journals. *Stat. Med.* **1998**, *17*, 2661–2674. [CrossRef]
16. Nieminen, P.; Virtanen, J.I.; Vähänikkilä, H. An instrument to assess the statistical intensity of medical research papers. *PLoS ONE* **2017**, *12*. [CrossRef] [PubMed]
17. Bland, M. *An Introduction to Medical Statistics*; Oxford University Press: Oxford, UK, 2015; ISBN 0199589925.
18. Pickering, R.M. Describing the participants in a study. *Age Ageing* **2017**, *46*, 576–581. [CrossRef] [PubMed]
19. Lang, T.A.; Altman, D.G. Basic statistical reporting for articles published in Biomedical Journals: "The Statistical analyses and methods in the published literature" or the SAMPL guidelines. *Int. J. Nurs. Stud.* **2015**, *52*, 5–9. [CrossRef]
20. Nieminen, P.; Kaur, J. Reporting of data analysis methods in psychiatric journals: Trends from 1996 to 2018. *Int. J. Methods Psychiatr. Res.* **2019**, *28*. [CrossRef]
21. Nieminen, P.; Vähänikkilä, H. Use of data analysis methods in dental publications: Is there evidence of a methodological change? *Publications* **2020**, *8*, 9. [CrossRef]
22. Thiese, M.S.; Ronna, B.; Ott, U. P value interpretations and considerations. *J. Thorac. Dis.* **2016**, *8*, E928–E931. [CrossRef]
23. Motulsky, H. *Intuitive Biostatistics*, 3rd ed.; Oxford University Press: New York, NY, USA, 2014; ISBN 9780199946648.
24. American Medical Association. *AMA Manual of Style: A Guide for Authors and Editors*, 11th ed.; Oxford University Press: New York, NY, USA, 2020; ISBN 978-0190246556.
25. Oberg, A.L.; Poland, G.A. The process of continuous journal improvement: New author guidelines for statistical and analytical reporting in VACCINE. *Vaccine* **2012**, *30*, 2915–2917. [CrossRef]
26. American Psychological Assiciation. *Publication Manual of the American Psychological Assiciation*, 6th ed.; American Psychological Assiciation: Washington, DC, USA, 2017; ISBN 978-1-4338-0561-5.
27. Gardner, M.J.; Altman, D.G. Confidence intervals rather than P values: Estimation rather than hypothesis testing. *Br. Med. J. (Clin. Res. Ed.)* **1986**, *292*, 746–750. [CrossRef]
28. Spector, R.; Vesell, E.S. Pharmacology and statistics: Recommendations to strengthen a productive partnership. *Pharmacology* **2006**, *78*, 113–122. [CrossRef] [PubMed]
29. ECMJE Recommendations for He Conduct, Reporting, Editing, and Publication of Scolarly Work in Medical Journals. Available online: http://www.icmje.org/recommendations/ (accessed on 25 May 2020).
30. Lang, T.A.; Altman, D.G. Statistical Analyses and Methods in the Published Literature: The SAMPL Guidelines. In *Guidelines for Reporting Health Research: A User's Manual*; John Wiley & Sons, Ltd.: Oxford, UK, 2014; pp. 264–274. ISBN 9780470670446.
31. Simundic, A.-M. Practical recommendations for statistical analysis and data presentation in Biochemia Medica journal. *Biochem. Med.* **2012**, *22*, 15–23. [CrossRef] [PubMed]
32. Mayo, D. *Statistical Inference as Severe Testing. How to Get beyond the Statistical Wars*; Cambridge University Press: Cambridge, UK, 2018; ISBN 978-1-107-66464-7.
33. Indrayan, A.; Malhotra, R.K. *Medical Biostatistics*, 4th ed.; CRC Press: Cambridge, UK, 2018; ISBN 1498799531.
34. Indrayan, A. Reporting of Basic Statistical Methods in Biomedical Journals: Improved SAMPL Guidelines. *Indian Pediatr.* **2020**, *57*, 43–48. [CrossRef] [PubMed]

35. Gwet, K.L. *Handbook of Inter-Rater Reliability*, 4th ed.; Advances Analytics, LLS: Gaithersburg, MD, USA, 2014; ISBN 9780970806284.
36. Glasziou, P.; Altman, D.G.; Bossuyt, P.; Boutron, I.; Clarke, M.; Julious, S.; Michie, S.; Moher, D.; Wager, E. Reducing waste from incomplete or unusable reports of biomedical research. *Lancet* **2014**, *383*, 267–276. [CrossRef]
37. *The Academy of Medical Sciences Reproducibility and Reliability of Biomedical Research: Improving Research Practice*; The Academy of Medical Sciences: London, UK, 2015.
38. Vetter, T.R.; McGwin, G.; Pittet, J.F. Replicability, Reproducibility, and Fragility of Research Findings-Ultimately, Caveat Emptor. *Anesth. Analg.* **2016**, *123*, 244–248. [CrossRef]
39. Smaldino, P.E.; McElreath, R. The natural selection of bad science. *R. Soc. Open Sci.* **2016**, *3*, 9. [CrossRef]
40. Shetty, A.C.; Al Rasheed, N.M.; Albwardi, S.A. Dental professionals' attitude towards biostatistics. *J. Dent. Oral Hyg.* **2015**, *7*, 113–118.
41. Hannigan, A.; Hegarty, A.C.; McGrath, D. Attitudes towards statistics of graduate entry medical students: The role of prior learning experiences. *BMC Med. Educ.* **2014**, *14*, 70. [CrossRef]
42. Batra, M.; Gupta, M.; Dany, S.S.; Rajput, P. Perception of Dental Professionals towards Biostatistics. *Int. Sch. Res. Not.* **2014**, *2014*, 1–6. [CrossRef]
43. Altman, D.G.; Goodman, S.N.; Schroter, S. How statistical expertise is used in medical research. *JAMA* **2002**, *287*, 2817–2820. [CrossRef]
44. Belia, S.; Fidler, F.; Williams, J.; Cumming, G. Researchers misunderstand confidence intervals and standard error bars. *Psychol. Methods* **2005**, *10*, 389–396. [CrossRef]
45. Moher, D. Reporting guidelines: Doing better for readers. *BMC Med.* **2018**, *16*, 18–20. [CrossRef]
46. Glonti, K.; Cauchi, D.; Cobo, E.; Boutron, I.; Moher, D.; Hren, D. A scoping review on the roles and tasks of peer reviewers in the manuscript review process in biomedical journals. *BMC Med.* **2019**, *17*, 1–14. [CrossRef] [PubMed]
47. Greenwood, D.C.; Freeman, J.V. How to spot a statistical problem: Advice for a non-statistical reviewer. *BMC Med.* **2015**, *13*, 1–3. [CrossRef] [PubMed]
48. Kyrgidis, A.; Triaridis, S. Methods and Biostatistics: A concise guide for peer reviewers. *Hippokratia* **2010**, *14*, 13–22. [PubMed]
49. Patel, J. Why training and specialization is needed for peer review: A case study of peer review for randomized controlled trials. *BMC Med.* **2014**, *12*, 1–7. [CrossRef] [PubMed]
50. Horbach, S.P.J.M.; Halffman, W. The changing forms and expectations of peer review. *Res. Integr. Peer Rev.* **2018**, *3*, 1–15. [CrossRef]
51. Hardwicke, T.E.; Goodman, S.N. How often do leading biomedical journals use statistical experts to evaluate statistical methods? The results of a survey. *MetArXiv Prepr.* **2020**, 1–29.
52. Hardwicke, T.E.; Frank, M.C.; Vazire, S.; Goodman, S.N. Should Psychology Journals Adopt Specialized Statistical Review? *Adv. Methods Pract. Psychol. Sci.* **2019**, *2*, 240–249. [CrossRef]
53. Overgaard, K.; Roberts, J.; Schaeffer, M.B.; Pessin, R. the Trenches. *Sci. Ed.* **2015**, *38*, 2015.
54. Curtis, M.J.; Alexander, S.; Cirino, G.; Docherty, J.R.; George, C.H.; Giembycz, M.A.; Hoyer, D.; Insel, P.A.; Izzo, A.A.; Ji, Y.; et al. Experimental design and analysis and their reporting II: Updated and simplified guidance for authors and peer reviewers. *Br. J. Pharmacol.* **2018**, *175*, 987–993. [CrossRef]
55. Fresco-Santalla, A.N.A.; Hernández-Pérez, T. Current and evolving models of peer-review. *Ser. Libr.* **2014**, *67*, 373–398. [CrossRef]
56. Vercellini, P.; Buggio, L.; Vigano, P.; Somigliana, E. Peer review in medical journals: Beyond quality of reports towards transparency and public scrutiny of the process. *Eur. J. Intern. Med.* **2016**, *31*, 15–19. [CrossRef]
57. Nuijten, M.B.; Hartgerink, C.H.J.; van Assen, M.A.L.M.; Epskamp, S.; Wicherts, J.M. The prevalence of statistical reporting errors in psychology (1985–2013). *Behav. Res. Methods* **2016**, *48*, 1205–1226. [CrossRef] [PubMed]
58. Vahanikkila, H.; Tjaderhane, L.; Nieminen, P. The statistical reporting quality of articles published in 2010 in five dental journals. *Acta Odontol. Scand.* **2015**, *73*, 76–80. [CrossRef] [PubMed]
59. Lukic, I.; Marusic, M. Appointment of statistical editor and quality of statistics in a small medical journal. *Croat. Med. J.* **2001**, *42*, 500–503. [PubMed]

60. Pouwels, K.B.; Widyakusuma, N.N.; Groenwold, R.H.H.; Hak, E. Quality of reporting of confounding remained suboptimal after the STROBE guideline. *J. Clin. Epidemiol.* **2016**, *69*, 217–224. [CrossRef]
61. Mokkink, L.B.; Terwee, C.B.; Patrick, D.L.; Alonso, J.; Stratford, P.W.; Knol, D.L.; Bouter, L.M.; de Vet, H.C.W. The COSMIN study reached international consensus on taxonomy, terminology, and definitions of measurement properties for health-related patient-reported outcomes. *J. Clin. Epidemiol.* **2010**, *63*, 737–745. [CrossRef]

# Permissions

All chapters in this book were first published by MDPI; hereby published with permission under the Creative Commons Attribution License or equivalent. Every chapter published in this book has been scrutinized by our experts. Their significance has been extensively debated. The topics covered herein carry significant findings which will fuel the growth of the discipline. They may even be implemented as practical applications or may be referred to as a beginning point for another development.

The contributors of this book come from diverse backgrounds, making this book a truly international effort. This book will bring forth new frontiers with its revolutionizing research information and detailed analysis of the nascent developments around the world.

We would like to thank all the contributing authors for lending their expertise to make the book truly unique. They have played a crucial role in the development of this book. Without their invaluable contributions this book wouldn't have been possible. They have made vital efforts to compile up to date information on the varied aspects of this subject to make this book a valuable addition to the collection of many professionals and students.

This book was conceptualized with the vision of imparting up-to-date information and advanced data in this field. To ensure the same, a matchless editorial board was set up. Every individual on the board went through rigorous rounds of assessment to prove their worth. After which they invested a large part of their time researching and compiling the most relevant data for our readers.

The editorial board has been involved in producing this book since its inception. They have spent rigorous hours researching and exploring the diverse topics which have resulted in the successful publishing of this book. They have passed on their knowledge of decades through this book. To expedite this challenging task, the publisher supported the team at every step. A small team of assistant editors was also appointed to further simplify the editing procedure and attain best results for the readers.

Apart from the editorial board, the designing team has also invested a significant amount of their time in understanding the subject and creating the most relevant covers. They scrutinized every image to scout for the most suitable representation of the subject and create an appropriate cover for the book.

The publishing team has been an ardent support to the editorial, designing and production team. Their endless efforts to recruit the best for this project, has resulted in the accomplishment of this book. They are a veteran in the field of academics and their pool of knowledge is as vast as their experience in printing. Their expertise and guidance has proved useful at every step. Their uncompromising quality standards have made this book an exceptional effort. Their encouragement from time to time has been an inspiration for everyone.

The publisher and the editorial board hope that this book will prove to be a valuable piece of knowledge for researchers, students, practitioners and scholars across the globe.

# List of Contributors

**Yuri Choi, In Ho Kwon and Jinwoo Jeong**
Department of Emergency Medicine, Dong-A University Hospital, Dong-A University College of Medicine, Busan 49201, Korea

**June-sung Kim**
Department of Emergency Medicine, Asan Medical Center, University of Ulsan College of Medicine, Seoul 05505, Korea

**Taerim Kim**
Department of Emergency Medicine, Samsung Medical Center, Sungkyunkwan University School of Medicine, Seoul 06351, Korea

**Su Min Kim**
Department of Digital Health, Samsung Advanced Institute for Health Sciences & Technology, Sungkyunkwan University, Seoul 06355, Korea

**Wonchul Cha**
Department of Emergency Medicine, Samsung Medical Center, Sungkyunkwan University School of Medicine, Seoul 06351, Korea
Department of Digital Health, Samsung Advanced Institute for Health Sciences & Technology, Sungkyunkwan University, Seoul 06355, Korea
Health Information and Strategy Center, Samsung Medical Center, Seoul 06351, Korea

**Jae-Ho Lee**
Department of Emergency Medicine, Asan Medical Center, University of Ulsan College of Medicine, Seoul 05505, Korea
Department of Information Medicine, Asan Medical Center, University of Ulsan College of Medicine, Seoul 05505, Korea

**Ling-Chien Hung**
Division of Neurology, Department of Internal Medicine, Ditmanson Medical Foundation Chia-Yi Christian Hospital, Chiayi 600, Taiwan

**Sheng-Feng Sung**
Division of Neurology, Department of Internal Medicine, Ditmanson Medical Foundation Chia-Yi Christian Hospital, Chiayi 600, Taiwan
Department of Information Management and Institute of Healthcare Information Management, National Chung Cheng University, Chiayi 621, Taiwan
Department of Nursing, Min-Hwei Junior College of Health Care Management, Tainan 736, Taiwan

**Ya-Han Hu**
Department of Information Management, National Central University, Taoyuan 320, Taiwan
MOST AI Biomedical Research Center at National Cheng Kung University, Tainan 701, Taiwan

**Chun-Tien Tai**
Department of Information Management and Institute of Healthcare Information Management, National Chung Cheng University, Chiayi 621, Taiwan
Chiayi Chang Gung Memorial Hospital, Chiayi 613, Taiwan
Department of Information Management, Shu Zen College of Medicine and Management, Kaohsiung 821, Taiwan

**Kuen-Liang Sue**
Department of Information Management, National Central University, Taoyuan 320, Taiwan

**Wen-Chien Ting**
Division of Colorectal Surgery, Department of Surgery, Chung Shan Medical University Hospital, Taichung 40201, Taiwan
Institute of Medicine, Chung Shan Medical University, Taichung 40201, Taiwan

**Horng-Rong Chang**
Division of Nephrology, Department of Internal Medicine, Chung Shan Medical University Hospital, Taichung 40201, Taiwan
School of Medicine, Chung Shan Medical University, Taichung 40201, Taiwan

**Chi-Chang Chang**
School of Medical Informatics, Chung Shan Medical University & IT office, Chung Shan Medical University Hospital, Taichung 40201, Taiwan

**Chi-Jie Lu**
Graduate Institute of Business Administration, Fu Jen Catholic University, Taipei 24205, Taiwan
Artificial Intelligence Development Center, Fu Jen Catholic University, Taipei 24205, Taiwan

**Sun Jung Lee and In Young Choi**
Department of Medical Informatics, College of Medicine, Catholic University of Korea, Seoul 06591, Korea
Department of Biomedicine & Health Sciences, College of Medicine, The Catholic University of Korea, Seoul 06591, Korea

**Sung Hye Yu and Jae Kwon Kim**
Department of Medical Informatics, College of Medicine, Catholic University of Korea, Seoul 06591, Korea

**Yejin Kim**
School of Biomedical Informatics, University of Texas Health Science Center at Houston, Houston, TX 77030, USA

**Jun Hyuk Hong and Choung-Soo Kim**
Department of Urology, University of Ulsan College of Medicine, Seoul 05505, Korea

**Seong Il Seo**
Department of Urology, Sungkyunkwan University School of Medicine, Seoul 06351, Korea

**Seok-Soo Byun**
Department of Urology, Seoul National University Bundang Hospital, Seongnam 13620, Korea

**Chang Wook Jeong**
Department of Urology, Seoul National University College of Medicine, Seoul 03080, Korea

**Ji Youl Lee**
Department of Urology, Seoul St. Mary's Hospital, College of Medicine, The Catholic University of Korea, Seoul 06591, Korea

**Afnan M. Alhassan**
School of Computer Science, Universiti Sains Malaysia, George Town 11800, Malaysia
College of Computing and Information Technology, Shaqra University, Shaqra 11961, Saudi Arabia

**Wan Mohd Nazmee Wan Zainon**
School of Computer Science, Universiti Sains Malaysia, George Town 11800, Malaysia

**Piotr Wąż**
Department of Nuclear Medicine, Medical University of Gdańsk, 80-210 Gdańsk, Poland

**Roberto Carlucci and Mario Ventura**
Department of Biology, University of Bari, 70125 Bari, Italy

**Vitoantonio Bevilacqua**
Department of Electrical and Information Engineering, Polytechnic University of Bari, 70125 Bari, Italy

**Juan de la Torre and Javier Marin**
IDERGO-Research and Development in Ergonomics, Biomechanical Laboratory, I3A-University Institute of Research of Engineering of Aragon, University of Zaragoza, 50018 Zaragoza, Spain

**Sergio Ilarri**
Computer Science for Complex System Modelling (COSMOS), I3A-University Institute of Research of Engineering of Aragon, University of Zaragoza, 50018 Zaragoza, Spain
Department of Computer Science and Systems Engineering, University of Zaragoza, 50018 Zaragoza, Spain

**Jose J. Marin**
IDERGO-Research and Development in Ergonomics, Biomechanical Laboratory, I3A-University Institute of Research of Engineering of Aragon, University of Zaragoza, 50018 Zaragoza, Spain
Department of Design and Manufacturing Engineering, University of Zaragoza, 50018 Zaragoza, Spain

**Byung Mook Weon**
Soft Matter Physics Laboratory, School of Advanced Materials Science and Engineering, SKKU Advanced Institute of Nanotechnology (SAINT), Sungkyunkwan University, Suwon 16419, Korea
Research Center for Advanced Materials Technology, Sungkyunkwan University, Suwon 16419, Korea
Department of Biomedical Engineering, Johns Hopkins University, Baltimore, MD 21218, USA

**Kathiravan Srinivasan, Nivedhitha Mahendran and Durai Raj Vincent**
School of Information Technology and Engineering, Vellore Institute of Technology (VIT), Vellore 632 014, India

**Chuan-Yu Chang**
Department of Computer Science and Information Engineering, National Yunlin University of Science and Technology, Yunlin 64002, Taiwan

**Shabbir Syed-Abdul**
International Center for Health Information Technology (ICHIT), Taipei Medical University, Taipei 110, Taiwan
Graduate Institute of Biomedical Informatics, Taipei Medical University, Taipei 110, Taiwan

**Agnieszka Bielińska**
Department of Quality of Life Research, Medical University of Gdańsk, 80-210 Gdańsk, Poland

**Dorota Bielińska-Wąż**
Department of Radiological Informatics and Statistics, Medical University of Gdańsk, 80-210 Gdańsk, Poland

**Giovanni Dimauro, Pierpasquale Colagrande and Danilo Caivano**
Department of Computer Science, University of Bari, 70125 Bari, Italy

**Hannah Inbarani H.**
Department of Computer Science, Periyar University, Tamil Nadu, Salem 636 011, India

**Pentti Nieminen**
Medical Informatics and Data Analysis Research Group, University of Oulu, 90014 Oulu, Finland

**Jothi G**
Department of Computer Science and Engineering, Sona College of Technology (Autonomous), Salem 636005, India

**Shun-Hsing Chen**
Department of Marketing and Distribution Management, Oriental Institute of Technology, New Taipei City 220, Taiwan

**Fan-Yun Pai**
Department of Business Administration, National Changhua University of Education, Changhua 500, Taiwan

**Tsu-Ming Yeh**
Department of Industrial Engineering and Management, National Quemoy University, Kinmen 892, Taiwan

**Christian Morbidoni, Alessandro Cucchiarelli, Sandro Fioretti and Francesco Di Nardo**
Department of Information Engineering, Università Politecnica delle Marche, 60100 Ancona, Italy

**Ahmad Taher Azar**
Robotics and Internet-of-Things Lab (RIOTU), Prince Sultan University, Riyadh 11586, Saudi Arabia
Faculty of Computers and Artificial Intelligence, Benha University, Benha 13511, Egypt

# Index

www.ingramcontent.com/pod-product-compliance
Lightning Source LLC
LaVergne TN
LVHW060542210926
848485LV00005B/1242